P9-DEQ-697

Handbook of
Paediatric
Intensive Care

Commissioning Editor: Deborah Russell
Project Development Manager: Kim Benson
Project Manager: Katharine Eyston
Designer: Jayne Jones

Handbook of Paediatric Intensive Care

Gale A. Pearson MBBS MRCP FRCPCH

Consultant Paediatric Intensivist (Head of Speciality)
Intensive Care Unit
The Birmingham Children's Hospital, Birmingham, United Kingdom

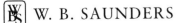 W. B. SAUNDERS

London   Edinburgh   New York   Philadelphia   St Louis   Sydney   Toronto   2002

W. B. SAUNDERS
An imprint of Elsevier Science Limited

© Harcourt Publishers Limited 2002
© Elsevier Science Limited 2002. All rights reserved.

Ⓡ is a registered trademark of Elsevier Science Limited

The right of Gale Pearson to be identified as author of this work has been
asserted by him in accordance with the Copyright, Designs and Patents Act 1988.

All rights reserved. No part of this publication may be reproduced, stored in a
retrieval system, or transmitted in any form or by any means, electronic,
mechanical, photocopying, recording or otherwise, without either the prior
permission of the publishers (Permissions Manager, Elsevier Science Limited,
Robert Stevenson House, 1-3 Baxter's Place, Leith Walk, Edinburgh EH1 3AF),
or a licence permitting restricted copying in the United Kingdom issued by the
Copyright Licensing Agency, 90 Tottenham Court Road, London W1T 4LP.

First published 2002
Reprinted 2002

ISBN 0702023469

British Library Cataloguing in Publication Data
A catalogue record for this book is available from the British Library

Library of Congress Cataloging in Publication Data
A catalog record for this book is available from the Library of Congress

Note
Medical knowledge is constantly changing. As new information becomes available, changes in
treatment, procedures, equipment and the use of drugs become necessary. The editors/authors/
contributors and the publishers have taken care to ensure that the information given in this text is
accurate and up to date. However, readers are strongly advised to confirm that the information,
especially with regard to drug usage, complies with the latest legislation and standards of practice.

Existing UK nomenclature is changing to the system of Recommended International
Nonproprietary Names (rINNs). Until the UK names are no longer in use, these more familiar
names are used in this book in preference to rINNs, details of which may be obtained from the
British National Formulary.

The
publisher's
policy is to use
**paper manufactured
from sustainable forests**

Printed in China by RDC Group Limited

Contents

ACKNOWLEDGEMENT

This book would never have been completed were it not for the support of my colleagues. I am particularly indebted to Andrew Tatman, Charles Ralston, Oliver Bagshaw and Steven Cray for their contributions, to David Barron for his illustrations and to Michael Marsh for proofreading the manuscript.

Dedication

To my loving wife Jennifer, my daughter Annie, my loving family and especially the inspiration and memory of my father.

PREFACE

Many junior medical staff rotate through the PICU during their training. Not all of these have career intentions in children's intensive care. This handbook is intended to be useful to those passing through as well as those training more formally in the discipline. The book is intended as both a memory aid and reference and therefore provides structured essays on general topics combined with an "organ-system structured" approach to paediatric intensive care. A relatively concise style has been adopted in the hope of helping quick reference in clinical situations. For similar reasons, extensive discussions of the "evidence base" behind what the author considers common practice have been avoided. Attention is largely focused upon pathophysiology and intensive therapy at the expense of the description of the diseases and their differential diagnoses, which are comprehensively covered in other texts. This is not therefore a textbook of general paediatrics. Nevertheless notes are included on some diagnoses which demand a specific pattern of approach from the intensivist. Their selection and coverage have been intentionally biased to include common causes of admission to PICU and instructive examples of its modus operandi.

1 An Introduction to PICU

- **Who comes to work in a paediatric intensive care unit (PICU)?**
- **Tips before starting work in a PICU**
- **A brief history of paediatric intensive care**
- **The role of the paediatric intensivist**
- **How big should a PICU be?**
- **Regionalisation of services**
- **Who should be referred to a PICU?**
- **Case mix**
- **Summary**

WHO COMES TO WORK IN A PICU?

Paediatric intensive care (PIC) is a unique environment; however careers within it can begin in a variety of disciplines, for example paediatric medicine, surgery and anaesthesia. Almost every new recruit arrives with a host of misconceptions about the post and about what it will entail. To achieve proficiency, all will require a sound grasp of paediatric physiology and will need to acquire a peculiar fusion of age-appropriate technical, diagnostic and interventionist skills.

The caricatures of two recruits are often described by recounting a telephone conversation that each has with their senior about their first admission (the same patient). One recruit is usually identified as an anaesthetist and the other as a paediatrician.

JUNIOR 'I've just admitted this baby who collapsed on the ward, they were just messing about with him! I don't think they knew what they were doing. Anyway I gave a rapid sequence induction, paralysed and intubated him, and put in central venous and arterial lines. I've started him on inotropes because he's hypotensive and didn't respond to volume and his gases are. . .'

SENIOR 'What do you think the problem is?'

JUNIOR 'I don't know – what are you asking me for?'

or alternatively, a different doctor with the same patient

JUNIOR 'I've just admitted this baby. He's a patient of Dr X's, and he collapsed on the paediatric ward. He's 3 kg, mum's first baby, the product of a full term pregnancy and his mother is otherwise well. He's 3 days old and he started to become unwell over the last 2 hours. His respiration is irregular, he is cold, greyish blue and poorly perfused. I think he's in heart failure because his liver is 5 cm palpable and on auscultation his second heart sound is single. I wonder if he has got a hypoplastic left heart. What do you think?'

SENIOR 'What have you done so far?'

JUNIOR 'A chest X-ray and I'm starting a septic screen.'

Clearly both these recruits have strengths and weaknesses in their approach. One has made attempts to support the patient without any idea of what he or she is dealing with. The other has a good idea of the diagnosis but has either got distracted or has failed to grasp the urgency of the situation. For whatever reason no attempt has been made to resuscitate the patient. Clearly neither candidate has responded adequately and both have a lot to learn.

TIPS BEFORE STARTING WORK IN A PICU

There are other lessons that it is nice to hear, if not learn, before crossing the threshold of the PICU.

You will encounter urgent situations where you will have to think and act quickly and calmly and you need to consider your temperament to be suited to such circumstances. That said, you should not think of the PICU as a stressful environment. A post on a PICU should not be considered daunting. Even for those with the right temperament, stress can occur and tends to result from doing too much. 'Too much' can either mean the sheer volume of work or its nature. Your trainers will be trying to make sure that you don't take on too much on your own or try to do things that you have not first been equipped and trained to cope with. You will certainly earn their confidence more quickly if you ask for help judiciously.

Remember that people referring patients to the PICU may well be stressed and will always need to be handled diplomatically. *Keep calm* from the outset and you will acquire the skills and confidence that will keep you calm. 'The first procedure at a cardiac arrest is to take your own pulse' (Shlemm). Do not lose sight of the urgency of situations however. Prioritise your clinical approach so that you resuscitate first and then diagnose and treat. Use your clinical skills and resist the urge to treat numbers in isolation. Treat causes in preference to effects and avoid generating chaos! For those who are not students of chaos theory this is probably worth explaining.

If you want a patient's central venous pressure to remain steady, you might be tempted to write orders such as these (lifted from a real doctor's orders sheet).

> If CVP >9 give 1 mg kg^{-1} of frusemide (furosemide), if CVP <9 give 10 ml kg^{-1} of 4.5% human albumin solution.

However this treatment is likely to have the opposite effect – instability. Choosing close limits as thresholds for action means that therapy changes quickly and repeatedly. Your chosen actions (frusemide (furosemide) or i.v. fluid) will cause the parameters that you have chosen to overshoot, precipitating a further reaction and large swings will result. The point is that you would have been better off tolerating a wider range in the original central venous pressure (CVP). Instead you have applied a rigid protocol with inherent feedback loops to a dynamic system. Decision trees that use 'fuzzy' rather than 'crisp' logic lead to smoother control. It is for good reason that *experienced clinicians respond to trends in preference to isolated values.*

A BRIEF HISTORY OF PAEDIATRIC INTENSIVE CARE

The recognition that children are a distinct group of patients with their own physical and emotional needs is not contentious. The evolution of paediatric intensive care is a simple consequence of combining this tenet with logic that has been recognised since the days of Florence Nightingale, namely the practical advantages of grouping together and treating patients distinguished by the severity of their illness. In modern times this theme was revisited during polio epidemics in the 1950s. Specialist cardiac units developed in the 1960s after the successful introduction of cardiopulmonary bypass techniques. In the UK this often occurred in 'infectious diseases' hospitals as thoracic surgeons extended their practice beyond pulmonary surgery for tuberculosis. Long-term intubation of children developed in the late 1960s and early 1970s as an alternative to tracheostomy, initially using rigid metal tubes in the treatment of tetanus. The most rapid growth of PIC medical and nursing expertise occurred in North America and Australia where demographics and geography favoured regionalisation of specialist units. Proper postgraduate training and certification soon followed. In the UK, specialist PIC nursing qualifications were introduced in the mid-1980s and specialist medical training started to become available in the late 1990s.

THE ROLE OF THE PAEDIATRIC INTENSIVIST

In different institutions and health care systems the manner in which health care is delivered can vary widely. For the sake of clarity throughout this text a 'paediatric intensivist' refers to an individual whose higher training has been in paediatric intensive care, who works exclusively in paediatric intensive care and who has control over the management, admission and discharge of patients to and from the PICU. An intensivist's non-clinical (adminis-trative, education and research) time is also devoted to the PICU. This definition identifies individuals whose input into patient care is focussed on specific periods of the hospital stay and whose responsibility for further follow-up is minimal. Throughout their hospital stay these patients will be under the care of other teams with broader remits. Historically these other teams may have provided intensive care without specific intensive care staff and the role of the latter has therefore had its validity questioned more than once. Intensive care units where referring doctors retain a high profile in patient management are sometimes termed 'open'. In contrast a 'closed' unit is one where the patient is 'taken over' and managed by the intensivist as the result of a referral, with the assistance of co-opted spe-cialists (where appropriate) and thence referred on to another, perhaps different, doctor at the end of the ICU stay. Although 'closed' units have been shown to function more effi-ciently in adult practice, they are less suited to the paediatric age group where the median length of ICU stay is short, confounding the benefits. Most PICUs run a 'shared' care approach some way between open and closed units.

As a consequence of the 'birth trauma' of the discipline of intensive care, a remarkable amount of evidence has been gathered to clarify the role and effect of intensivists in adult and paediatric practice. Virtually all the available literature reports a reduction in severity-adjusted mortality associated with the introduction of an intensivist. Inefficient use of ICU time is decreased. Inappropriate admissions (patients that are too well or beyond help) are reduced and potential early discharges are recognised and expedited. This allows the maximum benefit to yield from what is usually a scarce resource. The mean severity of illness at presentation to ICU tends to increase as the dilutional influence of low risk inap-propriate admissions is removed. Length of ICU stay falls but the mean level of intervention tends to rise. These effects are more noticeable in closed units.

HOW BIG SHOULD A PICU BE?

Big is better. The appointment of full time intensivists can only be justified in units of a certain size and throughput and such appointments have been shown to be associated with improved performance of the unit. However the intensivists cannot claim sole responsibil-ity for the improved performance. Their appointment is just one step in a more complex pos-itive volume:outcome association. Taken in combination, cross-sectional and longitudinal studies clearly show better outcomes in busy units and increases in patient volume lead to better outcomes in technological specialities such as paediatric intensive care. Large cen-tralised PICUs are also spectacularly more efficient and economical.

The idea that 'practice makes perfect' (rather than good units attract referrals) as an explanation of these effects makes good sense. High quality intensive care is about doing simple things well and overall results owe more to the strength of the weakest link in the chain than the strongest. Staff performance is enhanced if the staff can get sufficient expe-rience to train and then maintain their skills. There are caveats however. One study (Pollack 1994) has shown that the use of trainees to provide bedside care, as occurs in large train-ing institutions, imparts a negative influence on severity-adjusted outcome. Nevertheless this is still an argument *for* the use of specialist intensivists.

Similarly the nature of the volume:outcome relationship has never been well defined. Observational studies show good outcomes in large units and poor outcomes in data amal-gamated from small units (unit size is defined in terms of numbers of intubated child admis-sions per year). The best guess from the available evidence is that units should be admitting a minimum of about 600 intubated children per year (corresponding to about eight beds) and that below this value results are likely to suffer. Political consensus varies.

REGIONALISATION OF SERVICES

Only a small fraction of children in a given population will need PIC in a given year, there-fore the creation of large PICUs is part of a process of centralisation which is quite natural for a low volume, highly technical (and expensive) speciality. It is worth emphasising, however, that centralisation is more than just the creation of big units. It also requires appropriate communication channels and travel (retrieval and return) arrangements for patients using the PICU. Concerns are sometimes expressed about the alleged inequity of centralised intensive care, the assertion being that families are disrupted by having to travel large distances to receive intensive care. Such antipathy to a regional PICU is often reinforced by a resentment of the economic imperatives that support centralisation. However PICUs should clearly be sited in areas of population density, and in institutions which can supply the specialist paediatric support services that PIC entails. The 'equity' argument is turned on its head by studies showing the extent of the improved outcome of specialist care in tertiary hospitals and the excess death rates in areas with a decentralised infrastructure for PIC. Equity demands equal access to the best possible standard of care.

How many PICU beds does a population need?

Studies in western countries show remarkable consistency in the average numbers of PICU admissions required by a given population (1.2 admissions per 1000 children per year). The total PIC capacity required to accommodate these admissions depends upon the number of units into which the beds are divided and the efficiency with which those beds and units are used. Centralised care makes more efficient use of resources and is associated with shorter lengths of intensive care stay.

The number of PICU beds required for a given population has been modelled by Milne *et al.* (1994) by approximation to a Poisson distribution. Thus the number of beds (n) necessary to satisfy demand 95 per cent of the time can be calculated from

$$n = X + 1.64 \sqrt{X}$$

Where X =

$$\frac{(\text{number of children in the population}) \times (\text{rate of demand p.a.}) \times (\text{mean length of stay})}{365 \times \% \text{occupancy}}$$

To use this model if more than one unit is envisaged, the population should be regarded as being divided in a ratio matched by the relative size of each unit. In the worked examples below, the provision for a population of 1 million children can be seen to be provided 95 per cent of the time by four average-performing, eight-bedded PICUs or one peak-performing, fourteen-bedded PICU situated in a large children's hospital. Individuals responsible for the infrastructure should remember that 95 per cent cover such as this still means that 1 in 20

Worked examples

Using the model above to determine the required number of beds required for decentralised and centralised systems, assuming that both systems use beds as efficiently as each other, then in a population of 1 million children served by four PICUs, with each patient having an average length of stay of 4 days (assuming 80% occupancy), each PICU requires

$(250 \times 1.2 \times 4) \div (365 \times 0.8) = 4.1$ beds to satisfy demand 50% of the time, and $4.1 + (1.64 \times \sqrt{4.1}) = 7.4$, i.e. 8 beds to satisfy demand 95% of the time. Thus the population requires a total of 32 beds.

A single ICU to serve the same population would require

$(1000 \times 1.2 \times 4) \div (365 \times 0.8) = 16.44$ beds to satisfy demand 50% of the time, and $16.44 + 1.64 \sqrt{16.44} = 23.01$, i.e. 24 beds to satisfy demand 95% of the time.

However the increased efficiency of a centralised system with a PICU in a specialist centre involves a shorter length of stay. If we repeat the model and calculate the requirement taking this into account (lengths of stay taken from the Lancet 1997 349: 1213–17), in a population of 1 million children, each patient having an average length of stay of 2.1 days, and assuming 80% occupancy, one PICU requires

$(1000 \times 1.2 \times 2.1) \div (365 \times 0.8) = 8.63$ beds to satisfy demand 50% of the time, and

$8.63 + 1.64\ \sqrt{8.63} = 13.4$, i.e. 14 beds to satisfy demand 95% of the time.

referrals cannot be accommodated and statistically such instances are likely to cluster. One way to alleviate the problem is to plan to run the PICUs at an average of 80 per cent occupancy, which increases their ability to accommodate peaks in demand.

A more detailed theoretical cost utility analysis incorporating the effects of duplication of ICU infrastructure in a decentralised system was produced by Shann (*Which way forward for the care of critically ill children,* York University Press, 1994).

WHO SHOULD BE REFERRED TO A PICU?

Intensive care is used to provide organ system support for patients with potentially recoverable diseases who can benefit from closer observation with or without more invasive monitoring than is normally available on a paediatric ward. This may be because of impending or established organ system failure whether predicted as a result of a therapeutic intervention (such as cardiac surgery) or arising as the result of an acute illness.

The simplest and best model for paediatric intensive care is to arrange the transfer of any child to a large specialist PICU if the child's survival clearly depends upon it or (if they are expected to survive) if their ICU stay can be expected to last 24 hours or more. In this latter group one may reconsider referral if the transfer time to the PICU is likely to constitute more than 50 per cent of the total projected ICU stay. However this uncomplicated approach quickly runs into difficulties when there is inadequate overall provision of PIC beds.

Severity of illness, as assessed by mortality prediction models (see Chapter 4 Audit and Performance), can be used to model ICU populations. This includes retrospective analysis of whether ICU admissions were appropriate. For example inappropriate admissions can be defined as those with a low mortality risk who do not receive ICU dependent therapies (i.e. the patients were just observed) and delayed discharges can be similarly defined at the end of the ICU stay. However these models apply retrospectively to populations and are of *no use whatsoever* in prospective application to individual cases. They cannot be used to ration the provision of an ICU resource that is inadequate for the population being served. Indeed the mortality prediction models provide a mortality risk that assumes that the patient *receives* intensive care of a standard delivered to the population from which the model was derived.

A number of 'procedures' are conventionally recognised as being 'intensive care dependent' meaning that under normal circumstances it would be unacceptable to perform these procedures outside a critical care environment. Examples one might choose to include in local guidelines are given in Table 1.1.

Thus children should be referred to a PICU if:

- there is a reasonable anticipation, by subjective or objective clinical assessment, of the immediate or imminent need for an intensive care dependent procedure
- they have the potential to develop airway compromise
- they have symptoms or evidence of shock, respiratory distress or respiratory depression

Table 1.1 Procedures that are conventionally recognised as being intensive care dependent.

Nasopharyngeal and endotracheal intubation
Blind endotracheal suction
Continuous positive airway pressure (CPAP)
Artificial/mechanical ventilation
Continuous invasive cardiovascular monitoring (e.g. central venous or arterial line, or Swan–Ganz catheter)
Use of antiarrhythmic, inotropic or vasoactive drug infusions
Acute renal support (haemodialysis, haemofiltration, plasmafiltration and peritoneal dialysis)
Cardioversion or DC countershock
Acute or external cardiac pacing
Mechanical circulatory support
Intracranial pressure monitoring
Complex intravenous nutrition and drug scheduling
Complex anticonvulsant therapy
Frequent or pressurised infusions of blood products
Active or forced diuresis
Induced hypothermia
Balloon tamponade of oesophageal varices
Emergency thoraco- or pericardiocentesis

- they have an unexplained deteriorating level of consciousness
- they have required or are requiring some form of continuing resuscitation
- they have received a significant injury
- they have undergone prolonged surgery or any surgical procedure that is medium or high risk or of a specialist nature, even if this surgery is elective
- they have potential or actual severe metabolic derangement, fluid or electrolyte imbalance
- they have an acute organ (or organ/system) failure
- they have established chronic disease (or organ/system failure) and experience a severe acute clinical deterioration or secondary failure in another organ/system
- they require one-to-one nursing because of the severity of an acute or acute on chronic illness.

CASE MIX

PIC trainees can encounter a variety of different patterns of case mix (and clinical practice) depending upon where they choose to train. These patterns are affected by geographical, cultural, political and socio-economic influences. Additionally the whims of clinical referral patterns and the impact of medical reputations serve to amplify the variation. Nevertheless it is still possible to make broad predictions about overall PICU activity. Some 30 per cent of admissions are 'booked', i.e. planned after elective or scheduled surgery or other pro-

cedures. The rest (by far the majority) are unplanned emergencies occurring at all times of the day and night. Children of different age groups show different patterns of mortality that are reflected in the reasons for PICU admission. Congenital abnormalities figure prominently in young patients and malignancy and trauma in older patients.

Just under 40 per cent of admissions occur in the context of congenital heart disease. These may be new presentations, elective admissions after surgery or emergency admissions for other causes. Roughly 20 per cent occur in the context of respiratory disease although seasonal and geographical variations do apply. Major trauma accounts for about 15 per cent and neurological problems (other than trauma) make up less than 10 per cent. The composition of the remainder is more varied depending on the allocation of neonatal surgical patients and other services.

Despite the fact that the majority of admissions are unplanned emergencies, the turnaround time is remarkably short compared to adult or neonatal intensive care. The length of stay is a heavily skewed distribution with typical medians usually just over 24 hours. Crude mortality rates are low (approximately 6 to 8 per cent) but not all ICU survivors go on to survive to hospital discharge. Overall hospital mortality for patients that use the PICU during their stay averages 1–3 per cent higher than ICU mortality. The quality of survival however is usually high. Data from an ongoing cohort study in Melbourne, last reported in 1990, showed no relationship between length of PICU stay and outcome. Young children were more likely to die than older children, but young children who survived did not have an increased risk of handicap. Although 20 per cent of admissions had died by the time of long-term follow up, only 5 per cent of survivors had a severe handicap, and 17 per cent were functionally normal although still requiring medical supervision. 91 per cent of the survivors would be expected to go on to lead an independent life.

Despite the low mortality rate, short lengths of stay and good quality outcomes compared to other forms of intensive care (adult or neonatal), a career in paediatric intensive care is not a bed of roses. Paediatric intensivists see more child deaths than most paediatric practitioners do. Even though PICU admission should be precluded if death is inevitable, intensivists often have strong views about the 'quality' of death and extensive experience of palliative care.

SUMMARY

There are many routes for a professional to take to arrive at a career in paediatric intensive care. To work in PIC you need to keep your wits about you and keep up your clinical skills as well as your knowledge of physiology and technology. A PICU is a busy environment with a high turnover of patients. The work includes many urgent and emergency clinical situations but should not be considered stressful. It is a young medical speciality packed with enthusiasts and jobs are always likely to be confined to large centralised children's teaching hospitals where evidence suggests the best results are achieved and where intensivist appointments can be justified by the volume of work. The diversity of the clinical caseload and high quality results mean that job satisfaction and the psychological and emotional rewards of a career in PIC are high.

1 An Introduction to PICU

2 Resuscitation

- **The resuscitation team**
- **Resuscitate first!**
- **Recognition of the seriously ill child**
- **The systematic approach**
- **Advanced life support**
- **Trauma**
- **Short notes on common scenarios**
- **Parents**
- **Post-resuscitation care**
- **When to stop**

THE RESUSCITATION TEAM

A team approach to the running of any resuscitation is essential. Left to themselves, resuscitations tend to attract large numbers of people, lack organisation, direction or control and become increasingly chaotic. The effective application of resuscitation algorithms requires a team leader who assumes overall control. This individual coordinates the efforts of the participants leading to earlier achievement of key treatment goals.

Dedicated resuscitation teams should practice regularly with both didactic and interactive (scenario-based) training. Ward-based scenarios will often involve the 'arrest' team alone, whilst scenarios in the Accident and Emergency Department or PICU may involve other staff, often at a more senior level. The leader of a resuscitation team usually avoids participation unless their particular skills or experience are required. Other personnel should be assigned to manage particular aspects of patient care such as securing the airway and breathing, performing cardiac compressions or establishing intravenous access. The smooth running of a resuscitation is dependent upon several factors including strong leadership, a knowledge of protocols and confidence in dealing with the situation at hand. All these factors can be improved with appropriate training and regular practice.

RESUSCITATE FIRST!

When you encounter a critically ill child it is essential to prioritise your approach:

- **resuscitate** first, then
- **diagnose** the specific cause of the presentation, and finally
- **treat** the disease.

Resuscitation involves the recognition and treatment of one or more potentially life-threatening conditions that may not themselves constitute the primary diagnosis. These are prioritised in terms of their immediate threat to life rather than their relation to an underlying disease. By this definition, resuscitation may be anything from the application of a simple airway-opening manoeuvre in an unconscious patient to a team-oriented intervention in a complex, fulminating failure of multiple organ systems.

RECOGNITION OF THE SERIOUSLY ILL CHILD

Cardiac arrest

To enable effective resuscitation it is necessary to understand the mechanisms that lead to cardiac arrest in children. By the time arrest has actually occurred, the chances of successful resuscitation without morbidity are slim whereas recognition of the preceding symptoms

9

and signs allows time for urgent intervention. Spontaneous cardiac arrest is rare. Cardiac arrest is more commonly the end result of respiratory or circulatory failure that leads to intracellular (particularly myocardial) acidosis; the commonest cause is hypoxia.

The pathophysiological processes that lead to death are not as varied as the potential underlying diagnoses (although 'common' diagnoses are listed below). Hence you do not need to know the diagnosis to recognise the need for resuscitation and initiate it effectively. For example the mechanism of natural death from neurological disease is usually respiratory compromise such as loss of protective airway reflexes or apnoea. Prior to 'arrest', pre-emptive correction of the respiratory problem with interventions that provide effective oxygenation will usually lead to restoration of the circulation. In other situations detectable circulatory inadequacy precipitates first neurological, and then subsequent respiratory failure or leads to cardiac arrest directly.

COMMON CAUSES OF CARDIAC ARREST IN CHILDREN

- Sudden-infant death syndrome
- Trauma
- Sepsis
- Near-drowning
- Cardiac disease
- Foreign-body aspiration
- Hypovolaemia

Cardiac arrest on the PICU is a relatively uncommon event, occurring in less than 2 per cent of admissions. Abrupt cardiac arrest in the absence of significant premorbid disease is most likely to respond well. Similarly patients who require cardiopulmonary resuscitation (CPR) for less than 15 minutes tend to have a better outcome than those who require CPR for more than 30 minutes or who have multiple episodes of 'arrest'. There are very few conditions that justify longer CPR than this. Notable exceptions include patients with hypothermia (because of the possibility of cerebral protection) and some forms of poisoning (e.g. tricyclic antidepressants, anticonvulsants, phenytoin, β-blockers and calcium blockers) for whom case reports of exceptional outcomes occur reasonably regularly.

Since the brain is critically sensitive to the effects of circulatory inadequacy, the chance for intact neurological survival may have been lost by the time the heart stops. Care *must* therefore be directed at recognising the signs and symptoms of *impending* respiratory, circulatory or neurological failure to allow effective intervention.

IMPENDING COLLAPSE

Herald signs requiring urgent intervention should be sought in the respiratory, cardiac and neurological systems. Table 2.1 gives the normal values for cardiorespiratory variables in children of different ages (closer age divisions for cardiovascular variables are produced in the cardiovascular system chapter).

Adopting an Airway, Breathing, Circulation and Disability (Neurological) (ABCD) approach to critical illness, the signs and symptoms that need to be detected, identified or elicited are:

Table 2.1 Normal values for cardiorespiratory variables in children of different ages.

Age (years)	Respiratory rate	Heart rate	Systolic BP
< 1	30–40	110–160	70–90
1–5	20–30	95–140	80–100
5–12	15–20	80–120	90–110
>12	10–15	60–100	100–120

- Airway and Breathing – tachypnoea, bradypnoea, recession (intercostal, subcostal and suprasternal), accessory muscle use, nasal flare, **cyanosis**, **stridor**, grunting, wheeze, inadequate or unequal chest movement and breath sounds, or a **silent chest**.
- Circulation – tachycardia, **bradycardia**, pulse volume, capillary refill, skin colour and temperature, hypertension and **hypotension**.
- Disability – impaired or altered conscious level, coma, decorticate and decerebrate posturing, altered tone, abnormal pupillary signs, seizures.

(the more ominous and life-threatening signs are indicated in bold type).

The interaction between the various organ systems means that inadequacies in one will often have an impact on the others, for example a head injury with raised intracranial pressure may produce Cheyne–Stokes breathing, hypertension and bradycardia.

THE SYSTEMATIC APPROACH

Given that the situation that led to the cardiac arrest may pose a danger to the resuscitator and that resuscitation is easier with more than one provider working simultaneously, the **SAFE** approach should always be employed:

- **S**hout for help
- **A**pproach with care
- **F**ree from danger
- **E**valuate ABCD.

Evaluation of ABCD involves an initial check for responsiveness using both verbal and physical stimulation. The resuscitator should stabilise the head and gently shake the child on the shoulder or arm, while at the same time asking the question 'Are you alright?' If cervical spine trauma is suspected, plausible or possible, then the cervical spine should be immobilised as well as the head whilst interrogating the patient. A meaningful reply indicates that the airway, breathing and conscious level are all adequate.

Basic life support

The purpose of basic life support is to provide oxygenation, ventilation and perfusion from the time of collapse until there is a return of spontaneous cardiorespiratory function or until more advanced support can be provided.

The fundamental rule of the ABCD system and the source of its effectiveness is the preservation of the sequence. If a problem develops or there is a failure of response restart or check the sequence from the top. For example if the airway appears OK and artificial respiration is ineffective – recheck the airway.

(A)irway

Significant impairment of conscious level will compromise airway protection reflexes such as the cough and gag and may therefore be associated with signs of airway obstruction. A simple head tilt/chin lift manoeuvre in this situation may be all that is required to relieve the obstruction (Figure 2.1). Care should be taken in the infant, as the ideal head position is neutral, rather than the extended 'sniffing the morning air' position used in older children. Head tilt is contraindicated if cervical spine trauma is suspected.

A quick examination of the oropharynx at this time will detect the presence of gastric contents, blood or an obvious foreign body/material, all of which should be removed. A blind finger sweep is contraindicated, there is insufficient room for an adult finger to reliably remove a foreign body without pushing it deeper into the pharynx and it may traumatise the soft palate.

Having opened the airway a rapid assessment of breathing is made. This involves placing your ear in front of the child's nose and mouth, whilst looking down at the chest. It is then possible to *look* for chest movement, *listen* for breath sounds and *feel* for breathing.

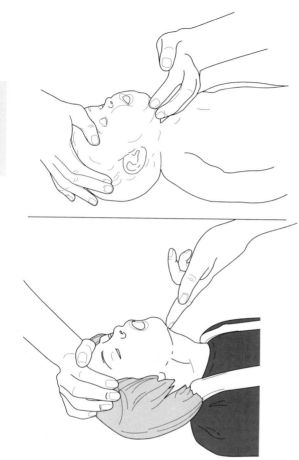

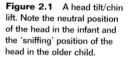

Figure 2.1 A head tilt/chin lift. Note the neutral position of the head in the infant and the 'sniffing' position of the head in the older child.

Occasionally the head tilt/chin lift manoeuvre may be ineffective or contraindicated. In such cases a jaw thrust manoeuvre should be employed (Figure 2.2). This involves keeping the head in the neutral position, whilst forcing the jaw forward by placing two or three fingers behind the angle of the mandible on each side and lifting the jaw upwards. Again, the *look, listen, feel* method of assessment of airway and breathing should be undertaken.

(B)reathing

If the look listen and feel suggests that breathing is absent or inadequate with a patent airway, then respiration should be supported. Initially *five rescue breaths* need to be given, of which at least two should be sufficient to cause the chest to rise. Slow breaths, using the minimum inflation pressure, will reduce the risk of gastric insufflation.

If the chest is not seen to rise then further adjustment of airway opening manoeuvres should be undertaken. Continued failure to ventilate the patient should raise the suspicion of a complete airway obstruction. A possibility, suspicion or history of foreign body should lead to manoeuvres to remedy choking. Other causes require more advanced airway manoeuvres (which are not basic life-support skills). Advanced airway-support techniques with increasing skill requirements of the operator vary from insertion of a Guedel airway to endotracheal intubation. If intubation is impossible and total airway obstruction persists then cricothyrotomy with retrograde intubation or jet insufflation of oxygen may be used. Ultimately a surgical airway, may be required as an emergency.

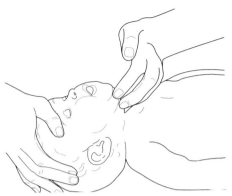

Figure 2.2 A jaw thrust.

(C)irculation

Following the five rescue breaths the circulation should be assessed by feeling for a central pulse for up to 10 seconds. In infants the brachial and femoral sites are recommended since the carotid may be deceptively hard for the inexperienced to feel. If the pulse is absent or the rate inadequate (less than 80/min in the newborn, less than 60/min in infants), then cardiac compressions should be commenced.

The optimal technique for cardiac compressions is a finger-breadth below an imaginary inter-nipple line in infants and two finger-breadths above the xiphisternum in older children. Compressions should be approximately one third the depth of the chest, irrespective of the age of the child. If at any time the chosen technique for the child is deemed to be ineffective, then an alternative technique should be employed to ensure an adequate cardiac output. The ratio of compressions to ventilation varies depending on the age of the child. In younger children the ratio is 5 : 1, whilst in the older child (over 8 years old) it should be 15 : 2. In children the ideal compression rate is 100 min^{-1}, equating to a compression:ventilation cycle rate of 20 min^{-1}. Neonates require a faster rate of approximately 120 min^{-1}. Cardiopulmonary resuscitation must be continued with the minimum of interruption until either there is a return of cardiac output and spontaneous respiration, or it is decided that support should be withdrawn. The complete basic life-support algorithm is shown in Figure 2.3.

At the start of basic life support the provider shouted for help. If no help has arrived then after 20 cycles (60 s) try again to get help – you can often carry the child with you and continue resuscitation as you go. If too few people, the wrong people or too many people arrive during the resuscitation then the situation should be corrected immediately. Voyeurs should be sent away and non-participant trainees should stay out of the way.

(D)isability

Conscious level is assessed by the stimulus required to elicit a response. The **AVPU** classification distinguishes patients who are **A**lert, respond to **V**oice, respond only to **P**ain or who are **U**nresponsive. This system is quicker than the Glasgow Coma Score (GCS) and can be applied across patient ages. The GCS is more well known but cannot be applied across the entire paediatric age range without adaptation for preverbal children. Burke *et al.* mapped AVPU by correspondence analysis to the GCS as shown in Table 2.2.

ADVANCED LIFE SUPPORT

If it is apparent that either basic life support is not sufficient to fully resuscitate the patient, or that the underlying condition will require more complex interventions to correct it, then advanced life-support (ALS) techniques should be employed. Advanced life support of the airway and breathing always includes the provision of 100 per cent oxygen if it is available. Access to the circulation should be gained after securing the airway breathing and cardiac

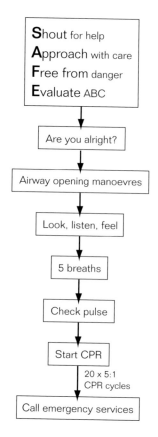

Figure 2.3 The BLS algorithm. Reproduced from APLS: The Pediatric Emergency Medicine Course, 3rd edn. 1998 American Academy of Pediatrics; p. 22.

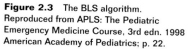

Table 2.2 Mapping AVPU to GCS				
	Alert	**Voice**	**Pain**	**Unresponsive**
GCS Eye component	4	3	2	1
GCS Motor component	6	5	2–4	1
GCS Voice component	5	3–4	2	1
GCS Total Score	15	11–12	6–8	3

compressions for pulseless patients. Attempts at venous cannulation should persist for no longer than 90 seconds, after which an intraosseous needle should be sited. Central venous cannulation or cut-downs can be used as supplements later.

Pulseless arrhythmias

See Figure 2.4. During basic life support in hospital, ECG monitoring should be applied (and is usually available from a defibrillator). The cardiac rhythms encountered in pulseless patients can be classified as non-ventricular fibrillation/ventricular tachycardia (Non-VF/VT) or ventricular fibrillation/ventricular tachycardia (VF/VT).

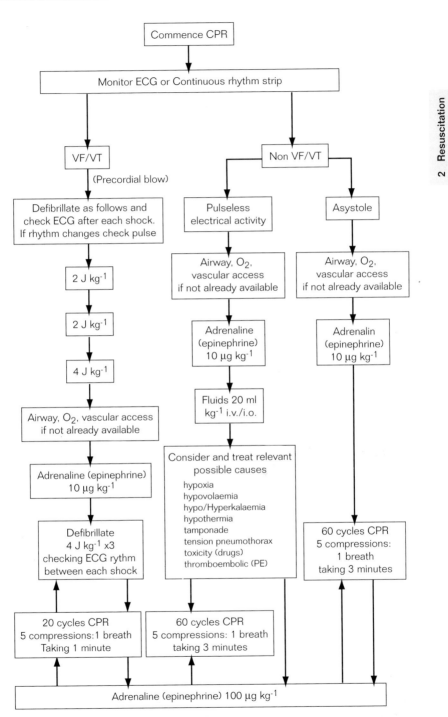

Figure 2.4 Pulseless arrhythmia resuscitation.

NON-VENTRICULAR FIBRILLATION/VENTRICULAR TACHYCARDIA (VF/VT)

This is by far the commonest situation likely to be encountered in a paediatric cardiac arrest. Approximately 70 per cent of paediatric patients suffering an out-of-hospital cardiac arrest will present in asystole, usually secondary to hypoxia. Prompt recognition and treatment are essential as outcome may be improved if the time between onset of arrest and initiation of ALS is minimised. Good basic life support with high-flow oxygen remains the mainstay of any resuscitation, allowing time to secure the airway and gain circulatory access.

In the absence of a spontaneous cardiac output, adrenaline (epinephrine) is administered in a dose of 10 μg kg^{-1} (0.1 ml kg^{-1} of 1 in 10 000). This should be followed by 3 minutes of CPR and reassessment of the circulation. If the cardiac output remains inadequate, then high-dose epinephrine at 100 μg kg^{-1} (0.1 ml kg^{-1} of 1 in 1,000) is administered. Adrenaline (epinephrine) can also be administered via the endotracheal tube if access to the circulation has not been established in which case the dose is 10 times the intravenous dose. Although controversy persists over whether high-dose adrenaline (epinephrine) does more harm than good, the arguments do not all apply to children, who tolerate it better than adults. As the cycle continues, endotracheal intubation should be undertaken if not performed earlier and consideration should be given to the use of bicarbonate and calcium in recalcitrant cases.

If an ECG rhythm (not VT) without a cardiac output is found on presentation, then the patient can be presumed to have pulseless electrical activity (PEA), formally known as 'electromechanical dissociation'. In this instance the basic and advanced life-support steps are the same as for asystole; special consideration should be given to specific causes often remembered as the four Hs and four Ts:

Hypoxia	Tension pneumothorax
Hypovolaemia	Tamponade
Hyper/Hypokalaemia	Toxicity (e.g. tricyclics)
Hypothermia	Thromboembolic

each of which requires targeted specific management. It is usually appropriate to administer a 20 ml kg^{-1} fluid bolus during the initial stages of treatment of PEA. Untreated PEA degenerates into asystole usually via an agonal rhythm of very broad slurred QRS complexes. Hence the list of causes can be useful in asystole as well.

VF/VT

In the unlikely event that the patient presents in either ventricular fibrillation or pulseless ventricular tachycardia, then the priority is to defibrillate without delay. This is why the distinction of VF/VT versus non-VF/VT is used. BLS need only be instituted if defibrillation cannot be undertaken immediately; otherwise it should follow on from the three initial shocks. The first two shocks should be approximately 2 J kg^{-1} and the third 4 J kg^{-1}. A pulse check need only be made between shocks if a rhythm change is noted on the monitor.

Safe practice should *always* be followed with the defibrillator. The paddles should never be allowed to touch, other staff members must be clear prior to discharge and the paddles must always be either on the patient or back on the machine. The standard paddles are 12 cm in diameter, smaller sizes are available for children (8.5 cm) and infants (4 cm) respectively. The largest paddles that can safely fit on the child's chest should be used to reduce the impedance to current flow. If only large paddles are available and the child is small then defibrillate with one on the anterior chest wall and one posterior. Unsynchronised shocks are preferred, even in the presence of pulseless VT, as otherwise difficulty with R wave recognition may lead to a significant delay in discharge of the defibrillator.

If the patient fails to revert to sinus rhythm following the initial shocks, then ALS should be commenced immediately. This includes securing the airway, oxygenating the patient, commencing cardiac compressions, and securing intravenous access. Adrenaline (epinephrine) is then administered in a dose of 10 μg kg^{-1} and CPR continued for 1 minute. Three further attempts at defibrillation should follow, but all at the higher energy level of 4 J kg^{-1}. If still unsuccessful then consideration should be given to specific, reversible causes such as hypothermia, electrolyte problems and poisoning. The administration of high-dose adrenaline ($100 \mu g \ kg^{-1}$) is also recommended. If the arrhythmia remains resistant to defibrillation, then the use of alkalinising agents and specific anti-arrhythmic agents, such as lignocaine (lidocaine), may be necessary. The role of bretylium tosylate in children is unclear and it is not recommended under the age of 12 years, or in doses greater than 5 mg kg^{-1}. However, rapid intravenous injection may be effective in resistant VF or VT, particularly following cardiac surgery or in the presence of hypothermia.

Resuscitation should continue with defibrillation attempts every minute, accompanied by further high-dose adrenaline (epinephrine) every 3 minutes, until either successful or resuscitation is abandoned. Hypothermic non-responders should be rewarmed to a core temp of at least 32°C during this process.

Arrhythmias with a pulse (see Figure 2.5)

SUPRAVENTRICULAR TACHYCARDIA → *give Adenosine !*

Supraventricular tachycardia (SVT) is the most common primary cardiac arrhythmia in children. Most cases are due to aberrant conduction whether in association with an accessory pathway or through the atrioventricular node. Characteristically the tachycardia is narrow complex, with a rate above 220 min^{-1}. The abnormal rhythm is usually well tolerated. Shock is rarely present but can be detected by assessment of the conscious level and the peripheral circulation. If shock is present then rapid termination of the arrhythmia is essential. The drug of first choice in this situation is adenosine given in incremental doses of 50 to 250 μg kg^{-1} which must be administered as rapid intravenous boluses. Failure to respond to adenosine should lead to synchronised DC cardioversion (0.5 J kg^{-1} increasing to 1–2 J kg^{-1}). However if the patient is not shocked and is otherwise stable then various vagal manoeuvres and drug treatments can be tried before elective DC cardioversion under sedation.

Confusion may arise if the SVT is associated with abnormal ventricular conduction, giving the appearance of a wide-complex tachycardia. In this situation the absence of shock and a slowing of the heart rate in response to adenosine helps to distinguish SVT from VT.

BRADYCARDIA → *1) Treat Hypoxia → 2) Epi ± Atropine*

Bradycardia severely compromises cardiac output, even to the point of mimicking cardiac arrest. It should always be assumed to be due to hypoxia, until proven otherwise, and treated accordingly. Other treatments include the use of adrenaline (epinephrine) as both a bolus dose (10 μg kg^{-1}) and infusion (0.05–1 μg $kg^{-1} min^{-1}$), and atropine (20 μg kg^{-1}) if vagal overactivity is suspected. If bradycardia persists then consideration should be given to an isoprenaline infusion or cardiac pacing (transvenous, external or oesophageal).

TRAUMA

ABCD (Primary survey)

The **airway** may be more likely to be obstructed by foreign matter, for example teeth, than in other scenarios and ascertainment of airway patency *must also involve control of the cervical spine*. If support is required for **breathing** in the context of trauma then intubation is likely to be indicated and necessary. Attention to the **circulation** should include steps to control haemorrhage and it is wise to site two large-bore cannulae for volume replacement and to cross match blood in accordance with the urgency of the situation in addition to any other blood tests. Although measurement of blood pressure is not a priority in acute resuscitation, hypotension from haemorrhage means that at least 25 per cent of the circulating blood volume has been lost. Having successfully got to **disability** dealing with problems along the way there should be no delay in giving analgesia.

Secondary survey

In a trauma scenario one must then **Expose** the patient to perform a secondary survey. Having said this the primary ABCD may have involved emergency surgery and all sorts of

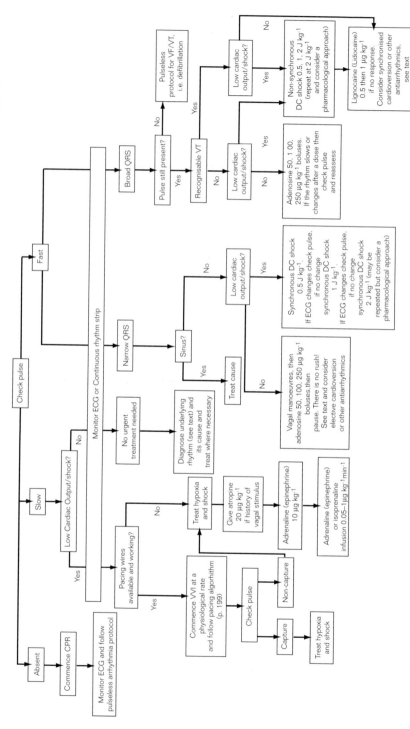

Figure 2.5 Arrhythmia resuscitation.

activities before the secondary survey is performed. If such a transfer is required then clearly document and hand-over the information that the secondary survey still needs to be performed. The secondary survey consists of a regional review of body parts (head, face, neck, thorax, abdomen, pelvis, spine (after log-rolling) and limbs/extremities). Try to limit the duration of exposure in children to avoid hypothermia.

Patterns of injury

Children are remarkably resilient. It is important not to lose sight of the fact that injuries almost trivialised by their medical descriptions must have entailed significant force. Always be aware of the possibility that an injury may be non-accidental or perpetrated on a child. Clues include a history that does not match the severity of the injury and 'characteristic' features of injuries that betray their causation. Unwitnessed severe injury raises questions about whether an inadequate standard of supervision afforded to the child put them at risk.

Head injury is more likely in children since their heads are relatively large, subject to weaker muscular neck control, and (being short people) are vulnerable to a variety of direct injuries less likely in taller people. During **'E'** look for evidence of a CSF leak, look at the fundi and test motor function. The ongoing priority is to prevent secondary brain injury. Shaking causes an acute diffuse axonal injury with cerebral oedema. Shaking (particularly recurrent shaking) may be associated with subdural haematoma. Associated 'slamming' impacts may cause more obvious external trauma or skull fracture (the principal indication for a skull X-ray).

Children's reduced respiratory reserve is an important factor in the management of chest trauma. Rib fractures and flail chest are very unusual in younger children whose ribs are very elastic, however the absence of these conditions does not exclude significant force in the injury. By far the most common cause of unilateral or asymmetric air entry after major trauma is malplacement of the ET tube. Thoracocentesis is only urgent if pneumo- or haemothorax is associated with hypoxia or shock.

Abdominal distension / tension has far more respiratory consequences than in adults and the viscera are differently proportioned. The liver and spleen are relatively exposed and vulnerable compared to older patients and the bladder is abdominal rather than pelvic. Laparotomy is often deferred since most intra-abdominal haemorrhage will tamponade (hence diagnostic peritoneal taps are less common). Rectal examinations should be performed once, and should be left to the person making the decision about laparotomy. Do not open the abdomen unless you are equipped to perform a hemi-hepatectomy. Double contrast computed tomography (CT) and ultrasound may give definitive information about the viscera.

SHORT NOTES ON COMMON SCENARIOS

It is common in paediatric medicine to be presented with a seriously ill child who is likely to need specific interventions in order to prevent deterioration and progression to a full cardiac arrest. Resuscitation should always be based on assessment and stabilisation of airway, breathing and circulation prior to definitive care. In some instances intervention can be so immediately effective as to mean that PICU admission is no longer warranted. However resuscitation is not over until the appropriate placement of the patient has been secured.

Anaphylaxis

BACKGROUND

The commonest causes of anaphylaxis in children are penicillin, latex, radiological contrast media and peanuts.

AIRWAY

If there is evidence of obstruction, give adrenaline (epinephrine) 10 µg kg^{-1} i.m. followed by 5 mg nebulised salbutamol. If obstruction progresses then intubation should be considered.

Complete airway obstruction demands intubation. Failed intubation with complete airway obstruction necessitates establishment of a surgical airway.

BREATHING

Apnoea demands rescue breaths and intubation must be attempted. If wheeze is present then give either parenteral adrenaline (epinephrine) if not already administered and /or nebulised salbutamol.

CIRCULATION

If the pulse is absent then BLS should commence immediately and an assessment of the cardiac rhythm should be made, followed by initiation of the appropriate protocol. If the patient is shocked then the adrenaline (epinephrine) should be followed by a fluid bolus of at least 20 ml kg^{-1}.

Hypovolaemic shock

BACKGROUND

It is most commonly due to severe dehydration, sepsis or trauma.

AIRWAY

Administer 100 per cent oxygen via a facemask.

BREATHING

Intubate and ventilate if significantly obtunded (GCS (<8), severely injured, requiring lines for invasive monitoring, or needing large volumes of resuscitation fluid (>40 ml kg^{-1}).

CIRCULATION

Wide-bore peripheral or intraosseous access should be established for volume replacement without delay. In traumatic shock at least two sites of access are necessary because of ongoing losses. As a rule of thumb:

- 22G cannulae for infants
- 20G cannulae for term infants and small children up to 2 years old
- 18G cannulae for children up to 6 years old
- 16 or 14G for older children.
- Give isonatraemic crystalloid fluid or colloid boluses of 20 ml kg^{-1}, reassess and repeat as necessary. Remember that crystalloid solutions may require a two to four times greater volume to produce the same effect as colloid. After 40 ml kg^{-1} of colloid it may be necessary to consider inotropic support (sepsis) or blood (trauma).

Burns

BACKGROUND

Approximately 50 000 children are treated for burns in Accident and Emergency departments every year, of whom about 10 per cent will require hospital admission and only 1 per cent of those (0.1 per cent of the total) will require intensive care if managed appropriately. Most cases are boys of pre-school age.

AIRWAY

Always give 100 per cent oxygen. Airway compromise is usually caused by either thermal injury with progressive oedema, or inhalational injury and not just by smoke. Hot, wet gases and steam deliver very serious thermal injuries. The airway needs to be secured early as later oedema may cause severe airway obstruction. Fire may have been associated with explosion – always consider the possibility of a cervical spine injury.

BREATHING

Breathing difficulty can result from inhalational injury, circumferential full-thickness burns, or other associated injuries. Look for laboratory evidence of carbon monoxide or cyanide poisoning, which may be betrayed by hyperventilation or acidosis in the presence of good oxygenation.

CIRCULATION

Hypovolaemic shock results from fluid loss across burned tissue and will therefore take several hours to develop. If shock presents early then other causes should be considered (i.e. associated trauma). If the presentation of the patient is delayed then the total fluid lost over that time ($1 ml\ hr^{-1}$ % $burnt^{-1}$ year of age^{-1}) will need to be replaced, either as crystalloid or more usually as fresh frozen plasma (FFP) or 4.5 per cent human albumin solution. There are a variety of eponymous fluid regimes for burns resuscitation. They usually use the patient's weight to approximate the total body surface area and so may underestimate it for small patients and overestimate it for large patients. The per cent burn is calculated by using the child's palm area as a measure of 1 per cent of the body surface area (BSA). Further maintenance fluid administration needs to take into account ongoing losses. Plan to give an additional 4 per cent of the maintenance rate for every 1 per cent BSA burned in the first 24 hours. Furthermore half of the total fluid requirement for the first 24 hours after the burn is normally given during the first 8 hours. The next quarter of the total is then given over the second 8 hours and the final quarter over the remaining 8 hours. In the second 24 hours plan to give an additional 2 per cent of the maintenance rate for every 1 per cent of the BSA burned and in the third 24 hours expect to need an additional 1 per cent of maintenance fluid for each 1 per cent BSA burned. Guidelines such as these should not be implemented without continuing to reassess the fluid requirement at frequent intervals.

Near-drowning

BACKGROUND

Near-drowning most commonly occurs in ponds and swimming pools but can occur anywhere that water is deep enough to cover the mouth and nostrils of a child lying face down. The incidence in the UK is 1.5 per 100 000 children with a mortality of about 50 per cent.

AIRWAY

The airway should be secured early because of the risk of regurgitation and aspiration of swallowed water. Assume the cervical spine is injured and immobilise.

BREATHING

Aspiration of water may lead to an acute lung injury, that is surfactant depletion, reduced lung compliance and hypoxaemia. Foreign debris may also be inhaled and should be cleared from the lungs with lavage and suction.

CIRCULATION

If the immersion time is significant then cardiac arrest may have already ensued, requiring BLS and the appropriate subsequent algorithm. Hypothermia may lead to intractable VF unless the patient is warmed to above 32°C. Rewarming leads to vasodilatation and creates a vascular space that if left unfilled results in hypotension. Optimal warming techniques include removing all wet clothing and drying the skin. External warming can then be achieved by using warmed or preferably heating blankets or a radiant heat source. External warming for colder patients, less than 32°C, runs the hazard of creating an oxygen demand in tissues that will be functionally ischaemic. Core rewarming is therefore necessary and can be achieved by:

- extracorporeal membrane oxygenation (ECMO) which warms from the core with oxygenated blood

- warm (42°C) peritoneal lavage (20 ml kg⁻¹ in and dwell for 10 min, out over 5 min and repeat) if ECMO or cardiopulmonary bypass not feasible or available
- warming intravenous fluids and ventilator gases to 39°C (for completeness).

Attempts at neurological assessment can only be made once the core temperature is at least 32°C.

Foreign body

BACKGROUND

Foreign bodies are most common in male toddlers, they are more common in males than females at any age, and more common in toddlers than in older children. Foodstuffs, small toys and coins are most commonly aspirated. A clear history is often absent.

AIRWAY

Attempt airway opening manoeuvres and avoid the blind finger sweep. If a foreign body is visible it can be removed with Magill's forceps.

BREATHING

Ventilation should be supported until the return of spontaneous respiration. If the object is stuck in the trachea this may prove impossible. Either removing the object or forcing it down a main bronchus may prove life saving.

CIRCULATION

This is rarely affected unless complications such as tension pneumothorax or hypoxic cardiac arrest ensue.

PARENTS

The trend in recent years has been for parents' advocates to assert their right to be present during the resuscitation of their child. Some appear to be grateful that they were able to witness the successful resuscitation of their child or indeed the comprehensive but unsuccessful attempts to revive them. Others eternally regret it, finding that it worsened their feelings of helplessness and describe it as the most traumatic aspect of the whole experience of their child's critical illness. The onus should not be put upon parents to stay. Those who choose to do so should be accompanied by a nurse and allowed to leave (with their nursing companion) whenever they wish. Allowing parents to stay and affording them such support seems a caring approach but little information is available on its value and it is up to the individual to judge. Inexperienced staff may feel under additional pressure and perform less well under parental scrutiny in which case they are duty bound to express their concerns and a senior doctor may need to take over tasks allocated to them. Even when surrounded by experienced staff there remain some aspects of advanced resuscitation which it would be foolish to invite parents to watch such as reopening the chest of a post-operative cardiac surgical patient.

POST-RESUSCITATION CARE

Resuscitation attempts do not stop with the successful return of spontaneous respiration and cardiac output. The precipitating condition should be diagnosed and treated and the affected organ systems will still require protection and support. For all but the most straightforward resuscitations the patient requires further management on an intensive care unit used to dealing with critically ill children.

Studies suggest that medically significant complications caused by CPR are rare (<3%). Those complications that have been reported include retroperitoneal haemorrhage, pneumothorax, pulmonary haemorrhage, epicardial haematoma and gastric perforation. The key to good post-resuscitation care is in fact the maintenance of homeostasis, with particular attention to oxygen delivery and cerebral protection. This includes:

- maintaining ABC
- provision of sedation, analgesia and muscle relaxation as required
- safe transfer to the PICU when stable
- adequate monitoring (e.g. ECG, blood pressure, SpO_2, temperature, urine output and blood gases) and linked to this
- insertion of appropriate lines of access (e.g. arterial, central venous, pulmonary artery) and monitoring (e.g. intracranial pressure bolt, oesophageal Doppler monitor)
- performing routine and further appropriate investigations
- and finally remember to *talk to the parents*.

WHEN TO STOP

The decision to stop resuscitating a child is always difficult, even when the situation appears futile. Expectations of success are always greater with children and the presence of parents can heighten the emotional charge of the situation. When significant underlying disease is present (which is comparatively rare) the doctors performing the resuscitation have no real opportunity to discuss limitation of resuscitative attempts and they are unlikely to be the individuals who have provided the preceding care.

In reality out-of-hospital paediatric cardiac arrests carry an appalling prognosis. Although the return of vital signs occurs in about two-thirds of patients, less than 15 per cent will survive to hospital discharge, with generally no survivors if more than two doses of adrenaline (epinephrine) are required or resuscitation takes longer than 20 minutes. Exceptions include patients who are significantly hypothermic or those who have taken cerebral depressant drugs. Similarly, cardiac arrests on the PICU may have a poor outcome as the aetiology is often different and the likelihood of a severe premorbid illness is high. The decision to stop should be taken by the person leading the resuscitation attempt. Under normal circumstances this will be a consultant.

3 Transport

- **Principles**
- **Who should perform PIC transport?**
- **The environment during patient transport**
- **The choice of vehicle**
- **Protocols for the transport team**

PRINCIPLES

Transport of patients within and outside hospital environments is a necessary routine that creates one of the biggest opportunities for entropy (chaos and disorder) within the ICU stay. The aim of patient transport is to provide as high a standard of intensive care as is available on the intensive care unit. This applies as much to the level of monitoring and drug and ventilatory support as to the access to appropriately skilled medical and nursing staff. In order to provide this level of care, additional staff are required over and above the resting establishment. Staffing a retrieval service is therefore likened to staffing a series of separate remote PICU beds.

PRIMARY TRANSPORT

This is the transfer of a patient from the outside world, for example the scene of an accident, into the hospital environment. Notwithstanding the essential elements of basic and advanced life support required at the scene, the essential feature of these transports is that the movement of the patient is frequently 'time-critical'. The advantages of receiving hospital dependent therapies within the 'golden hour' after injury (particularly head injury) may demand a 'swoop and scoop' approach to minimise delay. This priority can persist even when an experienced trauma medic or paramedic is at the scene or is part of the retrieval team. The result is that the patient is often transported at high speed with desperate urgency. However such an approach is rarely, if ever, appropriate for secondary transfers.

SECONDARY TRANSPORT

This is the transfer of a patient between hospitals or hospital environments. Such transfers are commonly required for movement of patients between hospitals to receive specialist intensive care (e.g. in a PICU). Similar principles also apply to the movement of patients from low dependency areas within the same hospital or for the transfer of intensive care patients to other hospital departments (e.g. radiology or the operating theatre). The theme is one of meticulous preparation and preparedness for adversity. In an acute situation this includes the resuscitation and stabilisation of patients at the site of referral, prior to transfer, described as the 'stay and play' philosophy. For secondary transport, the team may need to travel with urgency to the patient but the return trip should be far more controlled. Intensive care retrieval is almost universally a secondary transfer and should therefore be conducted methodically. Even so, all members of the team should be appropriately insured for the liabilities to which their role exposes them.

WHO SHOULD PERFORM PIC TRANSPORT?

The weight of evidence supporting the use of specialist retrieval teams to fetch intensive care candidates from referring institutions is impressive. The relative risk of an adverse event is up to ten times lower when specialist retrieval teams are used. 'Critical' incidents, morbidity and mortality are also reduced by as much as five times.

Transport and retrieval staff must, first and foremost, be skilled PICU practitioners. However transport requires specific additional skills which are not learned in the ICU environment. Team members must be familiar with the logistical difficulties they may encounter. They should calculate and meet the requirement for sufficient oxygen, fluids, drugs and equipment to cope with their needs. They must be familiar with the specific vehicle being used and the idiosyncracies of the purpose-built equipment that they carry. Such knowledge needs to be sufficient to lift them to a level of technical problem solving that would be delegated to others in a hospital environment. Additionally the transport team should carry sufficient 'kit' to deal with emergencies, although a degree of minimalism is essential to control the quantity, volume and weight of the 'transport' equipment and baggage.

THE ENVIRONMENT DURING PATIENT TRANSPORT

During routine intensive care transfers, the team may have to cope with circumstances that conspire to frustrate the aim of delivering the same standard of intensive care as that available in a PICU bed.

A cramped environment causes physical discomfort and further restricts access to the patient which may already be limited by clothing, blankets, incubator, strapping of medical accessories such as vascular access sites, drains, endotracheal tube, etc. When facing such limited access it is important to arrange seating and kit bags in advance so that they are still 'to hand' during transit. It is remarkable just how little common sense medical teams exhibit when addressing these problems for the first time. Cramped environments may be further exacerbated by low light conditions which further aggravate the sensory deprivation of the transport team.

The most common motion disturbance experienced during transport is coarse and relatively unpredictable, such as cornering in an ambulance or turbulence during flight; it causes nausea in susceptible individuals and aggravates fatigue. It can also dislodge patient, passengers, equipment and baggage which all need to be appropriately secured or harnessed to prevent unwanted movement during transit or emergencies.

Vibration or low-frequency, high-amplitude motion such as that produced by engines, also aggravates motion sickness and fatigue. More importantly it can disrupt many modes of patient monitoring such as oscillometric blood pressure determination, pulse oximetry and ECG. Solid-state monitoring equipment is more resistant to vibration artefact but is not immune to it. Vibration is often associated with noise which impairs communication, masks equipment alarms and prevents auscultation or the use of other auditory cues that one would normally rely on at the bedside.

Hazardous weather conditions may endanger the transport team and patient because of their effect on the mode of transport. Hypothermia is a particular problem in small patients, exposed patients or those who become wet during transfer to or between vehicles. Transport incubators struggle at low environmental temperatures which reduce the 'operative' temperature. Even in an incubator, patients may still need to be wrapped with covers that reduce radiant heat loss as well as that caused by convection and conduction. In cold conditions, gas cylinders may become difficult to open despite being tested before departure. Additionally cylinders of inhaled nitrous oxide (Entonox) deliver variable concentrations of anaesthetic when cold and after being exposed to low temperatures. As the temperature falls (to minus 7°C) more nitrous oxide separates as a liquid so that full cylinders discharge a higher fractional percentage of oxygen. Having done this they will subsequently contain and discharge purer nitrous oxide with less oxygen. Battery life is also significantly reduced by cold. Lead–acid batteries can function at lower temperatures than nickel–cadmium cells but are not immune to the phenomenon.

Altitude has significant physical and physiological effects that the transfer team needs to be aware of. Table 3.1 summarises gas tensions and volumes at different altitudes.

Solutions with high partial pressures of oxygen (e.g. blood after the oxygenator in an ECMO circuit) can experience decompression-type phenomena (oxygen coming out of solution) at altitude. This is a simple consequence of Henry's Law – the number of mole-

Table 3.1 Effects of changes in barometric pressure.

Altitude (ft)	Barometric Pressure mmHg (kPa)	Alveolar oxygen tension mmHg (kPa)	Alveolar carbon dioxide tension mmHg (kPa)	Alveolar water vapour tension mmHg (kPa)	Typical % saturation Hb (Adult Hb pH 7.4 Temp 37°C	Relative gas volume (to volume at sea level pressure)
0	760 (101.3)	103 (13.7)	40.0 (5.3)	47 (6.3)	97.5	1
5000	632 (84.3)	81 (10.8)	37.5 (5.0)	47 (6.3)	96	1.2
10 000	523 (69.7)	61 (8.13)	35.5 (4.7)	47 (6.3)	92	1.4
15 000	429 (57.2)	45 (6.0)	32.5 (4.3)	47 (6.3)	80	1.8
18 000	380 (50.7)	38 (5.0)	31.0 (4.1)	47 (6.3)	72.5	2
20 000	349 (46.5)	35 (4.7)	30.0 (4.0)	47 (6.3)	67.5	2.2

cules of gas dissolved in a liquid is proportional to the partial pressure and the temperature (though specific values vary for different pairs of liquids and gases).

The physical laws ascribed to Boyle, Charles and Gay-Lussac can be summarised as

$$PV = RT$$

Where P = pressure, V = volume, R is a constant and T = temperature. Thus as atmospheric pressure falls, the volume of a given quantity of gas rises proportionately (see Table 3.1). This is particularly important for a variety of medical considerations such as pneumothoraces, sinusitis, bowel obstruction, cuffed endotracheal tubes and the tidal volume delivered by pressure regulated ventilators.

The absolute tension of inhaled oxygen determines the partial pressure of oxygen in arterial blood (PaO_2). Since the barometric pressure falls at altitude then the inhaled oxygen tension also falls, necessitating a compensatory increase in the fraction of inspired oxygen (FiO_2). Falls in barometric pressure also increase the likelihood of fluid leak across the lung (pulmonary oedema). The high inhaled oxygen tensions that are required for ventilated patients at altitude can make it impossible to achieve a minimum alveolar concentration (MAC) with inhaled anaesthetic agents such as nitrous oxide. Vapourisers and flow meters do not read accurately at altitude. Furthermore low temperatures are associated with altitude even in hot climates.

Pressurised aircraft are usually designed to simulate an altitude of 4000 to 7000 ft inside the cabin. Greater pressures (up to sea level) can be achieved if essential but this may necessitate decreasing the range for the aircraft and the altitude, and risking more turbulence.

THE CHOICE OF VEHICLE

Ambulances, particularly those robust enough to transport large transport incubators, can be relatively slow and cumbersome vehicles. If there is an urgent component to the transfer it is usually related to the retrieval team reaching the patient. This may necessitate the use of a fast response car. The return journey is made after resuscitation and/or stabilisation of the patient and is a more sedate affair. The ambulance must allow room for the transport team to ride alongside the patient so that necessary interventions and monitoring are not impeded. A power supply and piped oxygen are added advantages.

Helicopters can operate over distances of 150 to 200 km (less than 125 miles) and can cross difficult terrain with ease. Flying at night is often precluded and they cannot fly in all weathers, particularly not through snow. In situations where helicopter transfer is common, protocols and availability are worked out in advance and a dedicated vehicle can be available within minutes to transport the retrieval team. The pick-up point can be sufficiently close to negate the need for intermediate transfer and patient transfer time can be minimised. However these advantages do not apply to the ad hoc use of aircraft. Facilities at the remote end of the transfer may be more limited, even in circumstances where the use of helicopters is routine. In such situations the length of time it takes to organise the transport has to be factored in to the choice of vehicle. A variety of craft have been used for ambulance work and there are very significant differences between them in terms of access to the patient during flight, payload capacity, and speed and manoeuvrability, all of which need to be taken into consideration. Vibration and noise can be particular problems.

Fixed wing aircraft require a runway and therefore usually the intermediate transfer of patient between hospital and airport at both ends of a retrieval. They subject the patient to marked acceleration and deceleration forces, which may have haemodynamic or regional effects, for example on cerebral blood flow. Unpressurised aircraft such as the Piper Navajo and Cessna 404 are piston engined and have a ceiling of about 10 000 ft; they are therefore more prone to turbulence. Pressurised turboprop aircraft such as the King Air and Cessna Conquest, fly high, quickly and smoothly and provide more room for the medical team and patient. At the lower end of the pressurised jet market, space may again be limited but speed and range are increased. Once airborne, the distance of transfer is largely academic, providing it is within the aircraft's normal operating range and the associated journey time has been judged appropriately and catered for.

PROTOCOLS FOR THE TRANSPORT TEAM

The person specification and job descriptions of the personnel considered qualified to staff a transfer team differ between health care systems. In the UK an experienced, intensive care and transport-trained paediatric intensivist accompanied by a similarly trained nurse would be considered essential. In the US airway competence and diagnostic skills are accredited to other individuals in addition to doctors and this is sometimes felt to expand the possibilities for available personnel. Technical assistants and paramedics may also be included. A clear hierarchy is necessary among the retrieval team with a single team leader. This individual is in charge of the patient, not the transport vehicle, and this is a particularly important feature of protocol for air transport. The amount of space available in the chosen transport vehicle limits the size of the transport team and despite the best intentions it is sometimes not practicable to include a parent in the same vehicle as the patient.

Irrespective of the composition of the retrieval team, each referral starts between doctors. It is vital that an experienced paediatric intensivist takes the call. A clear concise medical history is taken including details of patient's age, weight, diagnosis and relevant vital signs, investigations and procedures. Frequently the opportunity will be taken to give diagnostic and advanced life support guidelines to the referring team to assist management of the patient pending the arrival of the retrieval team.

Once the team arrives and has received an appropriate medical handover, they then assume complete responsibility and clinical charge over the patient. Preparation for transport must start with reassessment of the **ABCD** (airway, breathing, circulation, disability (neurological assessment)) and **E** (exposure). Expose the patient first for a full clinical examination including secondary survey in trauma patients. Then provide adequate wrapping for the outside environment. Interventions of all kinds are at best inconvenient and at worst impossible during transfer. It is not always possible to stop a vehicle or land an aircraft at the dictates of the medical team. Where at all possible, interventions should be performed pre-emptively before transport as part of the pre-transfer stabilisation. If you can anticipate problems and pre-empt them you will have fewer 'unlucky' experiences in your transport practice – 'chance favours the prepared mind'. For example patients in progressive or severe respiratory failure should be electively ventilated for the journey. Nasal intubation is far more stable than oral and is to be preferred unless there is a clear contraindication.

To reduce the tendency to entropy alluded to earlier, paralysis should be used in addition to sedation – this is particularly necessary to secure the intubation. Vascular access points should be well secured and the number of infusions kept to a minimum. Drips, infusion pumps and other 'spaghetti' should be clearly labelled and tracked together in a fascicular bundle or umbilical rather than allowed to spread. The number of infusions should also be minimised wherever possible. Invasive arterial monitoring is more reliable than a blood pressure cuff in the face of vibration and movement. Central venous lines are similarly useful and can be more reliably preserved than peripheral access.

Good judgement comes from experience but experience comes from bad judgement – seasoned veterans of intensive care transport in candid moments can often tell how they learned the lessons that made their practice safe. Failing access to this resource it is important to share one's experiences with colleagues and to audit transports with a formal log and procedure for critical incident reporting.

4 Audit and Performance

RANDOMISATION, MINIMISATION AND CASE MIX

The merits of paediatric intensive care have been described as 'unmeasured rather than uncertain' but this does not make PIC a futile exercise, nor does it challenge the 'specialty status' of the discipline. The statement merely reflects the restricted evidence base on which decisions about PIC admission must be made. One reason for this restriction is the prohibitive difficulty that researchers have experienced in contemplating randomised, controlled trials of (as opposed to within) PIC. For example, many would think it unethical to perform a trial where critically ill children were randomised to receive intensive care or to have it withheld. Similar difficulties prevent randomly assigning children to receive intensive care of differing standards.

Randomisation, blinding and minimisation are all methods used in clinical trials to 'control' bias. Randomisation and blinding should 'control' for virtually all bias whereas the process of minimisation only 'controls' for specific confounding factors that are known about in advance, although one can choose both potential and actual confounding factors as minimisation criteria. Without 'controlled' data of the sort that these techniques provide, it is difficult to compare groups of intensive care units or the same intensive care unit(s) over time. Any perceived differences could be caused by differences in the populations rather than in the unit(s) or the performance criterion. The question is how to control data on PIC outcomes without randomisation?

Children are not just small adults or overgrown premature babies. The distinction of paediatric intensive care from neonatal or adult intensive care is based upon conspicuous differences in 'case mix' and outcomes. There are large variations in case mix within the PICU population, not least in age (0–16 years) and diagnostic diversity. The service is low volume (and high cost) and presents particular challenges in terms of audit.

One substitute for the randomisation used in medical trials is to control the data using techniques of 'case-mix adjustment'. These techniques are used to create a frame of reference for each dataset, allowing valid comparisons to be made. 'Case mix' in this context is a generic term used to describe all of the confounding factors that could introduce bias or affect patient selection or the chances of a particular outcome.

THE ARGUMENT FOR A RANDOMISED CONTROLLED TRIAL OF PIC

As an aside it is worth disputing the facile dismissal of fundamental randomised, controlled trials. We have just made such a dismissal in the case of PIC, largely on the grounds that the potential mortality of a random assignment would be unacceptable. Such ethical dilemmas are not unprecedented in medical trials and do not universally preclude randomisation. An illustrative history is the evolution of neonatal ECMO. In the UK the potential benefits of this treatment were lost for as long as 10 years because of debate over the quality of the evidence that supported its efficacy. The situation was eventually resolved by a randomised controlled trial with death (or severe disability) as the potential end point. The trial revealed large reductions in mortality in the ECMO treated arm. During the 10 years of debate that preceded the trial, far more babies died without ever having a chance of ECMO referral than were ever randomised not to receive ECMO in the trial. Many of the delays in professional recognition of PIC as a specialty could perhaps have been avoided by a conveniently timed trial. However the opportunity has hopefully passed.

THE ARGUMENT FOR AUDIT

The ethical concerns that apply to interventional studies such as randomised controlled trials do not preclude observational studies. PICU admission policies, infrastructure, performance and organisation are all subjects within which data should be interrogated and hypotheses confirmed or refuted. Clinical audit may not yield results as persuasive as a large randomised controlled trial but the lack of opportunity to perform such trials encourages audit as a sort of compensatory mechanism. This is one reason why audit has become a standard of professional practice in paediatric intensive care. *Intensive care units that do not routinely audit themselves are not delivering adequate intensive care.*

THE LANGUAGE OF PIC AUDIT

Before exploring this area it is important to determine the context within which paediatric intensive care is to be judged and to determine the currency with which quality, efficacy, effectiveness, efficiency and outcomes are to be measured. In his thesis (*Outcome assessment of intensive care: principles and applications* (ISBN 90–393–0905 Utrecht University)) R. Gemke summarises the appropriate terminology and issues very clearly.

> **EFFICACY** – The result, or probability of benefit, of a health care programme under optimal circumstances. Efficacy addresses the core question, 'Can it work?'.
>
> **EFFECTIVENESS** – The result (benefit) of a health care programme for a defined population under average conditions in general daily practice where the benefits realised under strictly controlled conditions may no longer apply. After efficacy in a controlled clinical trial has been demonstrated, few studies address the question of effectiveness following the wider application of the technology to other health care centres. The core question to be answered is 'Does it work?' While efficacy and effectiveness of a medical technology may be established this does not imply that it will be employed efficiently.
>
> **EFFICIENCY** – The efficiency of a health care programme can be defined as the relation between the costs and consequences of that programme.
>
> The following is a hierarchy of efficiency analysis with increasing suitability of health output measures (and decreasing economic suitability).
>
> *Cost benefit analysis* assesses health outcome, converted to monetary revenues. As positive or negative changes in health are hard to express in monetary units and such an approach encounters numerous ethical problems, this method of comparison is used infrequently.
>
> *Cost utility analysis* measures the cost of a health care programme in comparison with its results, expressed in quality and duration of survival; usually expressed as quality adjusted life years (QALYs). Here quality of life is expressed as utility, i.e. the

preference, relative to perfect health on a scale from 1 (perfect health) to 0 (death), assigned by a random population to a given health state. The number of QALYs gained by a health care programme can be obtained from the number of gained life years multiplied by the relative preference of the health state under study. In this way the merits of a health care programme are expressed in a manner that enables them to be related to other programmes. Although perhaps preferable to wholly subjective analysis, QALY analysis has attracted much criticism. This is mainly because of implicit assumptions associated with their use, specifically the use of values in relation to human disability. For example, is a 40 year life expectancy for a severely disabled person whose health status has been rated as 0.25, really equivalent to 10 years of normal life? Less controversy is attracted when QALYs are used to compare outcomes of analogous technologies in homogenous patient groups.

Cost effectiveness analysis measures the results of a health care programme described in natural units (e.g. the number of pneumonias or number of headache periods prevented) in relation to the costs involved in achieving them. The term 'cost effective' should therefore really be reserved for those technologies that confer a reduction in cost *combined* with an equal or better health outcome in comparison with an alternative regime.

QUALITY ASSESSMENT – Can be defined as the critical appraisal of the measured results of a health care programme, in comparison with the formulated objectives. Hence quality assessment requires the formulation of standards (or guidelines) and subsequent evaluation to determine in what respect these are being met.

QUALITY ASSURANCE – Includes significantly more than quality assessment as it implies that action is being taken to improve performance when this is detected to be below performance guidelines. Moreover the term 'assurance' implies that this action is effective.

Another parameter that is often referred to in the interpretation of ICU audit studies is the 'EQUITY' of intensive care. All children have an equal humanitarian right to the same (i.e. highest) standard of intensive care. The reality however is that more often than not they receive intensive care of varying standards.

WHAT QUESTIONS SHOULD BE ASKED?

In order just to know what is going on in the PICU one needs to monitor patient flow through the unit, clinical activity and outcomes. To track patients we need to know how many patients there are? from where? with what diagnoses? staying how long? in how many beds? being discharged to where? and with what readmission rate? Data on clinical activity should also include monitoring what types of treatment they receive, the nature and number of interventions and the incidence and nature of adverse or critical events. In terms of outcome, death or survival to ICU discharge is the anchor to which most ICU assessment has been fastened. Even survival to hospital discharge has been less frequently explored because of the possible interplay of non-ICU related events. However outcome assessment should include morbidity as well as mortality. In paediatrics this argument is more persuasive because of low mortality rates and the additional impact of issues of growth and development as well as those of disability. Clearly all of these parameters need to be interpreted in the light of some assessment of the nature of the presenting patients and particularly the severity of their presenting illnesses.

Furthermore, how do we define quality care? What standards are recognised? How are they measured? What form of surveillance is involved? What are the impacts of changes in approach? And what about other outcomes? Does the unit recruit and retain staff easily or does everyone retire early through sickness, stress and depression? What quality of training is given to junior staff passing through the unit?

WHO SHOULD BE ASKED?

External assessment of PIC, whether quantitative or qualitative, is only one component of this analysis. The patients' or relatives' own perceptions are equally important. Severely ill patients may survive with significant emotional and psychological morbidity. Families may also be traumatised by the experience and their response will modulate the patient's perception and memories of intensive care. How do we assure the equity of intensive care? Does everybody have the same access to the same quality of care without discrimination? When one considers the depth and breadth of these issues, the approaches to ICU audit that have been used to date are as crude as they are brutal and direct.

THE TECHNIQUE OF RISK ADJUSTMENT

Most PIC research of this nature has centred on PIC mortality or survival to PICU discharge since such fundamental issues deserve priority over the wider considerations recounted above. Mortality is an unambiguous binary statistic that is easy to measure but on its own is unrefined and insensitive. One cannot argue on the basis of mortality that one ICU (or 1 year in an individual ICU) is worse than another if the patients are sicker. Furthermore the severity of illness after presentation is likely to have been influenced by the standard of intensive care received. A more discriminate account is necessary that at least takes account of the severity of illness at presentation if not other aspects of case mix.

Case-mix adjustment addresses the problem of the crude nature of raw mortality statistics. The broad definition of case mix encompasses all of the things that make individual cases different from each other but the focus is obviously upon the severity of the presenting illness. One (but not the only) way of comparing illness severity is by the 'risk of mortality' which can be expressed mathematically. Mathematical models derived from large populations of intensive care admissions are used to derive a mortality risk for each admission. For ease of interpretation these risks are then used to calculate the probability of death which provides a result with a linear relationship to outcome.

Limitations of mortality prediction models

The mathematical models that have been developed are extraordinarily useful in case-mix adjustment. However they have important limitations, most important of which is that they *cannot be used prospectively in the management of individual patients*. This is because:

- they only correct for those elements of case mix that contribute to the model
- they are only applicable to populations that are comparable to those from which they are derived
- they will not be as powerful or useful when applied to sub-groups within the population as they are to the population as a whole
- their utility is inherently affected by the way they are used
- models derived from an intensive care population make an *a priori* assumption that the patient receives intensive care.

For example one cannot expect to use a model derived from patients with sepsis to accurately predict the outcome of elective cardiac surgical patients. If the mathematical model yields a probability of death of 0.01 this means that approximately 1 per cent of patients this sick have died in the past. This does not mean that 1 per cent of patients like this will die in the future. Nor does it tell you in advance that a particular patient is one of the 1 per cent that die. If you consider this 1 per cent risk small, remember that the risk of mortality without intensive care may be 100 per cent. A good example is a child with severe croup or epiglottitis whose upper airway obstruction is not problematic once intubated on the PICU (hence models predict low mortality risk) but without that intervention, complete airway obstruction and death are quite probable. If you allow the predicted risk of mortality to affect your patient management you inevitably affect the utility of your mortality prediction model. If you do more or less to a patient as a result of the prediction you will either refute the predictor or make it come true, so that over time it appears to (and does) predict less or more accurately. This either makes the model less useful to you or it makes it a direct threat to the patient.

How mortality prediction models are generated

4 Audit and Performance

The mathematical technique used to generate these models is logistic regression analysis. This approach is chosen because the variables used to contribute to the predictor will often not bear a linear relationship to the outcome, making linear regression inappropriate. This could be a feature of the particular variables themselves (for example both high blood pressure and low blood pressure are dangerous) but it is also a consequence of the binary nature of the outcome lived/died which also precludes the use of linear regression. A further consequence of this outcome restriction is that the error of estimation is similarly confined. Nevertheless within these limits the principles of linear regression still apply.

The mathematics

In the model, a mortality risk y is assumed to be based upon n predictor variables (x_i) each weighted by a coefficient specific to it (b_i).

$$y = b_0 + b_1 x_1 + b_2 x_2 = \ldots + b_{n+1} x_{n+1}$$

The coefficients are derived from natural logarithms of the odds ratios (logits) relating the variable (or a simple mathematical translation of it) and the outcome. The expression of mortality risk (y) is the sum of these expressions and is therefore logarithmic itself.

The odds of death are regained from this logarithmic expression by taking the exponential value of y. Then, in the same way as the probability of a horse winning a race at odds of 2:1 against are 1/3 and not 1/2, the probability of death (POD) is obtained by converting from odds to probability using the formula

$$P = \text{odds} \div (1 + \text{odds})$$

Thus the probability of death (POD) is expressed as

$$POD = \exp(y) \div (1 + \exp(y))$$

There are two influences pulling at those who wish to design mortality prediction models for intensive care. On the one hand, the more variables in your model the more elements of case mix that you are taking account of. On the other hand once adequate predictive ability is achieved, any expansion of the model introduces unnecessary complexity. It is therefore customary during the development of these models to prune variables that are associated with each other. Such association may be because the particular variables are different measures of the same thing, or similar things. Alternatively it may be because of a more mathematical relation/association between the predictive nature of each. One can also choose to remove variables that do not enhance predictive power at all or do not make a statistically significant improvement to the models discriminative capability. In all cases the predictive abilities of a model are assessed in relation to the population as a whole and not to individuals within it.

Tuning the mortality prediction model

Before one uses a particular mortality prediction model, it should be calibrated and validated for one's own population. Typically two datasets are used in the development of such models; one as a learning or training dataset and a second as a testing dataset. This latter dataset may be a random sample of cases taken from the whole, or more preferably is

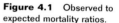

Figure 4.1 Observed to expected mortality ratios.

derived from a second prospective data collection. The process of calibration uses similar techniques to those used in analysing the testing dataset. One prospectively collects data, divides it into groups and then measures how close the observed mortality rate in each group is to that predicted by the mortality risk in each group (Figure 4.1). Typically the groups are defined by sorting the data into mortality risk strata using the mortality risk predicted by the model, although other criteria may be used. When such strata are used it is important to test the model across the entire potential range.

If the model provides a poor 'fit' to data from a subsequent test population then the problem may reside in the performance of the model, the performance of PICUs in that population or both. The subsequent clinical interpretation is rarely objective. The proliferation of mortality prediction models results in part, from a tendency on the part of clinicians to blame the model for their apparent poor performance, whereas perfect 'fit' tends to be magnanimously interpreted as validating the model as much as the performance of the test PICU(s). In fact systematic error is more likely (but not guaranteed) to result from differences in clinical rather than mathematical performance and the reverse is largely true for non-systematic errors. In order to avoid the risk of differences between populations being blamed on differences in the fit of the model, prospective comparative studies tend to derive their own internally consistent logistic regression models rather than using one 'off the shelf'.

Validation of a mortality prediction model also requires a test of its discriminatory ability. To explain how this is done let us first consider how to represent the performance of a particular test, whether it be a mortality prediction model or not. The first step is usually to generate a two-by-two 'decision matrix' linking proportions that test positive or not (in this context predicted to die or not) and those that actually have the outcome of interest (die or survive).

	Test +ve	Test −ve
Actually +ve	a	b
Actually −ve	c	d

In these terms; a represents the true positive and d represents the true negative whilst b and c represent false negative and false positive respectively. To evaluate the test:

the sensitivity of the test can be defined as $a/(a + b)$
the specificity of the test can be defined as $d/(c + d)$
the predictive power of a positive test will be $a/(a + c)$
the predictive power of a negative test will be $d/(b + d)$.

In the context of predicting death from our mathematical model we have to choose a value for the POD below which we are going to claim predicts survival and above or equal to which we are going to claim predicts death. One can then determine the sensitivity, speci-

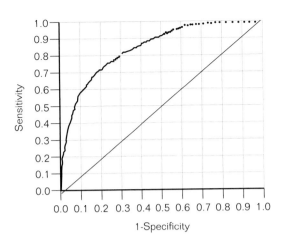

Figure 4.2 Receiver operating characteristic.

ficity and predictive powers of the test. The choice of the threshold for the POD depends upon the use to which you are going to put the test. For example a screening test needs to be highly sensitive but need not be too specific whereas if a clinical intervention is contemplated on the basis of the result then a highly specific but relatively insensitive value would be preferred. To 'discriminate' well the model must actually predict survival and death correctly across many different thresholds for the POD and in reality one chooses the appropriate value for the POD by looking for the desired sensitivity and specificity pair (likelihood ratio) first. To this end the mathematical model may be described by the relationship of its sensitivity and specificity without reference to the actual value of the POD. This representation is termed the 'receiver operating characteristic' (ROC) – a graph of sensitivity against 1-specificity. The 'characteristic', which has its origins in signal detection theory, can also be drawn as a curve. The 'ROC' (Figure 4.2) and the area underneath it, are measures of the discriminatory ability of the test.

The area under such a ROC is a useful numerical summary of the data contained in the graph. It is the most popular way of validating or comparing the discriminatory ability of models. However purists would say that comparing areas under the curves/characteristics is not a reliable substitute for examination of the graphs themselves. Different shaped characteristics describing indices of different utility over ranges of likelihood ratios may have areas of equal value underneath them. Chance prediction (coin tossing) yields an area of 0.5 under an ROC and perfect prediction yields an area of one. Clinically useful models have an area of 0.75 or greater. If a predictor has an area under the curve of 0.75 this means that a randomly selected actual non-survivor will have a higher value of POD than a randomly selected actual survivor 75 per cent of the time. It does *not* mean that prediction of death is associated with actual non-survival 75 per cent of the time.

HOW MORTALITY PREDICTION MODELS ARE USED

The POD bears a linear relationship with outcome and is therefore more meaningful as a comparative expression, than the sum of the logistic regression equation itself. Its most frequent use in monitoring a population of PIC patients is to calculate the expected death rate. If one calculates the POD for each admission then the expected death rate is the sum of these probabilities. Dividing the actual death rate by the expected death rate generates a ratio, the 'standardised mortality ratio' (SMR). Using the expected death rate in this manner effectively compares a unit's performance to a reference standard (the derivation dataset of the mathematical model). The significance of any differences (good or bad) between actual and expected death rates can be determined by other statistical techniques such as Flora's Z statistic. The amount of clinical information conveyed by the SMR is a contentious issue, as was implied when the calibration and the 'fit' of the model to subsequent data were discussed above. Although SMRs are not the whole story in comparative assessment, they are far less susceptible to confounding factors and bias than the crude mortality rate.

THE RANGE OF AUDIT TOOLS IN PIC

There are essentially two mortality prediction models of the type described above to choose from in paediatric intensive care; The **P**aediatric **R**isk of **M**ortality (**PRISM** – Appendix 2) and the **P**aediatric **I**ndex of **M**ortality (**PIM** – Appendix 1). The PRISM was derived from the **P**hysiologic **S**tability **I**ndex which itself was designed using an inclusionist approach (large number of variables). It has subsequently been revised so that PRISM III (Appendix 3) is the most up to date version (there is no PRISM II, only PSI, PRISM and PRISM III). The PRISM relies on extensive data collection in the first 24 hours of intensive care but has an established track record in studies of mortality risk assessment, cost containment and quality assurance. Its success in this regard has lead to the latest version becoming a commercial venture, which is also the reason that the dataset but not the algorithm are reproduced here. However the 'fit' of PRISM to ICU populations outside the US has been questioned. Independent research using a more reductionist approach (minimum number of fields to achieve the required predictive power) led to the publication of the PIM in 1997. Other scores are occasionally used for sub-group observational studies. These may be age specific (e.g. the **C**linical **R**isk **I**ndex for **B**abies or the **S**core for **N**eonatal **A**cute **P**hysiology) or disease specific.

An alternative approach that has been applied to adult intensive care and copied in PICU's relies upon the assertion that the sicker the patient, the more therapies they utilise at any one time. The **T**herapeutic **I**ntervention **S**coring **S**ystem (TISS) now exists in many adaptations. The number of interventions and the severity of illness are also related to the nursing dependency level. However nurse dependency encompasses additional factors and requires a different interpretation. For example the dependency of an agitated confused patient can be greater than that of a comatose one despite being less severely ill.

PATIENT–NURSE DEPENDENCY

In the UK a concept has been developed by the Paediatric Intensive Care Society of 'Levels of care'. These are defined by levels of intervention and nurse dependency and are used to calculate ideal nurse staffing levels. They are subject to considerable flexibility in interpretation.

Level I High dependency care requiring a nurse:patient ratio of 0.5:1

Close monitoring and observation required but not requiring assistance from 'life support' machines. Examples would include the recently extubated child who is stable and awaiting transfer to a general ward; the child undergoing close post-operative observation with ECG and pulse oximetry, receiving intravenous fluids or parenteral nutrition. Children requiring long-term chronic ventilation (with tracheostomy) are included in this category.

Level II Intensive care requiring a nurse:patient ratio of 1:1

The child requiring continuous nursing supervision who is usually intubated and ventilated (including endotracheal CPAP). Also the unstable non-intubated child, for example some cases with acute upper airway obstruction who may be receiving nebulised adrenaline. The recently extubated child. The dependency of a Level I patient increases to Level II if the child is nursed in a cubicle.

Level III Intensive care requiring a nurse:patient ratio of 1.5:1

The child requiring intensive supervision at all times, who needs additional complex therapeutic procedures and nursing. For example unstable ventilated children on vasoactive drugs and inotropic support or with multiple organ failure. In addition the dependency of a Level II patient increases to Level III if the child is nursed in a cubicle.

Level IV Intensive care requiring a nurse:patient ratio of 2:1

Children requiring the most intensive interventions such as unstable or Level III patients managed in a cubicle, those on ECMO, and children undergoing renal replacement therapy.

The utility of this approach depends in part upon an *a priori* assumption that the level of intervention being employed is appropriate, since one form of inadequate care occurs when clinicians fail to appreciate that it is necessary to escalate the level of intervention. In 1997 a UK governmental task force used these 'levels of care' to produce stipulations as to where PIC should be provided. Levels II and above were judged to represent 'intensive care' which should be provided in a PICU 'lead centre' admitting at least 500 children a year and conforming to nationally applied standards. Units providing care at Level I had to be capable of resuscitating sick children and initiating Level II care whilst awaiting appropriate transfer.

Within an intensive care unit some patients will be more sick than others. Some will be about to be discharged and should be comparatively well. By categorising the patients by 'level' on a shift-by-shift basis and using the associated nurse staffing stipulations one can calculate the mean dependency level of the PICU. It is then a simple matter to arrive at a number of nurses required to staff a unit to capacity or to its average level of occupancy.

CHOOSING BETWEEN MORTALITY PREDICTION MODELS

The choice of mortality prediction model is necessarily influenced by the ease of data collection. Ease of collection will improve the quality and completeness of the result. Data quality can also be significantly improved by employing dedicated data collectors rather than adding to the load of over-worked clinical staff. There are additional concerns however. Models that require data to be collected over the first 24 hours in intensive care may blur the differences between units. They may also be subject to bias as the condition of patients ameliorates or deteriorates in response to good or bad intensive care. This is particularly relevant because the early part of an intensive care unit stay is critical in terms of its effect on outcome. In PICU, experience shows that as many as 50 per cent of patients are discharged within 24 hours and that 40 per cent of the deaths occur within this time frame. Hence the extended 24-hour sampling period may add to predictive power by effectively recording outcome for these patients. Proponents of 24-hour data collection sometimes try to avoid this by ignoring data from the 'pre-terminal period' of patients who die. Nevertheless the effect still has to be taken into account when considering the differences in the discriminant power of different models as expressed by the area under the ROC.

In recent studies, premorbid or chronic health factors have been shown to have considerable influence on comparative outcome in PICU and are a significant component of the PIM but not the PRISM.

Another issue that is allied to the sample period for data collection is that of lead-time bias. This term refers to the potential effect of pre-ICU treatment or resuscitation leading to an underestimation of the severity of illness (or the reverse). Lead-time bias is of particular concern when the patient is first resuscitated by the PICU team in another environment (different department or hospital) and then transferred to the PICU. Although this potential bias has not been shown to have a consistent effect across the whole PIC population it is nevertheless wise to try and reduce its influence upon the mortality prediction model. The PIM attempts to reduce the impact of lead-time bias by defining the point of PICU admission as that when the PICU doctor takes over the patient's management rather than that when the patient physically crosses the threshold. Thus the model assesses the retrieval of patients as an integral part of their intensive care.

Methods have been described to calculate an updated mortality risk during the PICU stay using the PRISM score on the day of admission combined with that of the most recent day. Remodelled scores that revise risk assessment during the ICU stay have also been produced based upon adult risk adjustment tools such as the **A**cute **P**hysiology and **C**hronic **H**ealth **E**valuation (APACHE) and **M**ortality **P**rediction **M**odel (MPM). They are of interest in the sense that they often prove or quantify clinical axioms such as 'the patient whose condition does not improve is in fact deteriorating'. Nevertheless 'dynamic objective risk assessment' has not been widely applied and such updated risk assessments carry significant risks. For example knowledge of an evolving mortality risk at the bedside has a greater propensity for adversely affecting an individual's treatment.

MONITORING THE EFFICIENCY OF PICU

Standardised mortality ratios derived from mortality prediction models give some indication of the effectiveness of a particular PICU, as do morbidity and long-term outcome studies. By a similar token the efficiency of a PICU can also be expressed in terms that are enhanced by the inclusion of mortality prediction. Some precedent has been set in this regard by the authors of PRISM who used its precursor to identify inefficient admissions and potential early discharges. These were defined by having a low POD and receiving no ICU-dependent therapies on that day. Such an approach will however (like the TISS) interpret over-zealous intervention as an indication that the patients are sicker.

Shann (*Intensive care in childhood: a challenge to the future*, Update in intensive care and emergency medicine 25, D Tibboel, E van der Voort, Springer-Verlag, 1996) proposes an 'efficiency index' which one can quote separately for intubated and non-intubated patients. It is formulated along the following lines. An ICU is making efficient use of its resources if:

- it only has sick patients who need intensive care
- it has high bed-occupancy rates (an ICU that is usually empty is inefficient)
- it has short lengths of stay (an ICU that keeps patients longer than necessary is inefficient).

The efficiency index (EI) combines these three factors

$$EI = \text{mean POD} \times \% \text{ occupancy} \div \text{mean length of stay}$$

However since

$$\text{occupancy} = \text{mean length of stay} \times \text{number of admissions} \div \text{number of bed days}$$

the efficiency index can be redefined as

$$EI = \text{mean POD} \times \text{number of admissions} \div \text{number of beds}$$

The number of funded beds (as distinct from actual beds) is calculated in terms of the numbers of full-time equivalent nurses available to the unit

$$\text{Funded beds} = \frac{\text{nurse hours per week} \times \text{weeks worked per year} \times \text{number of FTE}}{(\text{days in a year}) \times (\text{hours per day}) + (\text{hours of handover})}$$

To provide a reference point for this index, Shann quoted a value of 7.62 for all PICU admissions at the Royal Children's Hospital in Melbourne in 1996 and the EI at the PICU in the author's institution has ranged from 6.2 to 8.6 in recent years.

DEVELOPING A BAYESIAN APPROACH TO PICU

Bayes theorem connects two entirely different probabilities that were outlined above in the consideration of the validation of the mathematical models. These were the probability of an outcome given the result of the predictor or test (the positive predictive power) and the probability of the prediction or test result given knowledge of the outcome (sensitivity). In odds ratio form the theorum can be expressed as

posterior odds = likelihood ratio × prior odds

The appeal of this theorum to the clinician is that knowing the relationship he/she can make informed judgements about many issues, including those considered in this chapter.

This chapter started with an account of the ethical difficulties that have prevented randomised controlled trials of PIC. A Bayesian perspective can provide the sort of relative risks that would otherwise have been derived from the results of such trials. The Bayesian approach can put a curious or comforting numerical slant upon clinical and ethical issues, depending on your viewpoint. For example, given the correct data one can answer the question 'When is it appropriate to admit a child to a PICU?' by using Bayes theorum to derive a numerical answer to the question 'How many deaths are equivalent to an unnecessary admission?'

Similar questions that would benefit from a Bayesian approach include 'When does the advantage of referral to a specialist unit override the risk of retrieval?' and 'When does intensive care treatment become futile?'

Appendix 1: PIM

Data collection

PIM is calculated from information collected at or about the time of the first face-to-face (not telephone) contact between the patient and the ICU doctor from the unit being audited. Use the first value of each variable measured within the period from the time of first contact to 1 hour after arrival on the PICU. The first contact may be in the PICU, emergency department, another ward in the same hospital or in a different hospital during a retrieval. Collect data on all children (less than 16 years old) admitted or retrieved to PICU. Readmissions are treated as separate patients.

DATASET

If information is missing record zero, except for systolic blood pressure which should be recorded as 120.

1 Booked admission to ICU after elective surgery or elective admission to ICU for a procedure such as insertion of a central line or monitoring or review of home ventilation. no = 0, yes = 1.
2 Is there one of the recognised underlying conditions (record the number in square brackets)?

Table A1.1 Premorbid conditions.

[0]	None	[5]	Cardiomyopathy or myocarditis
[1]	Cardiac arrest out of hospital	[6]	Hypoplastic left heart syndrome <1 month and requiring Norwood
[2]	Severe combined immune deficiency	[7]	HIV infection
[3]	Malignancy after completion of first induction	[8]	IQ probably < 35 (i.e. worse than Downs)
[4]	Spontaneous cerebral haemorrhage from aneurysm of AVM	[9]	Neurodegenerative disorder (progressive ongoing loss of milestones)

3 Response of the pupils to bright light. Both > 3 mm and both fixed = 1, other = 0, unknown = 0. The pupil reactions are used as an index of brain function; do not record an abnormal finding if this is probably caused by drugs, toxins or a local injury to the eye.
4 Base excess (mmol/L) in arterial blood (unknown = 0).
5 PaO_2 (mmHg) (unknown = 0).
6 FiO_2 at time of PaO_2 (unknown = 0).
7 Systolic blood pressure (mmHg) (unknown = 120).

Table A1.2 Logistic regression coefficients.

Elective admission yes/no	−1.552	$100 \times FiO_2/PaO2$ (mmHg^{-1})	0.415
Specified diagnosis yes/no	1.826	Absolute I SBP−120 I mmHg	0.021
Pupils fixed to light yes/no	2.357	Mechanical ventilation yes/no	1.342
Absolute I base excess I mmol/L^{-1}	0.071	Constant	−4.873

8   Mechanical ventilation at any time during the first hour (no = 0, yes = 1).

9   Outcome of ICU admission (discharged alive from ICU = 0, died in ICU = 1).

WORKED EXAMPLE

A child whose admission is not booked, first meets the intensive care doctor with pupils that react to light (pupils fixed = 0) has myocarditis (specified diagnosis = 5 = yes =1), is ventilated immediately (ventilation = yes = 1), has a systolic blood pressure of 40 mmHg (| SBP–120 | = 80), has a base excess –16.0 mmol L^{-1} (| –16 | = 16) and has an FiO_2 of 1.0 with an arterial oxygen tension of 60 mmHg ($PaO2$ = 60).

The PIM logit = $(2.357 \times 0) + (1.826 \times 1) + (-1.552 \times 0) + (1.342 \times 1) + (0.021 \times$ | 40 – 120 |) + (0.071 × | – 16 |) + (0.415 × 100 × 1.00/60) – 4.873 = 1.803

The probability of death (POD) (which should be quoted in preference to the PIM logit) is

POD = $e^{1.803} \div (1 + e^{1.803})$ = $2.7183^{1.803} \div (1 + 2.7183^{1.803})$ = 0.8585 or 86%

Appendix 2: PRISM

Data collection

PRISM is calculated from data collected during the 'admission day' – usually taken to mean the first 24 hours after physical admission to the intensive care unit. Readmissions are treated separately.

DATASET

Collect the following 26 data points for 18 variables

1　ICU outcome.
2　Age at admission (months).
3　Operative status (post-operative = 1, non-operative = 0).
4　Highest and lowest systolic blood pressure (mmHg).
5　Highest diastolic blood pressure (mmHg).
6　Highest and lowest heart rate (bpm).
7　Highest respiratory rate (breaths/min).
8　The occurrence of apnoea.
9　PaO_2/FiO_2 (PaO_2 in mmHg and FiO_2 as a decimal. Do not record in patients with intracardiac shunts or chronic respiratory insufficiency).
10　$PaCO_2$ or capillary PCO_2 (mmHg).
11　Glasgow Coma Score (only record if there is known or suspected CNS dysfunction. Do not record during iatrogenic sedation, paralysis, anaesthesia, etc.).
12　Pupillary reactions (normal, unequal or dilated, or fixed and dilated).
13　Prothrombin time (PT) or partial thromboplastin time (PTT) and the associated control.
14　Highest total bilirubin (do not record for neonates).
15　Highest and lowest serum potassium ($mEqL^{-1}$).
16　Highest and lowest serum calcium ($mgdL^{-1}$).
17　Highest and lowest plasma glucose ($mgdL^{-1}$).
18　Highest and lowest serum bicarbonate (use measured values).

Table A2.1　Scores for PRISM variables.

Systolic BP	Infants	Children	Score
	130–160	150–200	2
	55–65	56–75	
	>160	>200	6
	40–54	50–64	
	<40	<50	7
Diastolic BP	**All ages**		
	>110		6
Heart rate	**Infants**	**Children**	
	>160	>150	4
	<90	<80	
Respiratory rate	**Infants**	**Children**	
	61–90	51–70	1
	>90	>70	5
	Apnoea	Apnoea	

continued on next page　**45**

Table A2.1 Scores for PRISM variables.

Pao_2/Fio_2	**All ages**	
	200–300	2
	<200	3
$Paco_2$	**All ages**	
	51–65	1
	>65	5
Glasgow coma score	**All ages**	
	<8	6
Pupillary reactions	**All ages**	
	Unequal or dilated	4
	Fixed and dilated	10
PT/PTT	**All ages**	
	>1.5 × control	2
Total bilirubin (mg/dL) ($= \mu molL^{-1} \times 0.0585$)	>1 month >3.5	6
Potassium	**All ages**	
	3.0–3.5 6.5–7.5	1
	<3.0 >7.5	5
Calcium ($= mmolL^{-1} \times 4.008$)	**All ages**	
	7.0–8.0	2
	12.0–15.0 <7.0	6
	15.0	
Glucose ($= mmolL^{-1} \times 18.02$)	**All ages**	
	40–60 250–400	4
	<40 >400	8
Bicarbonate	**All ages**	
	<16 >32	3

The 'PRISM score' is obtained by adding the scores assigned to variables 4 to 18 in Table A2.1.

LOGISTIC REGRESSION

The mortality risk (r) is given by

$r = 0.27$ (PRISM score) $- 0.005$ (age in months) $- 0.433$ (operative status) $- 4.782$

The probability of death (which should be quoted in preference to the PRISM score or the mortality risk) is then given by

$POD = e^r \div (1 + e^r)$

Appendix 3: PRISM III

Data collection

For each variable in the dataset, record the highest and lowest values in the first 12 and 24 hours after physical admission to the ICU. Readmissions are treated as separate patients. Do not record data for patients:

- routinely cared for in other hospital locations
- staying in the PICU for less than 2 hours
- admitted receiving continuous CPR who do not achieve stable vital signs for 2 hours or more.

> Deaths of PICU patients occurring in the operating theatre are only included if the operation occurred during the PICU stay and was a therapy for the illness requiring PICU care.
>
> Terminally ill patients transferred from the PICU for comfort care are included as PICU patients for 24 hours after PICU discharge or, if receiving technologic support, until 24 hours after the technologic support is discontinued.

PRISM III weights variables differently for four categories of age defined as follows:

- neonate (0 < 1 month)
- infant (≥1 month–12 months)
- child (≥12 months–144 months)
- adolescent (>144 months).

Dataset

1 Non-operative cardiovascular disease: yes/no (includes acute cardiac and vascular conditions as the primary reasons for admission).
2 Chromosomal anomaly: yes/no and (if yes) acute/chronic!
3 Cancer: yes/no and (if yes) acute/chronic.
4 Previous PICU admission during this current hospital admission: yes/no.
5 Pre-ICU CPR (must include cardiac massage) during this current hospital admission: yes/no.
6 Post-operative (i.e. within 24 hours of a surgical procedure or a procedure taking place in an operating theatre): yes/no.
7 Acute diabetes: yes/no (includes acute manifestation of diabetes as the primary reason for PICU admission).
8 Admission from in-patient unit (excluding post-operative patients): yes/no (includes all in-patient locations except the operating or recovery areas).
9 Systolic blood pressure (mmHg).
10 Temperature (oral, rectal, blood or axilla).
11 Mental status: normal/stupor or coma. Do not assess within 2 hours of sedation, paralysis or anaesthesia. If there is constant paralysis and/or sedation, use the time period without sedation, paralysis or anaesthesia closest to the PICU admission for scoring. Stupor or coma is defined as GCS < 8 or stupor/coma using other mental status scales.
12 Heart rate (bpm) (Do not assess during crying or iatrogenic agitation).
13 Pupillary reflexes: one fixed and one reactive or both fixed. Non-reactive pupils must be > 3 mm. Do not assess after iatrogenic pupillary dilatation.

14 Acidosis: total CO_2 or pH (pH may be measured from arterial, capillary or venous sites). If total CO_2 is not measured routinely then use calculated bicarbonate values.

15 PCO_2 (mmHg) 1 kPa = 7.5 mmHg (may be measured from arterial, capillary or venous sites).

16 PaO_2 (mmHg) 1 kPa = 7.5 mmHg (use arterial measurements only).

17 Glucose (serum or whole blood). Whole blood glucose measurements should be increased by 10%.

18 Potassium (serum or whole blood). Whole blood potassium measurements should be increased by 0.4 mmol L^{-1}.

19 Serum creatinine.

20 Blood urea nitrogen (mmol L^{-1} × 6.006 = mg 100ml^{-1}).

21 White blood cell count.

22 Platelet count.

23 Prothrombin time (PT) or partial thromboplastin time (PTT) (seconds).

Logistic regression coefficients

The logistic regression coefficients for the PRISM III are not in the public domain. For its predecessor (PRISM) the logit included a summary 'score' derived by weighting the results for each variable. The rest of the logit was determined by age and operative status. PRISM III requests a similar weighting or score for each variable in the dataset. It is fair to assume that the scores will only form part of the logistic regression equation. Nevertheless they are listed in Table A3.1.

Table A3.1 Scores for PRISM III variables.

Systolic blood pressure (mmHg)	Score = 3	Score = 7
Neonate	40–55	<40
Infant	45–65	<45
Child	55–75	<55
Adolescent	65–85	<65
Else score = 0		
Temperature	Score = 3	
All ages	<33°C (91.4°F)	
	or >40°C (104.0°F)	
Else score = 0		
Mental Status	Score = 5	
All ages	Stupor/coma (GCS <8)	
Else score = 0		
Heart rate (bpm)	Score = 3	Score = 4
Neonate	215–225	>225
Infant	215–225	>225
Child	185–205	>205
Adolescent	145–155	>155
Else score = 0		
Pupillary reflexes	Score = 7	Score = 11
All ages	One fixed	Both fixed
Else score = 0	+one reactive	
pH	Score = 2	Score = 6
All ages	pH 7.0–7.28	pH <7.0
pH >7.55 score = 3,	or pH 7.48–7.55	
Else score = 0		

continued

Table A3.1 Scores for PRISM III variables.

Total CO$_2$ (mmol L^{-1}) All ages Total CO$_2$>34 score = 4, Else score = 0	Score = 2 5–16.9	Score = 6 <5	
Paco$_2$ (mmHg) All ages Else score = 0	Score = 1 50.0–75.0	Score = 3 >75.0	
Paco$_2$ (mmHg) All ages Else score = 0	Score = 3 42.0–49.9	Score = 6 <42.0	
Glucose (see dataset) All ages Else score = 0	Score = 2 >200 mg/dL (11.0 mmol L^{-1})		
Potassium (see dataset) All ages Else score = 0	Score = 3 >6.9 mmol L^{-1}		
Creatinine Neonate Infant Child Adolescent Else score = 0	Score = 2 >0.85 mg/dL or >75 µmol L^{-1} >0.90 mg/dL or >80 µmol L^{-1} >0.90 mg/dL or >80 µmol L^{-1} >1.30 mg/dL or >115 µmol L^{-1}		
Blood Urea Nitrogen Neonate All other ages Else score = 0	Score = 3 >11.9 mg/dL or >4.3 mmol L^{-1} >14.9 mg/dL or >5.4 mmol L^{-1}		
White blood cell count (cells mm^3) All ages Else score = 0	Score = 4 <3,000		
Platelet count (cells mm^3) All ages Else score = 0	Score = 2 100,000–200,000	Score = 4 50,000–99,999	Score = 5 <50,000
PT or PTT (s) Neonate All other ages Else score = 0	Score = 3 PT >22 or PTT >85 PT >22 or PTT >57		

5 Anaesthesia

- **History and background**
- **Anaesthesia and the critically ill child**
- **The process of anaesthesia**
- **Drugs commonly used in anaesthesia**
- **Drugs used to supplement anaesthesia**
- **Anaesthetic breathing systems**
- **Laryngoscopes and endotracheal tubes**
- **Anaesthetics in miscellaneous conditions**
- **Conclusion**

Trainees in intensive care are required to acquire anaesthetic knowledge and skills before undertaking clinical shifts on the PICU. This is best achieved by tuition during elective anaesthesia before working with critically ill children. Training in paediatric anaesthesia, which usually follows training in general anaesthesia, should also include exposure to the PICU. By approaching the PICU with some anaesthetic and paediatric skills potential pitfalls can be avoided – *a good anaesthetist gets into trouble less often*'. The intensivist is required to provide, maintain and reverse analgesia and anaesthesia for a variety of critically ill children. This involves handling anaesthetically challenging cases, including difficult airways, unstable haemodynamics, raised intracranial pressure, etc. Problems will inevitably occur at some point and experience is required to salvage the situation – '*an anaesthetist is best assessed by the way he/she gets out of trouble*'.

This chapter is intended as a brief overview of anaesthesia for the non-anaesthetic paediatric intensive care trainee in the pre-paediatric intensive care phase of their training.

HISTORY AND BACKGROUND

The introduction of anaesthesia to clinical practice has been attributed to William Morton who gave the first successful public demonstration of inhalational anaesthesia (using ether) in Massachusetts in 1846. The first recorded death caused by the administration of general anaesthesia occurred in 1848 (11 weeks after its introduction into clinical practice). It soon became clear that patient safety depended on:

- a thorough knowledge of the effects of anaesthetic agents
- the use of administration systems allowing their controlled delivery.

Anaesthetic training is now closely supervised, anaesthetic agents are becoming more refined and anaesthetic delivery and monitoring systems are increasingly more sophisticated and accurate. Nevertheless, anaesthesia-associated morbidity and mortality remain significant and it is widely recommended that anaesthetists do not undertake occasional paediatric practice. Anybody responsible for the administration of either inhalational or intravenous anaesthetic drugs must be familiar with their physiological and pharmacological effects and interactions and, most importantly, *must know how to manage complications arising from their use*.

ANAESTHESIA AND THE CRITICALLY ILL CHILD

Some 'golden rules' underpin the administration of anaesthesia to critically ill infants and children.

1. ORGANISE THE ENVIRONMENT

It is inadvisable to induce anaesthesia in an area where essential equipment is either unavailable or rarely used, for example ward areas and outpatient clinics. Most patients can be transferred safely to a more appropriate area (theatres, accident and emergency or the PICU) with careful airway control and oxygen therapy, prior to the induction of anaesthesia and continuing resuscitation.

2. CHECK AND ARRANGE THE EQUIPMENT

All emergency anaesthesia should take place in an area where the following (minimum) apparatus is immediately available and in serviceable condition:

- anaesthetic machine and gas delivery systems which comply with modern standards and are suitable for all ages of patients to be encountered
- tipping trolley or bed
- suction unit
- full range of endotracheal tube sizes, introducers, laryngoscopes and Magill forceps
- intravenous cannulae, fluids and administration sets
- resuscitation drugs.

As an absolute minimum the clinician must select, test and *have to hand* prior to inducing anaesthesia:

- two working laryngoscopes
- an appropriately sized and prepared endotracheal tube
- spare endotracheal tubes one size larger and one size smaller
- a wide bore Yankauer sucker (suction switched on)
- a pair of Magill forceps.

3. CALL FOR EXPERIENCED ASSISTANCE

If you retain insight and there is any doubt in your mind about your ability to deal with the situation safely, *call promptly for help* from a senior colleague. If you are inexperienced in anaesthesia or have ever been told that you lack insight (even if you didn't believe it!), call for help anyway.

Irrespective of the number of doctors present, it is desirable in any event that anaesthesia and intubation are initiated with additional immediate assistance from someone trained to assist. This should be from a member (or members) of the hospital staff *trained in*, and *familiar with*, the techniques to be employed and their application to children. This might include operating department practitioner, anaesthetic nurse, senior casualty staff or senior intensive care staff.

4. USE FAMILIAR TECHNIQUES

In the emergency situation, it is paramount to keep the process of induction of anaesthesia simple. Always pre-oxygenate and use agents with which you are confident and competent. Give clear instructions to your assistants.

5. AIRWAY, BREATHING, CIRCULATION

The paediatric intensive care trainee must have sound working knowledge of the effects of the anaesthetic method to be employed on the cardiorespiratory function of the critically ill child. In addition, he/she must be expert in basic and advanced paediatric life-support techniques.

Inadequate preparation and lack of attention to detail can make a relatively straightforward procedure unnecessarily stressful for the clinician and hazardous, or even lethal, for the child.

THE PROCESS OF ANAESTHESIA

As stated above the intensivist is required to provide both anaesthesia and analgesia to the critically ill child. This must be achieved in the course of advanced resuscitation and life-support techniques (including mechanical ventilation). During this process cardiovascular stability and optimum gas exchange must be preserved. All ICU patients should have ECG, pulse oximetry and blood pressure monitoring during induction.

INTRAVENOUS INDUCTION

Intravenous induction is an essential part of the 'Rapid Sequence Induction' (RSI) and the routine approach for many situations. However it is *contraindicated in situations where the airway is compromised* (e.g. acute upper airway obstruction) and/or those where endotracheal intubation may be difficult to achieve (e.g. lower face and jaw abnormalities).

1. ADVANTAGES

- Rapid – it is generally fast and easily accomplished (assuming intravenous access is straightforward).
- It is smoother in the presence of lung disease than inhalational induction.
- It allows prompt control in the emergency situation
- It usually reduces intracranial pressure.

2. DISADVANTAGES

- Most agents cause loss of vascular tone and a degree of myocardial depression. If the subject is incompletely resuscitated this will lead to sudden, severe hypotension
- May precipitate anaphylaxis or anaphylactoid reactions
- Loss of airway reflexes is immediate
- Apnoea is common, hypoventilation is the rule
- Low cardiac output states will slow the onset of anaesthesia – overdose in this situation is common, and may be lethal.

Rapid Sequence Induction ('Crash' Induction) should be performed in all situations where regurgitation and aspiration of gastric contents is judged to be possible (e.g. intra-abdominal pathology, multiple and severe trauma). **RSI requires the presence of a skilled assistant.**

The procedure entails:

1. PRE-OXYGENATION

It is necessary to replace air in the functional residual capacity (FRC) of the lungs with 100% oxygen, providing a reservoir of oxygen during apnoea. This provides the operator time to safely secure the airway (by endotracheal tube placement) without resorting to hand infla-tion by bag and mask.

Hand inflation during RSI is usually contraindicated because of the risk of promoting aspiration of gastric contents should regurgitation occur. Pre-oxygenation can *only* be ade-quately achieved by the application of a *close-fitting* facemask and delivery of 100% inspired oxygen through a properly assembled anaesthetic gas delivery system for a minimum of 4–5 minutes. The Laerdal resuscitation bag *with reservoir attachment* is a suitable alternative provided hand ventilation is occurring in synchrony with the patient's respiration.

2. ADMINISTRATION OF THE INDUCTION AGENT

Once pre-oxygenation is judged satisfactory, thiopentone is usually administered in a dose sufficient to induce anaesthesia (3–5 mg kg^{-1}) over a period of 10 to 15 seconds.

3. APPLICATION OF CRICOID PRESSURE (SELLICK'S MANOEUVRE)

A skilled assistant (familiar with this technique) applies *firm* backward pressure with index finger and thumb to the cricoid cartilage, *as soon as the child begins to lose consciousness*. The aim is to flatten the upper oesophagus by backward pressure applied to the cricoid ring and hence reduce the passage of regurgitant gastric contents. This requires significant pressure. *The order to relax cricoid pressure must **not** be given until the airway is secured by a properly positioned endotracheal tube (this includes cuff inflation where appropriate).*

4. ADMINISTRATION OF SUXAMETHONIUM

To date, suxamethonium is the muscle relaxant of choice for this procedure. As soon as anaesthesia is induced and cricoid pressure applied, a full relaxant dose (1–1.5 mg kg^{-1}) is rapidly administered. Following the subsidence of muscle fasciculation, endotracheal intubation can be achieved – usually within 30 seconds of administration.

INHALATIONAL INDUCTION

Inhalational induction is the method of choice during the management of acute upper airway obstruction and/or the (anticipated) difficult intubation.

1 ADVANTAGES

- It is gradual and allows safe airway control throughout the induction of anaesthesia.
- Airway reflexes are maintained for longer, and slowly diminish as the stages of anaesthesia progress.
- It can be safely performed without the immediate need for intravenous access.

2. DISADVANTAGES

- It requires experience and skill.
- The child may tolerate it poorly.
- It can cause hypotension secondary to peripheral vasodilatation and myocardial depression, though this is more gradual than that typical of i.v. induction.
- It is more difficult to perform in the presence of lung disease.
- It can elevate intracranial pressure by effects on cerebral blood flow.
- Volatile agents may trigger malignant hyperpyrexia, although this is rare.

The four stages of anaesthesia, first recognised by John Snow and enunciated by Guedel, are clearly seen during inhalational induction.

1. ANALGESIA

From beginning of induction to loss of consciousness.

2. EXCITEMENT OR UNINHIBITED RESPONSE

From loss of consciousness to onset of automatic breathing. This stage is often characterised by struggling, breath holding, coughing and swallowing. Vomiting may also occur – firm airway control is mandatory.

3. SURGICAL ANAESTHESIA

From onset of automatic breathing to respiratory paralysis. This stage may be conveniently divided into three planes:

- light anaesthesia – until the eyeballs become fixed
- medium anaesthesia – increasing intercostal paralysis
- deep anaesthesia – diaphragmatic respiration.

4. OVERDOSAGE

Increased deepening of anaesthesia leads to apnoea, loss of all reflex activity and death.

Direct laryngoscopy and endotracheal intubation is hazardous prior to stage 3, and in the absence of a muscle relaxant is most safely facilitated by the deep plane of surgical anaesthesia.

MAINTENANCE OF ANAESTHESIA

As a general principle, the *minimum* inspired concentration of oxygen required during general anaesthesia is 30%. This is necessary because of changes in the ventilation:perfusion ratio induced by anaesthesia and the potential influence of the volume of inhalational anaesthetic (particularly nitrous oxide) on the alveolar gas equation.

Anaesthesia is usually maintained in the operating theatre by continuous administration of a volatile anaesthetic agent (at the appropriate Minimum Alveolar Concentration (MAC)) in a carrying-gas mixture of oxygen enriched air or nitrous oxide. Alternatively, an infusion of a short-acting intravenous anaesthetic agent can be used to sustain anaesthesia. Combinations of intravenous agents are most commonly employed in the PICU but the preference for infusions of short-acting agents may be altered depending upon the context.

SEDATION OR ANAESTHESIA?

Most hypnotic drugs (e.g. benzodiazepines) and all intravenous anaesthetic agents will sedate the critically ill child, depending upon the dose administered. Opiates (e.g. morphine) and opioid drugs (e.g. fentanyl) provide narcosis and act synergistically with hypnotics to deepen sedation or anaesthesia. However they are not intrinsically sedative, acting predominantly on sub-cortical areas of the brain.

There is no practical scientific means of measuring the depth of anaesthesia. Similarly the adequacy of sedation in the PICU can only be judged by close observation of pupillary size and response, and by the manifestation of sympathetic discharge on the cardiovascular system, as well as other basic reflexes (e.g. swallowing, coughing, lacrimation). Clearly the level of sedation or anaesthesia required depends on the underlying condition of the infant or child and will be subject to both within-patient and between-patient variability. All clinicians practising intensive care must have a full working knowledge of the actions and side effects of all the agents they use in this situation.

AWARENESS

Awareness was unknown prior to the introduction of muscle relaxants into clinical practice. Their use enables lighter planes of anaesthesia during surgery, but can mask the delivery of inadequate amounts of anaesthetic. No muscle relaxant in current practice has any sedative or analgesic action whatsoever and therefore their use *must* be accompanied by drugs providing an appropriate level of sedation and analgesia.

DRUGS COMMONLY USED IN ANAESTHESIA

Intravenous anaesthetic agents

Sodium thiopentone

Thiopentone is often regarded as the 'gold standard' by which other intravenous agents are judged. As can be seen below it is far from the ideal agent! Used appropriately, however, it *does* provide a smooth and safe induction.

Thiopentone is the sulphur analogue of pentobarbitone and hence a derivative of barbituric acid. It is presented in single or multi-dose vials as a yellow amorphous powder. The sealed vials contain nitrogen and 6% anhydrous sodium carbonate to prevent breakdown to free acid. The powder is soluble in water (and alcohol) and in standard practice is reconstituted to form a 2.5% solution for clinical use. The solution can be left for 24 to 48 hours and re-used if necessary, but it is potentially unstable and should be discarded if not clear. It is highly alkaline (pH 10.7) and will precipitate with many compounds (e.g. vecuronium, suxamethonium).

ANAESTHETIC DOSE

This is 3–5 mg kg^{-1} but there is significant between-patient variability and the speed of induction will be affected by the cardiac output.

SYSTEMIC EFFECTS

CNS

- Cerebral activity is depressed causing sedation and clinical anaesthesia.
- Anticonvulsant.
- Reduced intracranial pressure.
- The relationship between cerebral blood flow and the metabolic consumption of oxygen is uncoupled. (This is the rationale behind barbiturate coma as part of cerebral salvage techniques).

Respiratory system

- Respiratory centre is depressed. Hypopnoea and apnoea are common.

CVS

- Myocardial depression.
- Dilation of venous capacitance vessels. This causes minimal or no problem in the normal circulation but can cause significant hypotension in the compromised patient.

METABOLISM AND EXCRETION

Thiopentone owes the short duration of its anaesthetic effect to redistribution. Plasma levels fall rapidly after intravenous bolus injection and the drug is redistributed to lean body mass (muscle) and fat. Metabolism is hepatic and excretion renal. Since it is extremely fat-soluble large amounts of the drug can be stored in body fat during prolonged infusion leading to persistence of effects long after termination of an infusion (e.g. barbiturate-induced coma).

COMPLICATIONS OF USE

- Extravasation – this is extremely painful as a result of the drug's alkalinity.
- Intra-arterial injection – causes severe burning pain and arterial and arteriolar spasm leading to thrombosis and tissue loss. If this occurs:
    - stop injection but leave cannula *in situ*
    - dilute effects by administration of saline down the cannula
    - consider direct vasodilator therapy (e.g. procaine hydrochloride 0.5% solution, or continuous tolazoline). Analgesia and anticoagulant therapy may also be necessary.
- Cardiorespiratory collapse
- Histamine release – often accompanied by arteriolar flare, urticaria and bronchospasm. This drug is contraindicated in severe asthmatics.
- Anaphylaxis – true anaphylaxis is fortunately rare, although when it occurs the mortality approaches 50 per cent.
- Porphyria – rare, but barbiturates may precipitate lower motor neurone paralysis and even death in these patients.

2,6 Di isopropyl phenol (propofol)

Propofol is available as 1% and 2% solutions (10 mg ml^{-1} and 20 mg ml^{-1} respectively) in a lipid emulsion. It is insoluble in water.

ANAESTHETIC DOSE

The anaesthetic dose is 2 to 4 mg kg^{-1}.

SYSTEMIC EFFECTS

CNS

- Cerebral activity is depressed.
- Intracranial pressure is reduced.
- Anticonvulsant.

Respiratory system
- Apnoea is common soon after induction.

CVS
- Hypotension, largely mediated by peripheral vasodilatation, may be profound.

METABOLISM AND EXCRETION
Propofol is rapidly redistributed, it is metabolised by the liver and does not accumulate. This combined with its relatively short duration of action makes it suitable for continuous infusion.

COMPLICATIONS OF USE
- Pain – propofol can be painful during intravenous injection, notably in small peripheral veins.
- Hypotension/apnoea.
- Hypersensitivity reactions – these have been reported but are not usually severe.
- Propofol infusions in the PICU – in recent years there have been reports implicating propofol infusions as a possible causative factor in the development of multi-system organ failure in some critically ill children. The case is far from proven, but it is currently not recommended for continuous infusion in patients under 3 years of age.

Ketamine hydrochloride
Generally speaking ketamine is a useful agent when there is a risk of hypotension at induction, or where analgesia or anaesthesia are required for short, painful procedures (e.g. burns, dressing changes). The side effects recounted below should not be underestimated however.

Ketamine is presented as a solution in concentrations of 10 or 50 mg ml^{-1}. It is a slow-acting agent, which uniquely provides good *analgesia* but only superficial sleep. It is related to phencyclidine and is a derivative of lysergic acid (LSD) and, as such, produces dissociation. It is an acidic solution and the higher concentration contains preservative. It can be administered by intramuscular or intravenous injection.

ANAESTHETIC DOSE
The anaesthetic dose is 1.5 to 2 mg kg^{-1} i.v. or 10 mg kg^{-1} i.m. A single dose may give up to 20 minutes anaesthesia and analgesia.

SYSTEMIC EFFECTS
CNS
- 'Dissociative anaesthesia'.
- Cerebral blood flow increased.
- Intracranial pressure increased.
- Hallucinations and nightmares may occur. When they do it tends to be on emergence from anaesthesia leading to later recall, flashbacks and distress.

Respiratory system
- Airway reflexes generally maintained although airway obstruction can occur.
- Increased salivation and bronchial secretions.
- Smooth muscle relaxation in the large airways can occur.
- Respiration is only depressed by large doses.

CVS
- Systolic arterial blood pressure increases.
- Cardiac output is unchanged or increased. These effects are blocked by verapamil and are probably related to an effect on myocardial calcium channels.
- Ketamine is not vagolytic.

METABOLISM AND EXCRETION

Metabolised in the liver to water-soluble products that are excreted in the urine.

COMPLICATIONS OF USE

- Emergence delirium may be severe but the effects can be reduced by concomitant administration of a hypnotic (e.g. benzodiazepines).
- Hypertension and arrhythmias can occur, particularly in overdose.
- Sensitises the heart to circulating catecholamines.
- Elevates intraocular and intracranial pressures.

Etomidate

Etomidate is an imidazole derivative seldom used in paediatric practice. The aqueous solution is presented in 35% propylene glycol and water.

ANAESTHETIC DOSE

The anaesthetic dose is 0.3 mgkg^{-1}.

SYSTEMIC EFFECTS

CNS

- Cerebral activity is depressed.
- Intracranial pressure is reduced.
- Abnormal limb and facial movements can occur on induction. These are transient and not related to seizure activity.

Respiratory system

- Hypoventilation and apnoea will occur.

CVS

- Etomidate is noted for its lack of detrimental cardiovascular effects.

METABOLISM AND EXCRETION

A single dose lasts 5–6 minutes. Etomidate is metabolised by the liver and the breakdown products renally excreted.

COMPLICATIONS OF USE

- Pain on injection – can be significant, notably in small veins.
- Infusions are contraindicated – Etomidate by infusion is associated with depression of cortisol secretion, which is particularly marked in the critically ill.

Inhalational anaesthetic agents

GENERAL PRINCIPLES

- All these agents are volatile liquids, which readily attain the vapour phase at relatively low temperatures.
- The depth of anaesthesia achieved is directly related to the partial pressure of vapour attained in the brain.
- The speed of onset and duration of anaesthesia is dictated by the blood/gas solubility coefficient of the agent.
- If there is low blood/gas solubility an alveolar partial pressure is rapidly reached which produces anaesthesia.
- The Minimum Alveolar Concentration (MAC) value for each agent is that fractional percentage concentration which ablates the reflex response to skin incision in 50% of subjects. It is therefore a measure of anaesthetic potency.
- Volatile agents are delivered via calibrated, thermostatically controlled vaporisers in a carrier gas flow containing a minimum of 30% oxygen, from purpose-built anaesthetic machines and delivery systems.

- All doctors using such machines should be trained in their use and understand routine checking procedures.

Halothane (MAC 0.75(%))

Blood/gas solubility is low, therefore uptake and recovery from halothane is rapid. It is non-irritant to the airway and is the agent of choice for inhalational induction during management of the difficult airway.

SYSTEMIC EFFECTS

CNS
- Cerebral blood flow increased. This effect is obviated by mild hypocapnia.

Respiratory system
- Pharyngeal and laryngeal reflexes are rapidly lost.
- Bronchial secretions are reduced.
- Relaxation of bronchial smooth muscle.
- Inhibition of cilial motility.

CVS
- Myocardial depression.
- Vasodilatation is the norm.
- Vagal bradycardia especially at deep planes of anaesthesia.
- Halothane sensitises the myocardium to catecholamines which causes arrhythmias (aggravated by hypercapnia).

METABOLISM AND EXCRETION

Twenty per cent of halothane is metabolised in the liver and excreted in the urine. The remainder undergoes pulmonary excretion.

COMPLICATIONS OF USE
- Cardiovascular effects – these are described above.
- Acute liver failure – this is an extremely rare complication. It appears to be related to the reductive metabolism of halothane, which explains the relative immunity of children to the problem.

Sevoflurane (MAC 1.9(%)) and Isoflurane (MAC 1.15(%))

These newer agents offer some advantages to halothane in certain circumstances.

- Isoflurane is less soluble and therefore more rapid in onset and recovery than halothane. In addition it undergoes minimal metabolism in the liver. It is less myocardial depressant but causes vasodilatation and reflex tachycardia in anaesthetic doses. It is irritant to the airway and so is poorly tolerated during inhalational induction.
- *Sevoflurane* is non-irritant and well accepted by most patients. In addition its low blood/gas solubility allows very rapid induction and recovery. During induction it can precipitate sudden apnoea but it is generally well tolerated from a cardiorespiratory viewpoint. The excretion of sevoflurane is entirely pulmonary and recovery can be so rapid as to represent something of a crash landing!

DRUGS USED TO SUPPLEMENT ANAESTHESIA

Muscle relaxants

GENERAL PRINCIPLES

These drugs exert their action at the motor end plate of the axons supplying *striated* muscle fibres. They can be divided into two groups of agents:

- depolarising drugs (e.g. suxamethonium)

- non-depolarising drugs (or competitive antagonists – e.g. vecuronium, pancuronium, atracurium, rocuronium).

As a general rule, infants are less sensitive to depolarising block (and need relatively higher dosage) and more sensitive to non-depolarising block than older patients.

Neuromuscular (NM) transmission is effected by an increase in the release of acetylcholine into the synaptic cleft of the neuromuscular junction. This occurs in response to the arriving neuronal action potential. Acetylcholine attaches to post-synaptic receptor sites on the muscle endplate and triggers ion shifts, which initiate sarcolemmal depolarisation and a muscle action potential. Under normal circumstances, the muscle stimulation is terminated by the action of acetyl cholinesterase (present in the synaptic cleft).

The neuromuscular junction is immature for the first 2 months after birth. Neonates exhibit slower contraction time, impaired train-of-four responses, tetanic fade, post-tetanic exhaustion, and lower tetanus to twitch ratios when compared with older children even without the administration of neuromuscular blocking agents. As a result they are more sensitive to non-depolarising muscle relaxants. However this effect is countered by the proportionately greater volume of distribution (a result of high extracellular fluid volume) so actual initial requirements vary little with age. Subsequent doses of most non-depolarising muscle relaxants should be lower than the initial doses and are required at longer intervals because of slower elimination.

DEPOLARISING DRUGS

Suxamethonium

Suxamethonium is the only one of this group in current UK practice. Structurally it resembles two linked acetylcholine molecules. When administered intravenously it depolarises the muscle end plate, causing immediate fasciculation followed by a refractory period involving muscle relaxation of variable duration.

DOSAGE

Administration of 1 to 1.5 mg kg^{-1} will provide complete relaxation within 30–45 seconds, lasting for 3–5 minutes.

SYSTEMIC EFFECTS

Neuromuscular block

- Profound and rapid onset. Suxamethonium is the current drug of choice for rapid sequence induction.

Respiratory system

- Complete respiratory muscle and diaphragmatic paralysis.

CVS

- Suxamethonium can cause a muscarinic (vagally mediated) bradycardia. Its use should therefore be accompanied by atropine.
- Hyperkalaemia-induced arrhythmias will occur in susceptible patients (see below).
- There are no direct myocardial effects.

GIT

- Salivary and gastric secretions can increase.

COMPLICATIONS OF USE

- Histamine release and anaphylaxis can occur.
- Cellular efflux of potassium – lethal tachyarrhythmias may be induced in patients suffering from
  - burns,
  - spinal cord injuries,
  - conditions associated with acute and progressive neuromuscular disease (e.g. muscular dystrophy, upper/lower motor neurone diseases),
  - renal failure.

- Increased intra-ocular pressure – suxamethonium should not be used where a penetrating eye injury is suspected.
- Malignant hyperpyrexia – suxamethonium is one of the most important trigger agents for malignant hyperpyrexia (1 in 100 000 uses).
- Abnormal metabolism – 'sux apnoea', neuromuscular block – 1 in 3000 of the normal population have an abnormal cholinesterase making them susceptible to a prolonged duration of neuromuscular block after a single dose. Block can last for up to 12 hours in severe cases. There is no mode of reversal and the subject should receive ventilatory support (and adequate sedation) until the block wears off. Sufferers of this condition should wear a Medic-Alert tag for life (it is hereditary and siblings should be tested for the condition).

NON-DEPOLARISING DRUGS

These agents are competitive antagonists to the action of acetylcholine at the post-synaptic receptor. Agents which potentiate this action of acetylcholine at the neuromuscular junction (e.g. neostigmine) can therefore reverse them. There are many non-depolarising muscle relaxants in current anaesthetic practice – only four are briefly described below. In general terms their onset of action is slower than that of suxamethonium and they have variable duration of effect.

Vecuronium, Rocuronium

These steroid-based agents have similar structures and pharmacological profiles.

DOSAGE

- Vecuronium 0.1 mg kg^{-1}.
- Rocuronium 0.5 mg kg^{-1} for intubation.

Infusion rates vary according to response.

SYSTEMIC EFFECTS

Neuromuscular block

Duration of block after single dose:
- Vecuronium 20–30 minutes
- Rocuronium 25–40 minutes.

Cardiovascular system

Both drugs have minimal adverse effects. Vecuronium and fentanyl together can provoke sinus bradycardia.

Respiratory system

- Complete respiratory paralysis occurs within 2 minutes.
- Rocuronium can provide conditions suitable for intubation within 60 seconds if given in larger dosage (e.g. 0.8–1 mg kg^{-1}), thus facilitating emergency airway control. The duration of block is accordingly prolonged however.
- Both agents can be reversed successfully 15 minutes after an intubating dose.

METABOLISM

These agents are metabolised in the liver and excretion is mainly renal. Accumulation of drug will therefore occur in the critically ill child.

SIDE EFFECTS

Clinically significant side-effects are rare and these agents are justifiably popular in anaesthetic practice. Histamine release is negligible, although anaphylaxis has been reported. Several types of antibiotics have been shown to enhance non-depolarising neuromuscular blockade. The effect is related to pre-junctional and post-junctional membrane stabilisation. Most prominent of the antibiotics are aminoglycosides, with neomycin and streptomycin being the most potent. Reversal of this element of blockade is inconsistent with calcium or anticholinesterases.

Atracurium, Cis-atracurium
DOSAGE
- Atracurium 0.5 mg kg–1.
- Cis-atracurium 0.1 mg kg–1 to achieve good intubation conditions.

SYSTEMIC EFFECTS
Neuromuscular block
- Duration of a single-dose block is 20 to 30 minutes.

Cardiovascular system
- Atracurium has been associated with histamine release and corresponding hypotension.
- Generally both agents have no detrimental haemodynamic effects.

Respiratory system
- Complete respiratory paralysis occurs within 1.5 to 2 minutes.

METABOLISM
These agents share a unique method of breakdown, Hoffman degradation, which is spontaneous and occurs at body pH and temperature. This gives them a useful role in patients with hepatorenal disease.

SIDE EFFECTS
- Minimal – though anaphylactoid reactions can occur.
- Laudanosine is the main breakdown product of atracurium and has been implicated as a cause of seizures in high concentration – *this is very rare* – but it is a potential problem obviated by the use of cis-atracurium. In addition, for similar reasons, cis-atracurium is said not to have accumulative neuromuscular blocking effects.
- Tachyphylaxis – atracurium particularly demonstrates this phenomenon during continuous infusions. Over time it may be difficult to sustain effective relaxation without significantly increasing dosage.

REVERSAL AND MONITORING OF NEUROMUSCULAR BLOCKADE
Neostigmine
Neostigmine will reverse the neuromuscular blockade caused by non-depolarising agents. It acts by inhibiting the action of anticholinesterase and therefore potentiates the action of acetylcholine at both nicotinic and muscarinic receptors. In overdosage it can cause depolarising blockade in its own right, and should always be administered in tandem with atropine to prevent muscarinic side effects.

DOSAGE
- Neostigmine 40–50 μg kg^{-1} i.v.
- Atropine 20 μg kg^{-1}.

Re-curarisation will occur if neostigmine is used in insufficient dosage, or too soon after the original dose of relaxant was administered.

Monitoring of neuromuscular block has traditionally been performed using a nerve-stimulator, which provides a small stimulating current to a large nerve at predetermined intervals and records the response of distal muscle groups (e.g. ulnar nerve and hypothenar muscles). Commonly a train-of-four (TOF) stimulus is used; this is four supra-maximal electrical impulses at 0.5 second intervals, and the twitch response of the muscle group is recorded simultaneously. The number of twitches recorded indicates the level of block:

- 0 twitches = 100%
- 1 twitch = 90%
- 2 twitches = 80%
- 3 twitches = 75%.

For a non-depolarising relaxant, the block has been completely reversed when all four twitches reach the same amplitude. However this can be difficult to assess without objective measurement such as that obtained using an accelerometer. A better test is the response to a tetanic stimulus. Fade during tetany indicates residual neuromuscular blockade. Absence of fade indicates adequate reversal of neuromuscular blockade. In addition if no twitches are present on the TOF, twitch might still be elicited if tried after 5 seconds of tetanic stimulation, in which case the successive subsequent number of twitches gives an indication of the likelihood of reversibility. Diminishing amplitude of twitch indicates persisting block and is known as 'post-tetanic fade'. It is again a characteristic of non-depolarising neuromuscular block and its presence again indicates residual curarisation.

Other drugs used to supplement anaesthesia

SEDATIVES

Benzodiazepines (e.g. midazolam, diazepam) and chloral hydrate are sedative agents commonly employed in the PICU. They are useful adjuncts that supplement the use of other drugs (such as opiates) but they are only capable of providing anaesthesia in impracticably high dosage.

Midazolam is a ubiquitous short-acting benzodiazepine that will obtund seizure activity, it is generally stable in terms of haemodynamic effects, and is useful in some situations as an infusion. Contrary to the product literature however, some of its breakdown products are active and emergence may not be as rapid as predicted. Its effects can be reversed by flumazenil but in mixed toxicity (e.g. with opiates) flumazenil administration is inadvisable.

Chloral hydrate is useful as a relatively short-acting sedative in infants. It can be given in doses ranging from 30 to 50 mg kg^{-1} via the nasogastric/oral route and is generally well tolerated. In susceptible infants hypotension can occur, however, and liver disease may prolong its duration of action.

ANALGESICS

Conscious children naturally use distraction and play as coping mechanisms for dealing with pain and distress. They can be encouraged in their efforts by diversional therapy. Children in pain do not necessarily appear unhappy, but stressed and anxious children are more distressed by painful experiences. Anything that can minimise stress, such as the presence of a parent, a full stomach or a degree of sedation is to be encouraged in the scary world of a PICU. Assessment of pain control may be difficult; first because of the patient's age and communication skills, and second because of appropriate sedation. Age-appropriate pain assessment tools may get round some of these difficulties but still cannot be relied upon in the sedated child. Sedation dulls the child's responses but does not provide analgesia. It is not the same as sleep. Also do not assume that because a child is asleep he/she is not in pain. Thus in many paediatric intensive care situations it is best to anticipate and assume that pain is present and to treat it accordingly. Morphine is the first-line analgesic in PICU, delivered by intravenous infusion. In older children up to 60 µg kg^{-1} hr^{-1} can be well tolerated without respiratory depression. Babies however, tend to accumulate doses higher than 20 µg kg^{-1} hr^{-1} and become narcosed, leading to difficulties in weaning ventilation. Patients with hepatic dysfunction may be more suited to alfentanil and there may be a niche for remifentanil.

Opiates, opioids (e.g. morphine, fentanyl, alfentanil)

Opiates are naturally occurring alkaloids related to the parent compound (morphine). Opioids are synthetically manufactured agents which are structurally similar (e.g. fentanyl). They act on a family of receptors distributed widely in body tissue, but have effects predominantly through the µ receptor in the brain and spinal cord. Depending on their receptor activity, they exhibit a range of effects including sedation, analgesia, nausea, pruritis, urinary retention and respiratory depression. The immaturity of the infant blood–brain barrier renders these patients more susceptible to μ-meditated effects. Therefore opiate drugs must be used in reduced dosage and with care in this situation – lethal apnoeas can be provoked by relatively small doses.

All these agents can be competitively antagonised and reversed by naloxone. It should be remembered, however, that the half-life of naloxone is approximately 20 minutes, and narcotisation can redevelop after that time. Naloxone has agonist effects in overdose and in some patients at normal doses.

ANAESTHETIC BREATHING SYSTEMS

The term 'breathing systems' includes all the technical elements of anaesthetic machines by which anaesthetic gas mixtures are administered to the patient. They include all the circuits commonly used during resuscitation, and in the intensive care setting.

The gas delivery (oxygen or oxygen-enriched air mixture) depends mainly on the breathing system's technical design and the fresh gas flow. It is also affected by certain patient ventilation parameters (including peak inspiratory flow rate and minute volume.)

Detailed analysis of these systems can be found in anaesthetic texts, but the two circuits most commonly used for manual ventilation in paediatric intensive care are the Jackson Rees modification of Ayre's T-piece, and the Mapleson C circuit (see Figures 5.1 and 5.2). These are both flow-controlled non-rebreathing systems. However, rebreathing (the accumulation and re-inhalation of exhaled carbon dioxide) can occur if these circuits are used incorrectly. Both circuits have a single (mixed) inspiratory and expiratory gas limb and rely on the pressure of the continuous incoming fresh gas flow to expel exhaled gas through the open-ended limb (T-piece) or the expiratory valve (Mapleson C) during the expiratory phase of ventilation.

The fresh gas flow rate (oxygen supply) is critical, and the *minimum* gas flow requirements are usually expressed in relation to the expected minute volume of the patient.

The Mapleson C circuit requires a minimum of 2 times the minute volume in spontaneous breathing and controlled ventilation. The T-piece requires a minimum of 1.5 times the minute volume in spontaneous breathing, and 1 to 2 times the minute volume in controlled ventilation. For technical reasons it is recommended that the *fresh gas flow through a T-piece should not be below 3 L min⁻¹ or exceed 8 L min⁻¹* (thus, it is not suitable for use in patients weighing more than 20 kg). Failure to use recommended gas flow rates can result in carbon dioxide retention or in the in-drawing of air into the breathing system, reducing the fractional inspired oxygen concentration (FiO_2).

CLINICAL EXAMPLE

10 kg child for controlled ventilation.

estimated minute volume = 100 ml (tidal volume) × 20 (respiratory rate)
= 2 L min⁻¹

Therefore

minimum fresh gas flow through the T-piece = 4 L min⁻¹ to prevent CO_2 rebreathing

LARYNGOSCOPES AND ENDOTRACHEAL TUBES

There are well-described differences between the infant airway and that of the older child or adult. Those most relevant to laryngoscopy and intubation are:

- the infant is edentulous and the soft tissues of the mouth and pharynx, including the tongue and epiglottis, readily obscure a clear view of the glottis
- the larynx is more anterior and two cervical vertebrae higher in position than in the adult
- the cricoid ring is the narrowest part of the infant airway, at puberty (about 12 years of age – equivalent to an airway size requiring a 6.0 to 7.0 mm internal diameter endotracheal tube) the vocal cords become the narrowest part of the airway.

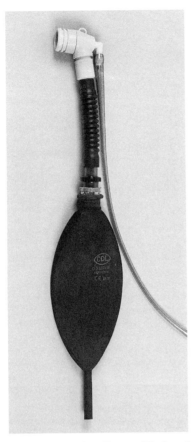

Figure 5.1 Jackson Rees modification of Ayre's T-piece.

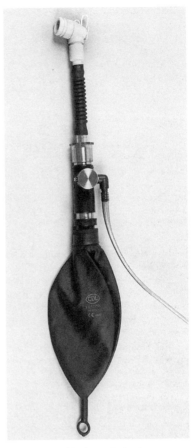

Figure 5.2 Mapleson C circuit.

As a result of these variations, infant airway management and intubation requires equipment and techniques that are significantly different to those in the older child.

Infant laryngoscopy

A **neutral head position** is vital for infants. Their shoulders should be flat on the cot surface with only moderate extension of the head on the neck, the occiput resting on the same flat surface. The blades used to facilitate the view are shorter and straighter than the adult counterpart, and usually of C-shaped cross-section (see Figure 5.3). Laryngoscopy involves passing the blade centrally over the tongue, beyond the epiglottis (often into the upper oesophagus) before lifting and gently withdrawing the blade to display the glottic opening above the oesophageal inlet, with the epiglottis held behind the distal part of the laryngoscope blade.

Child/adult laryngoscopy

Adult blades are designed to facilitate intubation of the more mature airway – the commonest blade used is the Macintosh (the blade on the left in Figure 5.3). Again, head position is vital to the technique. The neck should be flexed and the head extended, 'sniffing the

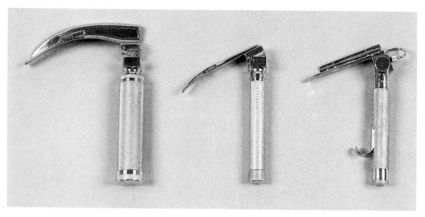

Figure 5.3 Laryngoscope blades.

morning air'. Support the head on a pillow with the shoulders (clear of the pillow) resting on the flat bed surface.

The blade is advanced over the right side of the tongue with the operator searching for the epiglottis. The tip of the blade is then inserted into the vallecula proximal to the epiglottis at the base of the tongue, and then the blade is *lifted* (not levered) elevating the supraglottic structures out of the line of vision and the glottis should come into view.

The anatomical transition from infant to child/adult airway conformation has significantly progressed by toddler age (18 months to 3 years) and should influence the technique and equipment used.

Endotracheal tubes

Paediatric tubes are generally uncuffed since a natural 'seal' is provided by the cricoid ring and any additional pressure from a balloon leads to mucosal necrosis. A small degree of leak is essential to reassure the operator that the tube is not oversize. The degree of leak will change if thoracic / pulmonary compliance decreases and airway pressures rise. As stated above by the age of 10 to 12 years (puberty) the airway conformation changes such that a cuffed endotracheal tube becomes necessary. For children of 1 year and over, the likely correct size for the internal diameter of the endotracheal tube is given by the formula

Table 5.1 Endotracheal tube sizes.

Age	Internal diameter (mm)	Length at lip (cm)	Length at nose (cm)	Sucker (FG)
Newborn (<1 kg)	2.5	5.5	7.0	6
Newborn (1–2 kg)	3	7.0	9.0	7
Newborn (2–3 kg)	3	8.0	10	7
Newborn (> 3 kg)	3.5	9	11	8
3 months	3.5	10	12	8
1 year	4	11	14	8
2 years	4.5	12	15	8

(age/4) + 4. Newborn babies require a size 3.0 to 3.5 and particularly small premature new-borns may require smaller tubes.

The ideal position of the tip of the endotracheal tube is at the level of the sterno-clavicular junction on the chest X-ray. For children of 2 years and over this position is usually achieved if the tube is positioned at a distance of (age/2) + 12 cm from the lips for oral intubation and (age/2) + 15 cm at the nose for nasal intubation. The position is more likely to be maintained if a nasal tube is used and if the tube is cut to size (allow-ing for the technique of external fixation). Babies require shorter tubes as summarised in Table 5.1.

ANAESTHETICS IN MISCELLANEOUS CONDITIONS

Anaphylaxis

Acute anaphylaxis involves massive histamine release and triggering of cytokines and other vasoactive mediators. The result is profound hypotension and an associated fall in capillary wall integrity. Cardiovascular collapse, acute bronchospasm and rapidly developing tissue oedema can be rapidly lethal. Management involves removing the trigger to the response (where possible) and an ABC approach. Most patients require endotracheal intubation, the administration of 100% oxygen and aggressive fluid resuscitation. Prompt administration of i.v. or i.m. adrenaline (epinephrine) is essential.

Malignant hyperpyrexia

This is a rare (1 in 14 000 child anaesthetics) complication of anaesthesia where an inherited predisposition, triggered by anaesthetic agents, leads to excessive and uncontrolled muscle spasm, the cause of which is calcium-stimulated tropomyosin complex formation in striated muscle fibres. Oxygen consumption is greatly increased and hypercarbia ensues in combi-nation with metabolic acidosis and a core temperature rise of 2°C per hour. If the condition is not reversed it is rapidly fatal. Halothane and suxamethonium are the best-recognised trigger agents.

Treatment involves removing the trigger agent, although the onset of symptoms may have been delayed for several hours after anaesthesia, and an ABC approach. Endotracheal intubation, administration of 100% oxygen, aggressive cardiovascular resuscitation and active cooling are mandatory. Active cooling requires the use of non-depolarising relaxants and may involve cold peritoneal lavage or even ECMO. Dantrolene sodium in incremental doses of 1 mg kg^{-1} up to 10 mg kg^{-1} will inhibit sarcolemmal calcium release and uncouple the excitation–contraction response in striated muscle, but active cooling may still be required for prolonged periods. Haemolysis, myoglobinuria and disseminated intravascular coagulation (DIC) can all occur as complications.

Regional anaesthesia

Numerous types of local anaesthetic block are available for anaesthesia and analgesia in the perioperative period or in the treatment of trauma. Local anaesthetic agents like bupivicaine, lignocaine (lidocaine) and ropivacaine are amide compounds. They interrupt action potential transmission through myelinated nerves by disrupting excitation in the gaps between the Schwann cells (nodes of Ranvier). Lignocaine (lidocaine) is the short-est acting of the three although the exact duration of action is dependent upon the nature of block employed and is susceptible to variability between patients. Their duration of action is also increased if the solution is alkalinised or if a mixture with adrenaline (epi-nephrine) is used. However the latter precludes their use in many distal sites.

Epidural anaesthesia

Local anaesthetic introduced into the epidural space (often by infusion) provides profound sensory and some motor anaesthesia in the surrounding nerve segments. The degree of spread can be enhanced by positioning the patient appropriately and elucidated by pinprick testing.

Associated autonomic nerve blockade can lead to hypotension. Reliable intravenous access, controlled fluid administration and cardiovascular monitoring are essential.

Asthma

Agents which encourage histamine release and mast cell degranulation provoke bronchospasm. These include thiopentone, suxamethonium, morphine and possibly atracurium.

Halothane and isoflurane have bronchodilator properties, while propofol, ketamine, fentanyl and vecuronium (or rocuronium) can all be used safely for anaesthetic induction during the management of a severe asthmatic incident.

Multiple trauma

Induction of anaesthesia in the patient suffering from multiple trauma requires skill and expertise. Airway management is vital. Airway integrity may be compromised by direct facial or neck trauma or by conscious level but the cervical spine must be kept immobile throughout even the most advanced manoeuvres. Chest/abdominal trauma may further hamper oxygenation and patients are frequently being resuscitated from hypovolaemia making them haemodynamically labile. In most circumstances a rapid sequence induction is the most appropriate approach because of the risk of regurgitation. The PICU trainee would be wise to call for senior assistance promptly in such circumstances.

CONCLUSION

Anaesthetic techniques are an essential part of the intensivist's armamentarium but training in intensive care does not make the intensivist qualified in anaesthesia. The trainee approaching paediatric intensive care from a background outside anaesthetics should become familiar with a range of drugs and basic techniques to enable him/her to safely manage critically ill infants and children. However *above all*, one should always recognise one's limitations and call for help early!

6 Neonatology

- **Minimal handling**
- **Temperature control**
- **Foetal and transitional circulations**
- **The first breath and respiratory physiology**
- **Jaundice**
- **Birth asphyxia**
- **Respiratory distress syndrome (RDS)**
- **Meconium aspiration syndrome**
- **Retinopathy of prematurity (ROP)**
- **Intraventricular haemorrhage**
- **Congenital diaphragmatic hernia**
- **Necrotising enterocolitis**
- **Neonatal ECMO**

Paediatric intensive care units admit newborn babies and hence share some common ground with neonatal intensive care units (NICU). In fact during PICU ward rounds the arguments that 'term babies are not premature' and 'children are not big babies' have to be invoked almost as frequently as 'children are not small adults'. This is not surprising since most paediatricians get their first intensive care training on a neonatal unit.

There is a lot of variation between countries and institutions in the way in which patients are distributed between the PICU and the NICU but neonates singled out for PICU tend to have a specific indication for referral. They generally constitute a cohort of comparatively mature infants with a requirement for specialist surgery or a specialist intensive care procedure such as ECMO. However the group includes occasional patients of more extreme prematurity and newborn infants delivered outside hospital presenting *de novo* to hospitals with a PICU but no maternity services. A background knowledge and experience of neonatal intensive care is essential amongst PICU staff. This chapter is intended as a brief primer for those lacking this experience.

MINIMAL HANDLING

Sick babies, especially premature infants, respond to stress by becoming hypoxic, peripherally shut down and bradycardic. The reasons for these reactions are elucidated below and elsewhere in the text but the point is that you must anticipate this response and minimise handling wherever possible. Do not persist in attempting a procedure unsuccessfully when a colleague could perform it more expertly later, when the child has recovered. Be particularly wary with babies that are receiving less invasive support (e.g. not ventilated) since they are more dependent on their own resources.

TEMPERATURE CONTROL

BABIES GET COLD QUICKLY

Babies have a high surface area to mass ratio and their heads account for a greater proportion of their surface area than in older children and adults. Heat is lost readily by convection, conduction and particularly by radiation onto incubator walls and external surfaces. Radiant losses are greatest near windows or in an open environment but are still significant when nursed in an incubator on the PICU. To reduce this effect, heat shields, **69** double glazing, reflective wrapping and clothing (including a hat) are used and the common shorthand of 'operative' temperature is employed. The operative temperature of an incubator is calculated by subtracting 1°C from the temperature measured in the incubator for every 7°C that environmental temperature is below it. This concept is particularly useful during transport.

WET BABIES GET COLD <u>VERY</u> QUICKLY

Water lost through immature skin or sweat in infants over 36 weeks gestation or applied from an external source, evaporates. The latent heat of vaporisation is drawn from the skin by conduction and heat travels away from the skin by convection assisted by the water vapour. This has a profound cooling effect which can be minimised by drying wet babies, increasing environmental humidity and avoiding air currents and exposure.

PREMATURE BABIES CANNOT REGULATE THEIR TEMPERATURE WELL

Mature neonates naturally conserve heat as a consequence of their flexed posture and they respond to cold with cutaneous vasoconstriction to conserve heat and by increasing heat production. Preterm neonates adopt a 'frog' posture that unfortunately maximises heat loss and whilst the sympathetically mediated vasoconstrictive response to cold is active, its effectiveness is limited by poor tissue insulation from their thin layer of subcutaneous fat and skin.

Neonates accomplish heat production by a generalised increase in metabolic activity, chiefly combustion of fatty acids and glucose. 'Non-shivering thermogenesis' is stimulated by noradrenaline (norepinephrine) and occurs in several sites, including brown adipose tissue which is rich in mitochondria, blood vessels and sympathetic innervation. Brown fat is present in the neonate, continues to develop in the early weeks after birth and recedes following infancy. It is poorly developed in the preterm neonate and is rapidly depleted during cold stress.

Babies also have a limited ability to reduce their temperature. The commonest cause of neonatal fever is exposure to a heat source (e.g. sunlight) or a high environmental temperature for some other reason, for example over-wrapping. Medical conditions such as infection or CNS injury are also possible.

COLD BABIES GET SICK

Thermogenesis increases oxygen consumption significantly as does fever. Lowering environmental temperature from 34°C to 24°C increases the neonate's oxygen consumption by about 50 per cent. Thermoneutral (non-hypoxic) environments for clothed and naked well babies have been usefully defined from experiments monitoring oxygen consumption (Figure 6.1).

Cold babies lose any ability to hyperventilate in response to hypoxia (an ability restricted to the more mature infants anyway) and both production and release of surfactant are severely impaired by hypothermia. Babies that sustain a cold injury suffer from severe respiratory distress syndrome (RDS), thrombocytopaenia, delayed weight gain, sclerema and have a higher overall mortality.

Cold infants can be surface warmed reasonably quickly using an overhead heat source. If a baby is cold in an incubator then the incubator temperature can be raised, the environmental temperature can be raised, a heat shield can be employed or the humidity in the incubator can be increased. Common practice would be to use a servo-regulated overhead warmer or warming mattress. When using these devices the patient's temperature dictates the amount of heat supplied by the warmer. Hence, when linked to a skin probe the devices work to ablate a core–peripheral temperature gradient and if successful may mask a problem of poor peripheral perfusion. Also if linked to a central temperature probe they will functionally cool a child with a fever by delivering less heat and this may mask the pyrexia (without necessarily increasing the toe–core temperature gap) and lead to increased oxygen consumption.

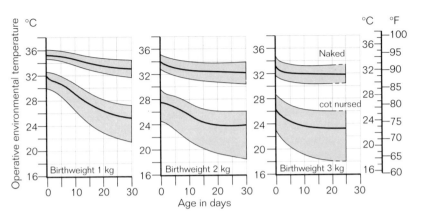

Figure 6.1 Thermoneutral temperature ranges for the newborn. The dark line indicates the optimum temperature (defined by minimal oxygen consumption). The shaded range represents that over which normal core temperature can be maintained – but not without a cost in terms of oxygen consumption. All figures relate to draught free environments, away from windows, at 50% humidity. (Reproduced with permission from Hey 1971. In: Recent Advances in Paediatrics, Gairdner, Hull, eds. Churchill, London; pp.171–216.)

FOETAL AND TRANSITIONAL CIRCULATIONS (see Fig 6.2)

In prenatal life the balance of systemic and pulmonary vascular resistance is reversed. The pulmonary vascular resistance is high, because the lungs are not inflated and the systemic vascular resistance is low, partly because the umbilical arteries link the systemic circulation to a low-pressure placental sump. A network of shunts allows blood to be diverted to the placenta for exchange of respiratory gases, nutrients, wastes, etc.

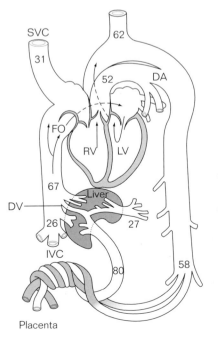

Figure 6.2 The foetal circulation.
DA – Ductus arteriosus
DV – Ductus venosus
SVC – Superior vena cava
IVC – Inferior vena cava
FO – Foramen ovale
RV – Right ventricle.
LV – Left ventricle.
Mean oxygen saturations are given as numbers in the relevant sites. (Adapted from Edward Baker 1993. Congenital heart disease in the neonatal period. In: NRC Roberton. A Manual of Neonatal Intensive Care 3rd edn. Edward Arnold; p. 167.)

Blood draining from the superior vena cava passes through the right atrium and almost all enters the right ventricle. The right ventricle ejects into the main pulmonary artery and thence via the ductus arteriosus to the aorta. There is little flow to the branch pulmonary arteries (< 10% of the right ventricle output). The majority of the oxygenated blood from the umbilical veins reaches the inferior vena cava (IVC) via the portal vein and ductus venosus but some traverses the liver and enters via the hepatic veins. At the IVC / right atrium junction a flap of tissue (the eustachian valve) inhibits flow from IVC to right ventricle. An atrial communication (the foramen ovale) allows about 30 per cent of the IVC blood across the atrial septum to join the small amount of pulmonary venous return. Despite mixing with this desaturated blood, the left ventricle still contains the most oxygen-rich arterial blood in the foetus and this blood perfuses the ascending aorta (i.e. brain and coronary arteries).

At birth the first breath expands the lungs. The direct effect of this expansion and the oxygen content of the inhaled air cause a fall in pulmonary vascular resistance. Lung blood flow increases, pulmonary venous return rises, the left atrial pressure is raised and the foramen ovale closes, but is not necessarily sealed. The sustained rise in arterial oxygen tension contributes to a further decline in pulmonary vascular resistance and hence pulmonary artery pressures over the first month. It also promotes closure of the ductus arteriosus.

PERSISTENCE OF THE DUCTUS ARTERIOSUS

Normal closure of the ductus arteriosus may not occur in sick, hypoxic or premature infants. This may have pathophysiological significance. When pulmonary vascular resistance is high it causes right–left (R–L) shunting and cyanosis (the so called 'persistent foetal circulation'). As pulmonary vascular resistance falls it allows L–R shunting producing a continuous crescendo–decrescendo systolic murmur, full pulses, low diastolic blood pressure and pulmonary oedema. The size of the duct can be assessed by echocardiography both in terms of its physical dimensions and patterns of blood flow. Doppler evidence of retrograde flow in the descending aorta during diastole implies a large left-to-right shunt and a steal of blood from the systemic circulation. An impression of the magnitude of pulmonary blood flow can also be obtained from the left atrial : aortic ratio. A left atrial : aortic ratio of greater than 2.5 : 1 because of a ductus usually requires treatment. In addition to treating pulmonary oedema there are two approaches towards ductal closure:

- **Medical therapy**
  Using cyclo-oxygenase inhibitors such as indomethacin. Potential complications include thrombocytopaenia and platelet inhibition, renal failure and intraventricular haemorrhage.
- **Surgical ligation**
  A comparatively safe procedure and frequently the preferred option, it can even sometimes be performed on the ICU. The duct is often larger than the descending aorta and the surgeon needs to delineate the anatomy carefully to avoid ligating the wrong vessel.

PERSISTENT PULMONARY HYPERTENSION OF THE NEWBORN (PPHN)

This can result from any perinatal hypoxic insult and occasionally appears to be idiopathic. Many of the ventilatory and cardiovascular support strategies that the intensivist uses for neonates are designed to control the balance of systemic and pulmonary vascular resistance (PVR) assuming that there are persistent foetal vascular connections. The most important factor in reducing PVR is adequate oxygenation, however optimal lung volume is also necessary and is hard to determine even in the absence of pulmonary hypoplasia.

THE FIRST BREATH AND RESPIRATORY PHYSIOLOGY

Foetal lung fluid is produced from about 12 weeks gestation and there is a net flow into the amniotic fluid assisted by foetal breathing movements. Absence of foetal breathing movements can be associated with failure of adequate lung development – pulmonary hypoplasia. During delivery, foetal lung fluid production decreases and at birth some drains from the upper airway but most is reabsorbed in lymphatics and pulmonary venous blood. The first breath generates negative inspiratory pressures as high as 40 cmH$_2$O and the lungs inflate rapidly. Spontaneous pneumothorax can occur. Poor clearance of foetal lung fluid, for example after Caesarean section, is associated with 'transient tachypnoea of the newborn'.

Primary apnoea – failure to establish *regular* respiration – is not excluded by the common presentation of a few feeble preceding respiratory efforts. It may be associated with acute asphyxia, depressant drugs, CNS trauma, prematurity, sepsis, muscle weakness, or congenital CNS or pulmonary malformation. Primary apnoea is often followed by a period of gasping which if effective or substituted by effective resuscitation leads to recovery. In the face of ineffective gasping or ineffective resuscitation, terminal apnoea supervenes.

A normal functional residual capacity is established within an hour but resting lung volume continues to rise over 24 hours as compliance continues to improve and airways resistance falls. Babies are obligate nasal breathers and half of the neonatal airways resistance is nasal, leading to a preference for orogastric rather than nasogastric tubes in distressed non-ventilated neonates. Lung perfusion is encouraged by falling pulmonary vascular resistance but ventilation perfusion mismatch is more prominent than in older children and is accentuated in the premature. The normal neonatal respiratory rate is 40 to 60 breaths per minute and is inversely related to lung compliance.

Neonates will marginally hypoventilate in hyperoxic environments. Hyperventilation in response to hypoxia is transient and unreliable in preterm infants. Term infants adjust their tidal volume in these responses whilst the preterm predominantly adjust their respiratory rate. The diaphragm is the principal ventilatory muscle and impairment of its function (phrenic palsy, gastric distension, etc.) leads to significant respiratory compromise. Problems involving the left hemidiaphragm being the most significant.

JAUNDICE

CAN BE NORMAL

Physiological jaundice is a reflection of the immaturity of the hepatic enzyme pathways for metabolising haemoglobin pigments. These enzymes are induced in response to a load that they experience for the first time postpartum. Thus physiological jaundice displays characteristic features:

- it is not evident at birth
- it appears after 48 hours
- the bilirubin is unconjugated (direct)
- it increases slowly and peaks by about 5 days
- it is usually gone by 10 days (14 in the preterm).

The rate of rise of bilirubin is determined by the natural breakdown of red cells after birth. Neonatal red cells have a short life span (40–70 days depending on the infant's maturity). Breast milk can contain steroid inhibitors of conjugation that can lead to persistent low level asymptomatic unconjugated jaundice in normal infants.

CAN BE ABNORMAL!

Abnormal unconjugated jaundice (i.e. hyperbilirubinaemia that occurs too early, rises too fast or too far, or persists for too long) requires explanation and treatment.

Investigation of unconjugated jaundice should start with:

- a full blood count to detect anaemia
- a direct Coombes test (as an interrogation of possible haemolysis) and determination of maternal and child's blood groups.

Table 6.1 Causes of unconjugated (indirect) hyperbilirubinaemia.

Intravascular haemolysis	Blood group incompatibility	Rhesus (Coombes +ve) ABO (often Coombes –ve) Other
	Red cell fragility	Spherocytosis, elliptocytosis
	Inborn errors of metabolism	G6PD, pyruvate kinase deficiency
Polycythaemia	Recipient of twin-to-twin transfusion Chronic hypoxia (e.g. with growth retardation) Placental transfusion	
Other blood breakdown	Bruising from birth injury (forceps, cephalhaematoma, breech)	
Conjugation	Inhibition	Breast milk
	Inborn error of metabolism	Gilberts, Dubin Johnson, Rotor or Crigler Najar
Other	Dehydration Sepsis	

Phototherapy can split unconjugated bilirubin in the skin and superficial blood vessels into water-soluble components which are excreted in urine and bile. Free bilirubin and its fragments commonly cause diarrhoea. Unconjugated bilirubin is bound to albumen in the blood but is not water-soluble. It precipitates at high concentrations (a process aggravated by acidosis). Precipitation within the brain causes kernicterus – permanent brain (basal ganglia) damage. Kernicterus is now rare but attempts to avert it in unconjugated hyperbilirubinaemia with signs of CNS irritability should include mild hyperventilation (to a $PaCO_2$ of approximately 4 kPa) with or without intravenous base and intravenous albumin. These can all be instituted whilst arranging the definitive therapy (not a cure) for extreme, early or rapidly increasing unconjugated hyperbilirubinaemia which is exchange transfusion, usually of two circulating blood volumes. Thresholds for such interventions are given in Fig 6.3.

CONJUGATED HYPERBILIRUBINAEMIA

Conjugated hyperbilirubinaemia (indirect) results from neonatal hepatitis or biliary obstruction. The priorities in such cases are to recognise hepatic failure (high ammonia, prolonged prothrombin time, acidosis and hypoglycaemia with or without raised transaminases) and extrahepatic biliary atresia. A degree of urgency stems from the fact that these are conditions that require specialist management and treatment options are lost if the diagnosis is made late. Extrahepatic biliary atresia can be excluded if the stools are a normal colour, abdominal ultrasound identifies a normal gall bladder and bile excretion scans are normal. A plethora of other causes of conjugated hyperbilirubinaemia are possible including many inborn errors of metabolism (see Chapter 10, p. 129). Not surprisingly diagnostic tests can become very involved. The following is a list of typical investigations which betray some of the differential diagnoses. The interested reader should refer to a textbook of paediatrics for discussion of differential diagnosis and the pattern of investigation. The list below is not comprehensive and the blood samples particularly should not all be taken at once for fear of exsanguinating the patient!

BASELINE

Liver function tests, split bilirubin, calcium, phosphate, urea, electrolytes, creatinine, laboratory glucose (galactose will discolour a glucose oxidase reagent strip), full blood count, reticulocyte count, clotting screen, ammonia.

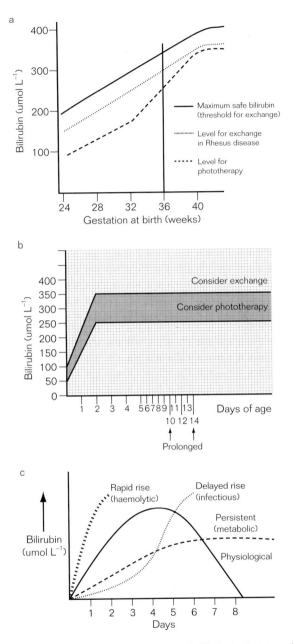

Figure 6.3 Neonatal Jaundice. Graph **a** shows recommended limits for decisions about phototherapy and exchange transfusion adjusted for the gestation at birth. To construct a graph of concentration against time (graph **b**) with decision ranges for an individual patient, start at 50 μmol L⁻¹ (lower limit for phototherapy) and 100 μ L⁻¹ (lower limit for exchange) at birth and rise to limits taken from graph 1, over 48 hours (example shown for a 36 weeks gestation infant). Remember the rate of rise is more important than the absolute level and the behaviour of the serum level may imply the underlying cause (graph **c**). (**a** adapted and **c** reproduced with permission from NRC Roberton 1993. Neonatal jaundice and liver disease. In: NRC Roberton. A Manual of Neonatal Intensive Care 3rd edn. Edward Arnold; pp. 240–241.)

INVESTIGATIVE SAMPLES

Blood group and Coombes test, galactose-1-phosphate uridyl transferase, thyroid function tests, 9 am plasma cortisol, alpha1-1-antitrypsin level and phenotype, serology for TORCH screen (congenital **To**xoplasma, **R**ubella, **C**MV, **H**erpes) and infective hepatitis (A, B, C), iron, ferritin, immune reactive trypsin, pyruvate, lactate, free fatty acids, 3 (OH) butyrate, amino acid profile, urine amino and organic acids, urine phosphate (simultaneous with blood to calculate tubular reabsorption of phosphate), urine protein creatinine ratio, urine reducing substances.

IMAGING

Abdominal ultrasound, bile excretion scan.

BIRTH ASPHYXIA

Chronic intrauterine asphyxia, for example from placental insufficiency, causes asymmetric growth retardation (preservation of head circumference) and polycythaemia. Birth asphyxia is different. The term refers to more acute insults during delivery and is the most common reason for a term infant to require neonatal resuscitation. Episodic asphyxia during labour can result from a variety of possible causes and the response to resuscitation is usually rapid. More severely asphyxiated infants develop hypotension, acidosis and organ-system failure that characteristically affects organs that otherwise benefit from preservation of blood supply in times of stress. CVS dysfunction manifests with hypotension, poor perfusion and sometimes overt cardiac failure with dilated cardiomyopathy or even myocardial infarction. Renal dysfunction usually manifests with haematuria and oliguria or more rarely anuria. If secondary renal injury through CVS dysfunction is avoided and fluid intake controlled, then renal replacement therapy (RRT) is rarely necessary. Electrolyte abnormalities can usually be controlled by conservative means but peritoneal dialysis is the preferred approach if RRT is necessary. The outcome most often depends upon the degree of neurological insult. Clinically three grades of post-asphyxial encephalopathy can be recognised.

- Grade 1: wide-eyed infants with marginal hypotonia but sometimes with differential tone in upper and lower limbs. They may have a mild metabolic acidosis but recover in 1–2 hours.
- Grade 2: accentuated features of grade 1 with poor feeding and seizures over first few days. The prognosis is generally good (approximately 75 per cent survive intact). Long-term anticonvulsant therapy is not normally necessary.
- Grade 3: comatose, profoundly hypotonic with recalcitrant seizures. Mortality is approximately 60 per cent.

Hypoxic ischaemic encephalopathy can also result from postpartum illness or can aggravate post-asphyxial encephalopathy associated with severe CVS dysfunction. Severe insults produce cerebral oedema, usually without raised intracranial pressure because the skull bones are not fused. The main thrusts of therapy are organ support, fluid restriction and control of seizures. Imaging may later demonstrate leukomalacia in the watershed regions of the brain. Infarction and cyst formation delineate over time. The watershed regions are periventricular in the preterm and sub-cortical in the term. The functional outlook in survivors depends upon the sites of worst brain damage.

RESPIRATORY DISTRESS SYNDROME (RDS)

The composition of surface-active material (surfactant) in alveoli, which is secreted by type II pneumocytes, is 90 per cent lipids. The vast majority of these are phospholipids – predominantly dipalmitoyl phosphatidyl choline. The hydrophilic phosphate-nitrogenous bases locate the molecules at gas/water interfaces and the hydrophobic fatty acid chains of the phospholipids project into the lumen of the alveoli. Surfactant lowers surface tension in a concentration-dependent manner (smaller alveoli experience a greater reduction in surface tension). It prevents atelectasis, maintains stability and uniformity of alveolar size and reduces the tendency of fluid to transudate into the alveolar lumen. It is the single most significant influence increasing lung compliance in all age groups.

Surfactant is produced from the beginning of the third trimester. Deficiency therefore occurs in preterm infants. Hypoxia, acidosis and hypothermia also impair surfactant production and release. Infants of diabetic mothers have delayed maturation of surfactant production (and may have abnormal surfactant composition). Antenatal steroids accelerate surfactant production in such infants and reduce the incidence of respiratory distress syndrome (RDS) by 50 per cent. Surfactant prophylaxis gives a further 50 per cent reduction. Bovine (Survanta®), Porcine (Curosurf®) and synthetic (Exosurf®, Alec®) surfactants are available.

Surfactant deficiency causes RDS, a generalised lung disease associated with reticulogranular X-ray appearances and an air bronchogram. The reduced pulmonary compliance causes respiratory distress (tachypnoea, intercostal, subcostal, sternal recession, nasal flaring and grunting) within 4 hours of age, which deteriorates over 24 hours. Surfactant synthesis then occurs and symptoms should start to ameliorate by 4 to 5 days. Failure to improve at this point may be because of secondary infection or intermittent positive pressure ventilation (IPPV) injury, which may take the form of pulmonary interstitial emphysema or later chronic lung disease of prematurity (bronchopulmonary dysplasia). Pulmonary improvement is often heralded by a spontaneous diuresis as the capillary leak starts to resolve.

Mechanical ventilation is indicated pre-emptively for respiratory failure or for evidence of a degree of respiratory work that will lead to exhaustion, especially as oxygen requirement rises. Early institution of ventilation or CPAP is likely to reduce the tendency to atelectasis. Most units still use continuous flow, pressure regulated, time cycled ventilators for neonates although this is also the group in which there is most experience with high-frequency oscillation. With the conventional ventilator, the restrictive defect and characteristics of the mode of ventilation lead to the use of a 'square' pressure waveform to achieve the highest mean pressure for the lowest peak inspiratory pressure. The short time constant in RDS allows the use of rates up to 100 breaths per minute without a reduction in tidal volume. Particular care is required with IPPV during the deterioration and amelioration phases of the illness as changes in lung compliance lead to covert changes in tidal volume if one is using a traditional ventilator. RDS may be complicated by pneumothorax, pulmonary haemorrhage and pulmonary hypertension, all of which should be addressed directly.

The disease is often associated with secondary capillary leak, ileus and, what in effect is, systemic inflammatory response syndrome. Intensive care levels of monitoring are required. The risk and consequences of hypotension (mean blood pressure < 35 mmHg or < 30 mmHg for the extreme very low birth weight infant) demand arterial (umbilical) pressure monitoring. It can be hard to assess intravascular volume in neonates but efforts to reduce tissue oedema and optimise lung function lead to fluid restriction and a low threshold for intravascular volume supplementation in the face of hypotension. Electrolyte abnormalities are common. Many units will administer antibiotics until there is proof that a severe congenital bacterial pneumonia is not masquerading as RDS and nasogastric feeds are delayed in the presence of ileus.

MECONIUM ASPIRATION SYNDROME

Mature (and especially post-mature) infants have often opened their bowels before delivery. If this has occurred long before delivery then the meconium breaks up and is little more than a stain in the liquor at delivery. However, bowel opening is a pre-terminal event in distressed, hypoxic babies as it is in distressed hypoxic individuals generally. Fresher meconium in the liquor which has been aspirated as part of foetal breathing movements or premature gasping during foetal distress, can cause enormous difficulties with ventilation. A mixed lung disease results, with areas of collapse (airway occluded by meconium) and hyperexpansion (airway partially occluded by meconium that is obstructing expiration) compromising any adjacent unaffected lung. Typically the chest X-ray shows mottled hyperexpanded lungs and there is a major risk of pneumothorax during IPPV. Approaches to ventilation have to be gauged by the individual's response but the aim with a conventional ventilator has to be to minimise airway pressure. Large mature babies are often working much harder than the physician realises. When relaxants are administered, mechanical ventilation may have to be dramatically escalated (this is not an argument against elective paralysis). In the absence of barotrauma / infection, the disease is self-limiting but can still be complicated by PPHN. For the extreme cases the results of venoarterial (VA) ECMO are dramatic since, provided early referral is made, all that is really needed is time for the meconium to clear and secondary IPPV-aggravated lung injury can be avoided.

RETINOPATHY OF PREMATURITY (ROP)

Retinopathy of prematurity is a disease of the immature retina exacerbated by high oxygen levels, which in the premature infant with RDS are most likely to occur in the first four hours or on the fourth to fifth day. Normal outward growth of retinal vessels is arrested and subsequent abnormal vascular proliferation occurs forwards into the vitreous humor. Infants less than 30 weeks gestation or who weigh less than 1300 g (regardless of whether or not they have had oxygen administered) and all premature infants less than 35 weeks gestation or birth weight less than 1800 g who have required supplemental oxygen, are routinely screened for ROP at intervals until they reach the equivalent of 'term' i.e. 38 to 40 weeks.

Retinopathy of prematurity has been classified by consensus and is described by its location, extent and stage. The location refers to the position relative to the optic nerve. The closer to the edge of the retina the more mature and less vulnerable the vessels.

- zone I is centred on the optic disc and extends beyond the macula
- zone II is concentric to zone I and extends to the nasal limit of the retina
- zone III is the remaining crescent on the temporal side of the retina.

The extent of ROP is described by how many clock-hours of the retina are involved and the stages are:

- stage 1 is characterised by a demarcation line between the normal retina and the non-vascularised peripheral retina
- stage 2 has a ridge of scar tissue and new vessels growing at the demarcation line
- stage 3 shows an increased size of the ridge caused by extending vessels and scar formation
- stage 4 includes a partial retinal detachment caused by contraction of the scar
- stage 4 is further stratified into (a) and (b) depending upon whether or not the macula is detached
- the term 'stage 5' is sometimes used when a complete retinal detachment (blindness) has occurred.

Both screening and treatment are the realm of paediatric ophthalmic surgeons.

INTRAVENTRICULAR HAEMORRHAGE

Intraventricular haemorrhage (IVH) affects a quarter of very low birth weight infants (< 1.5 kg). Although it can be spontaneous in very small infants (< 1 kg birth weight) it is widely regarded as a complication of severe illness that has typically involved hypotension, hypoxia and acidosis. Thus it may occur with or without RDS and the risk is increased by sudden deteriorations such as apnoea or pneumothorax. The haemorrhages are classified by their ultrasound appearances. Grades I to III arise from the germinal matrix on the floor of the lateral ventricles – a feature of the foetal brain that does not persist to term. Grade I does not extend into the ventricular cerebrospinal fluid (CSF) while grade II extends into the CSF but without causing ventricular distension; these two grades account for 80 per cent of IVH, they typically occur in the first 3 days of life and are asymptomatic. Grade III haemorrhage is associated with ventricular distension and is often symptomatic. Systemic collapse with apnoea, acidosis, hypoxia and hypotension is more likely than neurological signs but seizures may occur. The appearance of grade IV haemorrhage is that of grade III but with echogenicity in the periventricular white matter, probably caused by venous occlusion rather than parenchymal extension of the haemorrhage. There is no treatment for IVH and the emphasis is upon prevention by avoiding known precipitants and minimal handling. Secondary hydrocephalus is usually 'communicating' and may require external drainage and later shunting.

CONGENITAL DIAPHRAGMATIC HERNIA

In congenital diaphragmatic hernia (CDH), embryological persistence of the pleuroperitoneal canal results in a defect in (or absence of) the diaphragm. The incidence is 0.25 per 1000 live births, 90 per cent are left sided and mortality is 50 to 60 per cent in most series. There is a spectrum of cardiorespiratory compromise presenting at or after birth and for which one may be prepared by an antenatal ultrasound diagnosis. Otherwise the clinical diagnosis is usually made during neonatal resuscitation as a result of recognising a scaphoid abdomen and displacement of the apex beat away from the hemithorax with reduced breath sounds. Given this scenario, elective paralysis, endotracheal intubation and passage of a nasogastric tube to allow decompression of the gut are essential. Subsequently the severity of illness depends upon the interaction of:

- the degree of pulmonary hypoplasia caused by *bilateral* pulmonary compression in utero
- persistent pulmonary hypertension caused principally by the imposition of hypoxia upon the transitional circulation
- pulmonary compression from the unreduced hernia potentially aggravated by gaseous distension of the gut or pneumothorax on either side.

Surgery is delayed until cardiopulmonary stability has been achieved and the high neonatal pulmonary vascular resistance has had a chance to fall. It involves reduction of the hernia and closure of the defect, which may require a patch. Postoperatively a tight abdomen can impair ventilation by splinting the diaphragm/patch. Conversely a loose patch can move paradoxically during respiration and mechanically impair breathing on the affected side. Recent advances such as surgical repair on the foetus and tracheal ligation (leading to overgrowth of the hypoplastic lungs as they distend with foetal lung fluid) have yet to be adequately evaluated.

For many years one of the most topical features of the care of babies with CDH has been the recognition of irretrievable patients or the selection of candidates who may benefit from more novel or aggressive therapies such as ECMO, high-frequency oscillation, liquid ventilation, etc. Any patient who has achieved a preductal PaO_2 more than 10 kPa should be considered potentially viable. Bohn *et al.* (1987, *Journal of Pediatrics*, 111(3):423–31) were able, retrospectively, to distinguish patients who died using the $PaCO_2$ value combined with a ventilation index and proposed this as a predictive tool. In truth no predictor is good enough to apply prospectively to individual cases and the percentage of cases that are borderline (i.e. can only be saved with ECMO or an exotic therapy) is probably small.

NECROTISING ENTEROCOLITIS

The incidence of necrotising enterocolitis (NEC) is between 1 and 5 per cent of all NICU admissions with considerable variation between units. It is predominantly a disease of premature infants the cause of which is unknown but for which the mortality is 30 to 40 per cent. The presentation is usually at 3 to 10 days of age and postulated causes include infection, enteral feeds and vascular compromise/reperfusion injury. Although the majority of premature infants who are enterally fed do not develop NEC, 90 to 95 per cent of all infants who develop NEC have been enterally fed. A beneficial effect of breast milk against the development of NEC has been identified. Occasional epidemics imply an infective origin but most cases are sporadic.

Early signs of NEC are indistinguishable from 'sepsis' and include abdominal distension, ileus, bile-stained vomits, bloody stools, recurrent apnoea and shock. Examination may reveal abdominal wall erythema, tenderness, guarding or a mass. However, physical findings may be minimal even in infants with perforation. Laboratory evaluation reflects systemic inflammation and emulates sepsis. Abdominal X-rays may show gas in the bowel wall (pneumatosis coli) or gas in the portal venous system. Free gas or gas in the falciform ligament, indicates visceral perforation.

Treatment consists of:

- vigorous resuscitation from shock with intravenous fluid (and inotropic support) and respiratory support when necessary
- bowel rest with nasogastric decompression and intravenous feeding
- treatment of potential or proven septicaemia with broad spectrum antibiotics
- frequent review for signs of intestinal perforation.

Multi-organ system failure can occur in association with NEC or as a consequence of the severity of illness. Neutropaenia is common in severely stressed neonates, representing an inadequate marrow response/suppression. DIC, thrombocytopaenia and haemolysis can occur during NEC, the latter being sometimes related to exposure of T-antigen on red cells.

Surgical approaches range from peritoneal drainage under local anaesthesia to colectomy with defunctioning ileostomy/jejunostomy. Surgical intervention may be prompted by failure of resolution of multiorgan system failure (MOSF) or other features of the disease. More specific indications include evidence of perforation or persistent fixed dilated loops on abdominal X-ray. It is wise to seek a surgical opinion early. Late complications such as stricture also require surgical intervention and patients with extensive resections may be left with short-gut syndrome.

NEONATAL ECMO

The haemodynamics, gas exchange and other practicalities of ECMO are covered in the respiratory and cardiovascular chapters of the text. Three randomised controlled trials have vindicated its application to neonates who are the group most responsive to this intervention. In severe neonatal cardiopulmonary failure, survival is at least twice as likely with ECMO compared to alternative treatments and the quality of survival in terms of neurological outcome is high. Patients are selected according to the prospects of a successful outcome using the following criteria:

- IVH no higher than grade I
- no hypoxic ischaemic brain damage
- more than 34 weeks gestation
- weighing more than 2 kg

and the severity of illness. Since standard mortality prediction models are not sufficiently organ or patient-specific for this process, the oxygenation index (OI) has been used to select ECMO candidates for many years. Its validation includes historical controls and the randomised controlled trials alluded to above. Experience shows that neonates with a value of 40 or more should receive ECMO and that this value distinguishes neonates with high mortality (approximately 80% in historical controls and 59% in the UK ECMO trial) for ECMO treatment (> 80% survival in ELSO data and 68% survival in the UK ECMO trial). The oxygenation index is not a physiological parameter as much as a contrived tool that relates the degree of hypoxia to the inspired oxygen tension. It is calculated according to the formula

$$OI = \frac{(MAP\ (cmH_2O) \times FiO_2(\%))}{post\text{-}ductal\ PaO_2(mmHg)}$$

where MAP is the mean airway pressure. For given 'maximal' ventilator settings at around the threshold value of 40, the index bears an almost linear relationship to the PaO_2. At low levels of PaO_2 the calculated oxygenation index rises sharply. Similarly at high PaO_2 changes in oxygenation have less effect on the oxygenation index. This behaviour of the oxygenation index (to amplify the significance of a low PaO_2) is probably the source of its utility rather than a drawback. A rigorous statistical justification of the oxygenation index using prospectively gathered data has not been performed. Consistency in the origin of the blood gas data is important because of the effects of ductal shunting which can be included (post-ductal samples) or excluded (pre-ductal samples). In the presence of such a shunt and using preductal oxygenation indices, the threshold value for starting ECMO should be much lower than 40.

In recent years the numbers of neonates treated with ECMO and their survival statistics have declined; the result of promulgation of the technology out of specialist centres and the evolution of a culture whereby, to graduate for ECMO, one must first have failed a succession of less invasive but novel and less well-proven therapies. In the overall analysis, the very real benefits of high frequency oscillation and nitric oxide for some individuals have to be balanced against the negative effect of late ECMO referral in the population as a whole.

6 Neonatology

7 Fluids, Electrolytes and Blood

- **Water**
- **Electrolytes**
- **Blood**
- **Colloid balance**

WATER

Total body water and its distribution

Humans have been described as 'bags of mostly water' and the description is fairly accurate, more so for babies than it is for older children and adults. The 'total body water' accounts for 80 per cent of mass at birth and this percentage falls to 60 per cent by 1 year of age. The change is the result of a disproportionate increase in cell mass compared to the volume of extracellular fluid.

The relationship between total body water and body weight is linear over short time scales within an individual but there is considerable variation between individuals. This is largely accounted for by variation in the amount of adipose tissue (which contains < 10% water). For this reason post-pubertal females with more subcutaneous fat have lower total body water (55% of total mass) than males and prepubertal females.

Figure 7.1 shows the major compartments within which the total body water and its solutes are distributed. Within each, the changing balance of water and electrolytes is manifested by changes in volume and composition (concentration of solutes). In describing these the term 'osmolarity' is used which refers to the osmolar effect in a fixed mass of solution. In comparatively dilute solutions such as body fluids this approximates to the 'osmolality'. This latter term however refers to the activity of the solutes added to a fixed volume of water and is therefore independent of temperature and their 'volume in solution'. Quantitatively, physiological osmotic pressures exert enormously powerful effects on water movement when compared to hydrostatic forces.

The age-related changes in the relative volumes of the major fluid compartments are shown in Figure 7.2. In the following text the standard abbreviations shown will be deployed with the suffix 'v' to denote volume:

- total body water – TBW
- intracellular fluid – ICF
- extracellular fluid – ECF
- interstitial fluid – ISF.

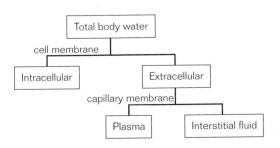

Figure 7.1 Fluid compartments. 83

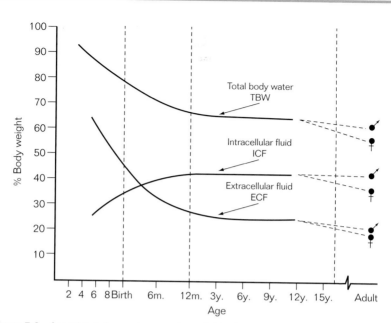

Figure 7.2 Age related changes in compartment fluid volumes. (Reproduced with permission from Winters RW 1973. The Body Fluids in Paediatrics. Little Brown, Boston; p. 100.)

Intracellular fluid

The ICFv is not easily measured directly but it can be inferred from TBW–ECFv. The two main influences upon the ICFv are:

- the composition of the ECF
- the integrity of active homeostatic systems such as the Na^+/K^+ ATPase.

An osmotic effect reducing ICFv is created by Na^+/K^+ATPase (see p. 271). The ICF accounts for an increasing percentage of TBW from foetal life up to 1 year of age, but this is mostly a reflection of the reduction in ECFv. The predominant cation in intracellular fluid is potassium and the predominant anions are phosphate and proteins.

Extracellular fluid

The ECF has many components since it includes plasma and ISF which itself includes CSF and fluid spaces such as peritoneum, pleura, ocular, synovium, etc. Gastrointestinal fluid is also extracellular but topologically is extracorporeal. Dilutional techniques can be used to measure ECFv but the results depend upon which marker solute is used, as their volumes of distribution differ. ECFv is greater than ICFv in the foetus but decreases as described over the first year. Both total ECFv and the distribution of fluid between ECF compartments vary widely in disease. The distribution is dictated by the interplay of hydrostatic, oncotic and osmotic forces, and membrane permeability. Transcapillary exchange is discussed further under multi-organ system failure – the intensive care situation where it is most deranged (page 271 onwards). Composition of the various extracellular fluids vary as described in Table 7.1.

Serum sodium, potassium and water balance fluctuate so rapidly in the critically ill that crystalloid fluid balances (intravenous infusions and enteral fluids versus urine output and enteral losses) are reviewed hourly by the bedside staff. Most PICUs also use blood gas analysers that routinely measure electrolytes so that the internal 'milieu' is kept under close scrutiny.

Table 7.1 Composition of solutes in body fluids.

	Na$^+$(mmol L^{-1})	K$^+$(mmol L^{-1})	Cl$^-$(mmol L^{-1})	HCO$_3^-$(mmol L^{-1})
Plasma	135–145	3.5–5	98–110	18–25
ISF	145	4.1	117	27
ICF	10	159	3	7
Saliva	10–25	20–35	10–30	2–10
Gastric	20–80	5–20	100–150	0
Jejunal	130–150	5–10	100–130	10–20
Ileal	50–150	3–15	20–120	30–50
Diarrhoeal	10–90	10–80	10–110	20–70
Sweat (normal)	10–30	3–10	10–35	0
Sweat (CF)	50–130	5–25	50–110	0
Burn exudate	140	5	110	20

Includes 30–50 g L^{-1} of protein

Water balance

Water intake is normally regulated by thirst which arises in response to changes in both the osmolality and volume of the plasma. Insensible water losses across the skin and respiratory tract are largely obligatory but are not fixed (see Table 7.2). Of the sensible water losses, the principal physiological control is over the volume and content of urine production. This is reduced by antidiuretic hormone (ADH), which works on the collecting duct and is increased by atrial naturetic peptide (ANP), which is released from the heart when the ECF is expanded. ANP inhibits sodium reabsorption in the distal nephron and increases glomerular filtration rate (GFR) by increasing blood pressure and the filtration fraction. There are, however, obligatory water losses in the urine – the volume required to excrete the solute load – which are higher in babies. ADH release occurs in response to osmoreceptors in the hypothalamus and baroreceptors (really stretch receptors) in the circulation. The osmoreceptors are by far the more sensitive, enabling fine control over plasma osmolality but the ADH response that they initiate is muted compared to that caused by a fall in plasma volume. Strong releases of ADH occur in response to reduced plasma volume, irrespective of the tonicity of the plasma. Water balance naturally fluctuates with the dictates of sodium balance (renin–angiotensin system). The urine sodium content can be used to differentiate oliguric states. Normal responses to hypovolaemia make urine sodium content low (< 20 mmol L^{-1}) whereas in acute tubular necrosis it usually exceeds 40 mmol L^{-1}.

Water balance must be monitored meticulously on the PICU. Children need higher water and electrolyte intakes than adults making them more susceptible to dehydration. Their increased water losses are due to:

* caloric expenses of a high metabolic rate
* high insensible loss (high minute ventilation, high surface area : volume ratio, immature epidermis in premature babies)
* decreased ability to concentrate urine.

However babies are also less able to excrete a water load because of renal immaturity (< 1 year of age) and have a tendency to high ADH levels. The most common error in fluid management is actually *water overload* which can very rapidly result in symptomatic hyponatraemia for patients receiving intravenous fluids. Treatment is principally by fluid

Table 7.2 Maintenance fluid requirements for children.

		Fluid regime/adjustment
Baseline	1 day of age	50 ml kg^{-1}day^{-1}
	2 days of age	75 ml kg^{-1}day^{-1}
	≥ 3 days of age	100 ml kg^{-1}day^{-1}
	< 10 kg	100 ml kg^{-1}day^{-1}
	10–20 kg	1000 ml day^{-1} + 50 ml kg^{-1}day^{-1} for every kg over 10 kg
	> 20 kg	1500 ml day^{-1} + 20 ml kg^{-1}day^{-1} for every kg over 20 kg
Factors that decrease requirement	humidified gases	× 0.75
	paralysed	× 0.7
	high ADH (e.g. IPPV or coma)	× 0.7
	hypothermia	−12% per °C core temp is < 37°C
	high ambient humidity	× 0.7
	renal failure	× 0.3 (+ urine output)
Factors that increase requirement	full activity and oral feeds	× 1.5 / free fluids
	fever	+ 12% per °C core temp is > 37
	room temp over 31°C	+ 30% per °C
	hyperventilation	× 1.2
	preterm neonate (<1.5 kg)	× 1.2
	radiant heater	× 1.5
	phototherapy	× 1.5
	burns day 1	+ 4% per 1% of body surface area affected
	burns day 2+	+ 2% per 1% of body surface area affected

restriction with the provisos covered under 'Hyponatraemia' (see p. 88). Diuretic therapies are usually avoided for fear of reducing serum sodium further.

Oedema is common in ventilated patients even without water overload. As a consequence, fluid regimes are frequently standardised and comparatively restrictive. As can be seen in Table 7.2, baseline 'maintenance' fluids are a considerable over-estimation of water requirement for most hospitalised patients. Indeed unrestricted baseline fluid administration is probably only prescribed in enterally fed patients where the volume is required for caloric reasons. Mandatory reductions to baseline fluids apply for patients receiving intravenous fluids, nursed in bed, paralysed, breathing humidified gases or being nursed in a humidified environment. All fluids administered must be taken into account including drugs, flushes for intravenous and intra-arterial lines etc. Serial weight measurements are the most scientific approach to fluid management but they may be impractical in very sick or very small patients.

Dehydration

Weight loss is the best method to determine the extent of dehydration. However in many clinical circumstances a recent appropriate weight is not available. In these circumstances clinical signs must be used such as urine output, fontanelle fullness, skin turgor and moistness of mucous membranes. A common clinical shorthand is to measure the serum urea. Urea rises in dehydration when the ECF contracts to a degree sufficient to reduce the glomerular filtration rate (relative to the rate of urea production). Patients who are protein depleted may therefore not display a rise to markedly abnormal levels during dehydration.

Similarly, types of dehydration in which water is preferentially lost from the ECF are more likely to reduce GFR and will be associated with greater rises in serum urea.

Classically the degree of dehydration is mapped to a three-point scale – mild, moderate or severe. At the midpoint of this scale evidence of shock becomes apparent. There is evidence that physicians tend to overestimate the degree of dehydration and percentage points of 3, 6 and 9 per cent may be more appropriate (shock becoming evident at 6%) than the more commonly described 5, 10 and 15 per cent. Nevertheless there should be no confusion in the clinical approach to rehydration provided one distinguishes the treatment of shock from rehydration.

Three classes of biochemical derangement are distinguished in dehydrated patients.

HYPEROSMOLAR DEHYDRATION

In this condition the net loss of water has been more than that of solute (e.g. when fluid replacement has occurred with hypertonic solutions). The hyperosmolal plasma equilibrates with the intracellular environment which experiences a greater fluid loss than in other forms of dehydration. This means that compared to other forms of dehydration, more of the total body water is lost for the same degree of haemodynamic compromise. More importantly, rehydration involves re-expansion of the ICFv and carries a high risk of cerebral swelling. It should therefore be performed slowly (over at least 48 hours). Hyperosmolarity is usually, but not exclusively, recognised by hypernatraemia. It is also present in hyperglycaemic dehydration due to diabetic ketoacidosis.

ISO-OSMOLAR DEHYDRATION

In this condition equivalent quantities of salt and water have been lost.

HYPO-OSMOLAR DEHYDRATION

In this condition there has been more net loss of salt than water (e.g. when fluid replacement has occurred with excessively hypotonic solutions). The predominant water loss is from the extracellular (hence including the vascular) space and so hypotension and shock are an earlier feature of this form of dehydration. Relative preservation of intracellular turgor may increase the risk of cerebral ischaemia during hypotension.

> In all forms of dehydration, shock, acidosis and hypoglycaemia are treated aggressively but rehydration should be more controlled using normal saline initially, irrespective of the serum sodium.

Thus salt is replaced in hypo-osmolal dehydration and in hyperosmolal dehydration the serum osmolality is sustained during the early stages of rehydration – reducing the risk of cerebral oedema. A policy of aiming to replace water deficit over at least 48 hours in all forms of dehydration protects against the common tendency to overestimate the water deficit. The patient's fluid (and electrolyte) regime has three components:

- normal maintenance requirement
- replacement of the deficit over 48 hours
- replacement of continuing losses which should be closely monitored and replaced throughout rehydration. In conditions of profuse water loss (such as hyperglycaemia) the rate of replacement may need adjusting on an hourly basis. The appropriate electrolyte content of the replacement fluid can be judged from Table 7.1 or from urinary or stool electrolytes as appropriate.

Recovery from dehydration is sometimes described as proceeding in four phases.

1   Phase I – restoration of blood volume (i.e. treat shock) – 1 to 2 hours.
2   Phase II – restoration of ECF (replace water and sodium deficit) – 48 hours.
3   Phase III – replacement of body potassium stores (see p 89–90) – several days.
4   Phase IV – replacement of body fat ands protein stores – weeks.

ELECTROLYTES

Sodium

Sodium is the principal cation of the ECF and normal requirements are 2 to 4 mmol kg^{-1} day^{-1}. It is absorbed actively from the jejunum and is lost in urine, sweat and faeces. Control is mediated over absorption and excretion by the renin–angiotensin system. The critical point of balance is the degree of reabsorption in the distal convoluted tubule despite the fact that most of the sodium in the glomerular filtrate has been reabsorbed before this point.

Hyponatraemia

This can be falsely diagnosed in the presence of hyperlipidaemia where anhydrous lipids occupy a significant proportion of the plasma volume and the laboratory report the sodium concentration per litre of plasma rather than water. Sodium loss is usually associated with a concomitant water loss and the resultant serum sodium depends upon the balance between the two. Hyponatraemia causes ileus, listlessness and ultimately cerebral oedema and convulsions, the extent of the symptoms is more closely related to the rapidity of change in serum sodium than the absolute value. Hyponatraemia can occur in the face of normal total body sodium (SIADH, glucocorticoid deficiency, water overload, etc.), raised total body sodium (heart failure, cirrhosis, nephrotic syndrome and sequestration) or decreased total body sodium (increased losses, diuretic therapy, inadequate intake). Hyponatraemia is common in preterm infants because of their high urinary losses and it is associated with inadequate sodium intake if fed breast milk exclusively.

The term 'syndrome of inappropriate ADH secretion' (SIADH) is used when influences other than plasma volume or tonicity cause ADH release. The most common causes (from a long list of possible candidates) are CNS injury and bacterial pneumonia. Whether such a physiological reaction is 'inappropriate' may be equivocal. Although SIADH is more common in paediatric than in adult medicine the reader will not be surprised, bearing in mind the comments made above about routine fluid restriction in the critically ill, to learn that most cases of SIADH are aggravated by SIAD (syndrome of the inappropriate administration of dextrose). Secretion of ADH in critical illness has clear evolutionary advantages that did not anticipate an intravenous infusion. The production of ADH during SIADH is similar to that induced by volume depletion. The diagnosis is made when one can confidently exclude hypovolaemia and yet find evidence of high urine osmolarity when one would expect it to be low because of low plasma osmolarity.

Rapid correction of hyponatraemia is justified in circumstances where severe symptoms have resulted from a rapid fall in serum sodium. If a good history is not available, symptoms are severe and serum Na$^+$ is < 120 mmol L^{-1} a rapid initial correction may be justifiable to values of 125 mmol L^{-1} the rest being achieved more gradually with fluid restriction. In all other circumstances slow correction is advisable by fluid restriction alone and the provision of normal rather than increased sodium supplements.

Hypernatraemia

This can occur in association with low total body sodium, in which case the salt loss has occurred in the context of a greater water loss (e.g. osmotic diuresis, vomiting and diarrhoea). When losses are predominantly water, total body sodium balance may be normal (e.g. fever, radiant heater, phototherapy, diabetes insipidus) as is the case when the ISFv expands at the expense of the plasma volume (e.g. capillary leak). True excess of sodium can also occur (e.g. iatrogenic – especially when intravenous sodium bicarbonate is used to correct acidosis, or when incorrectly reconstituted formula is given). In all hyperosmolar states, water moves from ICF to ECF and so the ICF is dehydrated. Neurological symptoms predominate (irritability, seizures and coma). The loss of volume of brain cells can even cause cerebrovascular disruptions and bleeding. Treatment of hypernatraemia should be aimed at the primary cause and any necessary rehydration should be slow because of the risks of cerebral oedema. True sodium overload without dehydration requires removal with diuretics or renal replacement therapy as required.

Table 7.3 Causes of diabetes insipidus.	
Central	Congenital
	Trauma
	Infections
	Tumours
	Demyelination (Guillain–Barré)
	Hypoxia
	Post-neurosurgery
	Vascular
	Miscellaneous
	Brain death
Nephrogenic	Congenital
	Chronic renal failure
	Drugs

Like SIADH, diabetes insipidus may be caused by a variety of conditions and drugs. In intensive care the acquired forms predominate. The diagnosis is inferred by a therapeutic response to DDAVP® (urine osmolality rises to greater than that of plasma) in polyuria. Continuous infusions of vasopressin need to be titrated against the serum sodium rather than the urine output.

Potassium

The range of normal potassium levels in babies is wider than that in older children and adults (4.5–7.2 mmol L^{-1} in pre-term and 3.6–6.4 mmol L^{-1} in term infants). Potassium is the principal cation of the ICF, extracellular potassium represents only 2 per cent of the total body content. Normal requirements are 1–2 mmol $kg^{-1}day^{-1}$ and absorption is principally in the duodenum and jejunum. Like sodium, the balance is critically mediated by control of excretion in the kidney where the majority of potassium is absorbed along with water in the proximal convoluted tubule and fine tuning is performed by the distal nephron. Filtrate entering the distal convoluted tubule already contains less potassium than plasma. Potassium is secreted into the filtrate in the distal convoluted tubule and cortical collecting duct in exchange for sodium or hydrogen ions. Hence the relationship between alkalosis and hypokalaemia.

The distribution of potassium between the ICF and ECF is heavily dependent upon the action of the Na^+/K^+ ATPase. This latter enzyme imports $2 \times K^+$ from the ECF and exports $3 \times Na^+$ from the ICF. Electrical neutrality may be preserved by the efflux of a chloride ion, which adds to the osmotic effect leading to a reduction of the ICFv. The balance of potassium across the cell membrane otherwise contributes to the resting membrane electrical potential. Acid–base status, insulin and catecholamines all exert effects upon the distribution of potassium across the cell membrane. Acidosis causes an efflux of potassium from the cell and alkalosis the reverse (Figure 7.3). The greatest effect occurs with mineral acids rather than lactic or keto acids where the cell is more permeable to the accompanying anions and the effects on potassium levels lag behind those of pH.

Hypokalaemia

Hypokalaemia without a true deficit in potassium can result from redistribution into the cells in response to a β adrenergic stimulus, alkalosis, excess insulin or rarer causes like familial hypokalaemic periodic paralysis. Hypokalaemia with a deficit in potassium can result from inadequate intake, or increased renal (diuretic) or gastrointestinal losses introducing a host of potential diagnoses. Hypokalaemia has cardiovascular, neuromuscular and metabolic consequences including a propensity for dysrhythmias, ileus, muscle weakness and effects on carbohydrate and protein metabolism. Potassium replacement has to be given into the

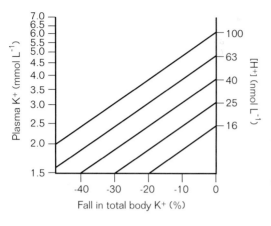

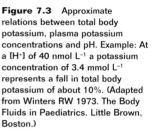

Figure 7.3 Approximate relations between total body potassium, plasma potassium concentrations and pH. Example: At a [H+] of 40 nmol L^{-1} a potassium concentration of 3.4 mmol L^{-1} represents a fall in total body potassium of about 10%. (Adapted from Winters RW 1973. The Body Fluids in Paediatrics. Little Brown, Boston.)

ECF even though the principal destination is the ICF. Infusion rates should never exceed 0.5 mmol kg^{-1} hr^{-1} for fear of deranging myocardial membrane potential causing lethal arrhythmia. Adequate replacement may take days (phase III of rehydration). Potassium supplements or replacement should not be routinely given in the presence of oliguria or anuria without regular monitoring of serum levels.

Hyperkalaemia

Hyperkalaemia without true overload (or even deficit) may result from measurement error (e.g. haemolysis in the sample), acidosis, insulin deficiency, or drugs such as digoxin, β-blockers and depolarising muscle relaxants. There is also a hyperkalaemic form of familial periodic paralysis. High serum potassium occurs in instances of increased load (e.g. iatrogenic infusion, tissue destruction, gastrointestinal bleed, tumour lysis, etc.) or decreased excretion (renal failure, mineralocorticoid deficiency, congenital adrenal hyperplasia, etc.). In acute renal failure hyperkalaemia may be dramatic, because of other simultaneous injury to other organs and tissues increasing the load. In chronic renal failure GFR has to get down to 5 to 10 per cent before hyperkalaemia results although the 'renal reserve' for potassium excretion is reduced before this. The most severe consequence of hyperkalaemia is cardiac arrest, which can occur at any point in the progression of the ECG abnormalities and arrhythmias. If the problem is detected before cardiac arrest then possible emergency therapeutic measures include:

- intravenous bolus of calcium (0.1 mmol kg^{-1}) reduces risk of dysrhythmia
- correction of acidosis
- salbutamol administration (1–5 mcg kg^{-1} min^{-1})
- glucose and insulin. (0.1 U kg^{-1} of insulin with 2 ml kg^{-1} of 50% Dextrose)

A slower response can be obtained using ion exchange resins.

Calcium and magnesium

Calcium and magnesium homeostasis are closely linked to phosphate levels. Interpretation of total calcium levels must also be put into context with the serum albumin although it is more physiological to look directly at the ionised (free) component. Parathyroid hormone (PTH) increases calcium by promoting bone reabsorption, increasing calcium reasorption from the renal tubule and increasing vitamin D activation, which increases enteral absorption of calcium and phosphate. Calcitonin is secreted in the thyroid and thymus in response to hypercalcaemia, and it lowers both calcium and phosphate levels.

Hypocalcaemia is common in sick infants because of high levels of PTH antagonists such as glucocorticoids and calcitonin. It may also be caused by intravenous bicarbonate therapy or the use of citrated blood products. If persistent in the newborn it may be caused by DiGeorge syndrome, maternal vitamin D deficiency, feeding of cows' milk or magnesium deficiency. It causes jittery symptoms in babies, multifocal clonic convulsions and, rarely, ECG abnormalities, dysrhythmias or heart failure. Normal requirements are 0.3 mmol kg^{-1} day^{-1} increased to 1 mmol kg^{-1}day^{-1} when treating deficiency. Calcium infusion has vasoconstrictive and inotropic effects of greater significance in children than adults. Vasoconstriction predominates in hypomagnesaemic states and it opposes the negative inotropic effects of hyperkalaemia.

Hypomagnesaemia usually occurs in the context of parenteral nutrition because of solubility problems caused by the concurrent administration of phosphate. Clinical problems are rare until levels fall below 0.5 mmol L^{-1} but do include lethal arrhythmias such as VF/VT and torsades de pointes. Deficiency also reduces cardiac contractility but during infusion magnesium salts are reasonably potent vasodilators and will drop the blood pressure. Magnesium has also been used to treat pulmonary hypertension and asthma. Hypocalcaemia and hypokalaemia may not respond to supplementation if concurrent hypomagnesaemia is not corrected.

Hypercalcaemia is rare (unlike in adult ICUs) but it occurs; in the recovery phase of acute renal failure, a variety of endocrine diseases, hypervitaminosis D and granulomatous disorders. Idiopathic hypercalcaemia is a feature of Williams syndrome – these patients often pass through the PICU after surgery on their cardiac defects. Most cases of hypercalcaemia are iatrogenic however. Symptoms include CNS (hypotonia, seizures and coma), CVS (tachyarrhythmias and in chronic cases hypertension.) Many patients will be volume depleted at presentation and respond to resuscitation followed by diuretic therapy. Severe cases are treated by solute-orientated renal replacement therapy (haemodialysis or haemofiltration with a high ultrafiltration rate). Hypermagnesaemia occurs when excessive administration (cathartics or enemas) coincides with renal failure. Symptoms are similar to hypercalcaemia but include bradyarrhythmias with first degree block and a broad QRS complex. Treatment is again focussed on enhanced excretion. Serious arrhythmias may respond to calcium.

Phosphate

Phosphate is the principal anion of the ICF. Normal serum levels are 1 to 1.8 mmol L^{-1} (up to 2.6 mmol L^{-1} in the preterm) but like serum potassium these are a poor guide to total body levels. Plasma levels fluctuate as the result of shifts between ECF and ICF, and are also closely linked to ionised calcium levels. False low values/assay interference occur after mannitol administration or in the presence of lipaemia, free haemoglobin (haemolysis) or bilirubinaemia. Phosphate excretion involves free filtration at the glomerulus with passive reabsorption of 80 per cent in the proximal convoluted tubule as a symport with sodium. Although PTH results in phosphate release from bone and increased phosphate absorption from the gut, its net effect at high levels is to decrease plasma phosphate because it inhibits its renal tubular reabsorption. The foetus is however relatively hypoparathyroid in response to active calcium influx across the placenta.

Hypophosphataemia

Hypophosphataemia occurs in circumstances of:

- inadequate intake (e.g. breast-fed preterm infants)
- impaired gastrointestinal absorption, for example as a consequence of antacids containing calcium, magnesium or aluminium (sucralfate)
- cellular redistribution, for example alkalosis, therapy for diabetic ketoacidosis, β_2 adrenergic stimulation
- carbohydrate infusions and other forms of hyperalimentation can lead to hypophosphataemia by stimulating insulin release (phosphate moves into cells with glucose in response to insulin)

- successful stimulation of an anabolic state after critical illness can be associated with a profound and symptomatic hypophosphataemia
- excessive losses, for example as a consequence of diuretics, steroids, cytotoxic regimes or paracetamol poisoning
- trauma (including burns)
- hereditary hypophosphataemic rickets.

The most important feature of phosphate physiology in the ICU is the formation of ATP. Symptomatic hypophosphataemia causes muscle weakness that aggravates respiratory failure and causes a reduction in myocardial contractility. When necessary, phosphate supplementation should aim to provide a dose of up to 1 mmol kg^{-1} day^{-1} (maximum 20 mmol) but be aware that proprietary supplements frequently have a high potassium content.

Hyperphosphataemia

This occurs in neonates fed cows' milk or inadequately adjusted formula feed, or with tumour lysis syndrome and renal failure, severe haemolysis, hyperthyroidism, acromegaly hypoparathyroidism or phosphate poisoning. Symptoms are those of the consequent hypocalcaemia and deposition of hydroxyapatite crystals in cornea, lungs and heart. Treatment includes resuscitation to restore ECFv. In the absence of renal failure, phosphate binders and alkaline diuresis may be used. Tumour lysis syndrome is discussed further in Chapter 15 (Renal System) since failed preventive measures (allopurinol, uricozyme and prehydration) usually entail PICU admission for renal replacement therapy.

BLOOD

Neonatal blood volume varies from 50 to 100 ml kg^{-1} depending on the volume of the placental transfusion at birth. This is half completed within a minute of delivery if the umbilical cord has not been transected and can boost the blood volume by as much as 60 per cent. Mean neonatal haemoglobin levels are 14.5 g dL^{-1} at 28 weeks but by term are 16.6 to 17.1 g dL^{-1} with a 95 per cent range of 13.7 to 20.1 g dL^{-1}. The practice of blood sampling by heel-skin prick can lead to overestimation of haemoglobin by as much as 4 g dL^{-1}. The decrease in plasma volume over the first 6 hours of extrauterine life can be associated with a rise in haemoglobin concentration of as much as 6 g dL^{-1}.

Blood volume in ml kg^{-1} decreases over the first year in association with a reduction in haematocrit and plasma volume, although the proportion of the blood occupied by plasma rises (40% of 80 ml kg^{-1} changing to 60% of 65 ml kg^{-1}). Nucleated red cells form part of the normal blood film (0.5×10^9 L^{-1} at term but up to 1.5×10^9 L^{-1} in the preterm). The normal neonatal decline in haemoglobin concentration continues into infancy and reaches its nadir at 8 to 12 weeks of age by which time nucleated red cells are unusual. Trough haemoglobin levels are usually above 11 g dL^{-1} in term infants but are lower (7–8 g dL^{-1}) for preterm deliveries. The subsequent rise is heralded by a rising reticulocyte count (to > 2%). The production of adult haemoglobin starts before birth but foetal haemoglobin persists until half way through the first year of life, longer in the presence of haemoglobinopathy.

Transfusion regimes

When faced with an anaemic patient it is important to elucidate the cause (see Table 7.4 for examples) which may take time. From a patient management perspective the more critical decision is whether or not to transfuse. During critical illness at any age and irrespective of variations in measured value, an acceptable haemoglobin concentration can only really be defined in terms of the adequacy of oxygen delivery. Thus it depends on the context, evidence of oxygen extraction and knowledge/inference of the cardiac output and oxygen delivery ($\dot{D}O_2$). In situations where $\dot{D}O_2$ is likely to be critical, the target haemoglobin concentration should be more than or equal to 14 g dL^{-1}. The threshold for intervention (transfusion) is similarly context sensitive but depends more on trends than absolute values. Patients

Table 7.4 Causes of anaemia.

Increased loss

Haemorrhage or occult bleeding
  In neonates remember foeto-maternal or from placental haemorrhage, twin-to-twin transfusion, or excessive blood sampling of extreme low birth weight babies
  gastrointestinal tract
Intravascular haemolysis
  Blood group incompatibility
    incompatible transfusion
    materno-foetal incompatibility – rhesus ABO, Coombs positive, Coombs negative
  Red cell defects
    spherocytosis, elliptocytosis, PNH
  Inborn errors
    G6PD deficiency
  Arteriopathy / red cell stress
    haemolytic uraemic syndrome
    cardiac valve defects (e.g. VSD / regurgitant flows impinging upon valve apparatus)
    cardiac prosthesis
    vasculitis
  Toxin
    water – hypotonic intravenous fluids, fresh water drowning
    envenomation
  Infection
    malaria, clostridial infections, neuraminidase-positive infections
Extravascular haemolysis
  Autoimmune
    normally sequestered antigen or abnormal antibody, warm and cold agglutinins
  Haemoglobinopathy
    sickle cell and to some extent thalassaemia
  Hypersplenism

Inadequate production

Dietary deficiency
  Iron – microcytic hypochromic
  B_{12} folate – macrocytic
  Vitamin C – macrocytic
  Copper – microcytic
Defective haem synthesis
  Porphyria
  Lead poisoning (microcytic)
Defective globin synthesis
  α Thalassaemia (usually hydrops foetalis)
  β Thalassaemia / trait
  Haemoglobin S, C, D, E, etc.
Chronic disease
  Liver, kidney, malignancy, any chronic infection or inflammation can cause relative bone marrow failure
Abnormal marrow
  Infiltrated
  Congenital hypoplasia of red cell precursors (Blackfan Diamond)
  Aplastic

Dilutional
  Non-red-cell colloid administration

with known sources of continuing blood loss (haemorrhage or haemolysis), high oxygen requirements or known problems with oxygen delivery should be transfused sooner. Patients for whom viscosity issues are more important (e.g. after liver transplantation or cardiac patients with Blalock–Taussig shunts and small pulmonary arteries) should be maintained at lower haematocrits. Packed red cell transfusion to an appropriate target haemoglobin will require a 4 to 6 ml kg⁻¹ g⁻¹ rise in haemoglobin concentration, depending principally on:

- the haemoglobin concentration in the packed red cells supplied
- changes in circulating blood volume during the transfusion
- the rate of any ongoing blood loss.

Most incompatible transfusion 'accidents' in hospital arise because of problems with incorrect labelling of crossmatch samples or patient identification prior to administration. Whenever possible, donor and recipient should be ABO and rhesus matched. However AB positive patients can, if necessary, receive A, B or O because of their 'universal recipient' status. Non-crossmatched O rhesus negative blood should be immediately available in sites within the hospital where emergencies are anticipated. The blood is usually comparatively old and therefore may have a high extracellular potassium content. The red cells of ABO and rhesus 'type specific' blood will be compatible with recipient plasma in 98 per cent of cases and can be made available in an emergency within 15 to 20 minutes. A full crossmatch however takes 45 minutes to 1 hour (longer if atypical antibodies are detected).

Blood products

The treatment of donated blood is fairly standardised. It is normally screened for hepatitis B surface antigen, antibodies to hepatitis C, HIV and *Treponema pallidum* (syphilis) and grouped by ABO and rhesus antigens. Some blood is also screened for cytomegalovirus (CMV) antibodies in order to provide a supply of CMV-negative blood for immunocompromised patients. The plasma from most donations is removed and pooled. The red blood cells are then resuspended in saline with adenine, glucose and mannitol (SAGM) making transfusion problems caused by donor haemolysins very unlikely with these units. Use of SAGM also reduces patient exposure to citrate.

Whole blood is convenient for transfusion in acute massive blood loss. It has a packed cell volume of 0.35 to 0.45 and flows quickly through rapid intravenous infusers. Unless requested as 'fresh' it can be assumed to be deficient in coagulation factors V and VIII but not necessarily the other coagulation factors. Factor VIII activity has a half-life of 24 hours in vitro and factor V levels fall to 50 per cent within 2 weeks of donation. Even so, the consumption of all coagulation factors and platelets during large-scale haemorrhage makes it necessary to administer fresh frozen plasma and platelets during such transfusions. Fresh 'walking donor' blood transfusions are not screened and difficult to defend although they once had their proponents when citrated (ACD) preserved red cells were routinely supplied. Filtered red cells are available for patients at risk of human leucocyte antigen (HLA) immunisation or non-haemolytic transfusion reactions. Irradiated products are used for patients at risk of graft-versus-host disease. Washed red cells (and, in extreme cases, frozen and thawed red cells) can be used for very rare blood groups or unusual transfusion reactions. Red cell transfusions should be filtered during administration and warmed if of a significant volume or if the recipient weighs less than 10 kg. Two types of blood filters are available. Leucocyte specific filters will remove virtually all the white cells and platelets and are used for patients who have had multiple transfusions and who may be, or are, HLA or platelet sensitised. Microaggregate filters are less fine and remove the larger aggregates of white cells, platelets and fibrin that can accumulate in stored blood.

Fresh frozen plasma (FFP) is plasma that has been separated from freshly donated blood or drawn by plasmaphoresis from plasma donors and frozen. It is used as a transfusable source of coagulation factors the half-lives of which vary according to the specific factor and its rate of consumption. Consumption is exponentially increased in disseminated intravascular coagulation. However normal half-life varies from 4 hours (factor VII) to up to 4 days (fibrinogen). Slow thawing of FFP produces a 'cryoprecipitate' that can be fractionated to manufacture factor concentrates (although recombinant sources are preferable). It is a high concentration source of, among other things, fibrinogen, Von-Willebrand factor and factor VIII. Cold ethanol fractionation is used to manufacture immunoglobulin concentrate and human albumin solution from the 'cryosupernatant'. Donated pooled plasma was principally used as a colloid but has largely been replaced by human albumin solution.

Blood substitutes

In this context 'blood substitute' means a solution that is retained in the vascular space and can deliver significant quantities of oxygen to the tissues. No practicable clinical role has been established for any of the current candidates although the potential advantages in avoiding donor exposure are growing. Free haemoglobin suspensions are associated with poor oxygen delivery. Unless pyridoxylated and polymerised they have low haemo-globin concentrations (7 g dL^{-1}) in order to maintain a physiological osmotic/oncotic pressure. Also the P_{50} is low because the haemoglobin dissociation curve is left shifted in the absence of 2,3-diphosphoglycerate. Concerns about possible nephrotoxicity from haemo-globinuria have not been entirely put to rest although renal problems are not as severe as they are in the presence of in vivo haemolysis because cellular stroma does not accumu-late in the glomerulus. Polymerisation of the haemoglobin also reduces nephrotoxicity. Stable perfluorocarbon emulsions can dissolve more oxygen than water or plasma which carries approximately 2 vol% of oxygen at a FiO_2 of 1. With high proportions of fluorocar-bon in the circulation and an FiO_2 of 1 the oxygen-carrying capacity can be raised to a quarter of that of whole blood (i.e. up to 5 vol%). For any given dilution of fluorocarbon the oxygen content has a linear relation with the PO_2 and therefore the inhaled oxygen tension must be kept high.

COLLOID BALANCE

In situations where intravascular volume loss is proven or likely, for example postoperative patients, it is often useful to consider colloid balance independently of crystalloid balance although both must be taken into account when considering overall fluid balance. Colloid losses may be measurable in the presence of haemorrhage or drain losses but may have to be inferred in the presence of covert bleeding or capillary leak. It would be impossible to produce a comprehensive list of indications for intravascular volume expansion here. However generically these situations include:

- clinical evidence of shock or hypovolaemia, which includes tachycardia, poor peripheral perfusion, a low measured cardiac index (< 3 L min^{-1} m^{-2}), altered mental state or oliguria
- a measurement implying reduced preload (low CVP, left atrial pressure (LAP), pul-monary capillary wedge pressure (PCWP)) in the context of a known source of volume loss (haemorrhage, capillary leak, polyuria, diarrhoea, etc.) or change in the capacitance of the circulation (e.g. rewarming from hypothermia or administration of a vasodilator).

The usual volume of intravenous bolus for the treatment of shock is 20 ml kg^{-1} since this volume represents roughly 25 per cent of the circulating blood volume (in a baby) and the maximum acute loss that can be compensated without hypotension.

If there is an indication for giving red cells such as active haemorrhage, anaemia or any other circumstance of critical tissue oxygen delivery (shock, MOSF, etc.) then the choice is clear – red cell transfusion. In controlled circumstances packed red cell transfusion is the most appropriate.

If a procoagulant effect is desired, give FFP or platelets as indicated. Remember that a normal platelet count is not a guarantee of normal platelet function (especially during or after the use of an extracorporeal circulation) and that cryoprecipitate and specific clotting factors are used as supplements, not for volume expansion.

If neither red cells nor clotting factors are required then a choice exists between 'crys-talloid' and 'colloid'. The large molecules in colloid solutions lead to their temporary reten-tion in the circulation where they exert oncotic pressure and thereby further expand the plasma volume. The volume of fluid required to resuscitate a patient with colloid is less than that of other types of fluid. There is a historical preference for colloid administration during resuscitation. Although the effect of intravascular volume expansion lasts significantly longer than with crystalloid solutions, the latter are still acceptable for resuscitation in an acute setting provided they are isonatraemic; they are even preferred by some as they are cheap and relatively inert. However the volume of distribution of crystalloid (throughout the whole ECF) means that it requires at least twice as much volume to provide the same degree of resuscitation and the extravascular accumulation of fluid can be problematic. The use of crystalloid solutions in situations of fluid maldistribution (e.g. capillary leak) is counterintuitive, although during such situations the constraint of colloids to the vascular space is also reduced. The protein content of oedema fluid depends more on the integrity of the capillary endothelium (the degree of capillary leak) than the choice of volume replacement. Crystalloids are not suitable for the selective expansion of plasma volume in controlled settings. Their rapid distribution throughout the whole of the ECF is associated with hazards including pulmonary and cerebral oedema. In paediatric practice the usual colloid administered is human albumin solution and this situation persists because to date there has been no reliable evidence on which to base a change.

Albumin

This is a human blood product. Prolonged heat treatment during its manufacture virtually eliminates the risk of blood-borne virus (but not prion) transmission. It has a strong negative charge but binds both charged and covalent species avidly. It has potential advantages as a buffer and free-radical scavenger and binder of other acute-phase reactants. These advantages are not proven to be clinically significant in terms of influencing disease outcome. With an intact capillary membrane, transfused albumin persists in the circulation with a half-life of 16 hours. Albumin degradation products diffuse more easily and are osmotically active. Two-thirds of transfused albumin eventually distributes to interstitial fluid even under normal circumstances. Albumin degradation products are also lost in the urine. Patients with interstitial oedema of presumed high protein content (e.g. after capillary leak) have sometimes been treated with intravenous boluses of albumin and diuretics, the fanciful theory being that a temporary boost in serum oncotic pressure shifts water from the interstitial to the vascular space and that this water is then lost by diuresis. Irrespective of the diuresis (which can cause intravascular volume depletion) this albumin also redistributes

Table 7.5 Composition of colloid replacement solutions (adapted from British Journal of Hospital Medicine, 1995 54(4): 155–9).

Colloid	Solute concentrations in mmol L^{-1}					Distribution 24 h after administration and overall survival in blood			
	[Na$^+$]	[K$^+$]	[Cl$^-$]	[Ca^{2+}]	%Colloid	Plasma	Urine	Extravascular	Overall survival in blood
Urea linked gelatin (Haemaccel)	145	5.1	145	6.2	3.5	13%	71%	16%	168 hours
Succinylated gelatin (Gelofusine)	154	0.4	125	0.4	4	12%	62%	26%	168 hours
Hydroxyethyl starch	154	0	154	0	6	10%	47%	43%	6 weeks
Dextran 70	150	0	150	0	6	29%	38%	33%	4–6 weeks

to the interstitial space and leads to fluid retention. More reliable factors that promote the clearance of such oedema include

- time
- relative fluid restriction
- natural repair of the capillary endothelium
- muscular activity.

The choice of colloid solution other than albumin consists of dextrans, hydroxyethyl starch and gelatins, see Table 7.5. Experience of the use of these solutions in children is severely limited.

Dextrans

Dextrans are solutions of glucose polymers with a range of molecular weights and therefore a complex metabolism. The two common preparations are dextran 70 and dextran 40, the latter having smaller molecules, shorter half-life in plasma and greater oncotic effect. Dextran preparations with lower molecular weight can cause or aggravate renal failure by precipitation within the tubules when the GFR is low. They cause a dose-related defect in platelet adhesion and aggregation, and other coagulation problems limiting their use to a maximum of 2 g kg^{-1}day^{-1} (on day 1) and 1 g kg^{-1}day^{-1} (on subsequent days).

Hydroxyethyl starch

This is a modification of amylopectin (a branched glucose polymer). It is also a heterogenous mixture of molecule sizes with a complex metabolism, which includes uptake by the reticuloendothelial system. The thrombocytopaenia and elevated activated partial thromboplastin time associated with its use can be problematic and there is little published experience of its use in paediatrics.

Gelatins

Gelatins are manufactured by chemical treatment of bovine collagen. Two principle commercial products are succinylated (Gelofusine®) and urea linked (Haemaccel®). Dose-related coagulopathy is a dilutional effect.

8 Nutrition

- **Introduction**
- **Definitions**
- **Nutritional requirements**
- **Inadequate nutrition and malnutrition**
- **Nutritional assessment**
- **Enteral feeding**
- **Parenteral feeding**
- **Conclusion**

INTRODUCTION

Nutrition is essential for activity, growth and maintenance tissue repair. Many factors contribute to poor nutrition in intensive care patients including:

- poor intake (anorexia, fluid restrictions, 'nil by mouth' orders)
- poor absorption (ileus, diarrhoea, gastric stasis)
- increased losses (diarrhoea, large burn areas, drain losses)
- increased metabolic requirements (pyrexia, sepsis, burns)
- increased activity (work of breathing)
- pre-existing debilitating disease (cystic fibrosis, chronic heart failure, etc.)

Failure to compensate for imbalances between requirement and provision may lead to acute protein energy malnutrition, which results in:

- poor wound healing
- impaired host defences
- increased risk of infection (both number of episodes and their severity)
- growth failure
- and ultimately increased mortality.

> These effects occur in previously healthy, well fed and even obese patients as well as in previously malnourished patients.

Conversely, inappropriate hyperalimentation (nutrition in excess of normal requirements) may lead to fluid overload, acidosis, increased work of breathing, diarrhoea, azotaemia, lipaemia and increased risk of sepsis. It is therefore important to assess and calculate patients' nutritional requirements to ensure adequate, controlled provision.

DEFINITIONS

In this chapter the terms 'metabolic rate' and 'energy expenditure' are used interchangeably.

BASAL METABOLIC RATE

The basal metabolic rate (BMR) is defined in terms of energy (calorie) consumption at 'rest'. 'Rest' being an idyllic state of comfort with absent muscular activity, in a thermoneutral, non-hypoxic environment, the only drawback being the additional requirement for a post-absorptive intake state (i.e. after an overnight fast). BMR usually accounts for 60 to 70 per cent of total energy expenditure. It decreases with age (Table 8.1) and, in post-pubertal children it is lower in females (who have proportionately more fat). The Harris–Benedict equations approximate for these effects and then predict BMR based on size, judged by both height and weight males $BMR = 66.5 + 13.8W + 5.0H - 6.8A$

females $BMR = 655 + 9.6W + 1.8H - 4.7A$

Table 8.1 Basal metabolic rates per kg by age.	
1 year	55 kcal kg^{-1} day^{-1}
5 years	45 kcal kg^{-1} day^{-1}
10 years	38 kcal kg^{-1} day^{-1}
adult	26 kcal kg^{-1} day^{-1}

Table 8.1 where W = weight in kg, H = height in cm and A = age in years.

The metabolic rate changes with temperature. Pyrexia causes a 10 per cent increase per 1°C above 37°C. Stresses, such as trauma, burns and sepsis also increase the metabolic rate. The metabolic rate is low during hypothermia although attempts to generate and conserve heat during exposure to cold increase energy expenditure. Other factors that reduce metabolic rate include analgesia/sedation (5% to 10% fall) and neuromuscular blockade (40% fall). These factors must all be taken into account during the calculation of metabolic requirements but note that in order for them to affect the metabolic rate for a 24 hour period, they must apply to the whole of that period. A spike of fever increases the metabolic rate only during the spike. The underlying effects of sepsis or trauma persist for longer.

RESTING METABOLIC RATE (RMR)

Resting metabolic rate is a term usually coined to describe a baseline for comparison against a subsequent change. It is frequently used when reference measurement conditions cannot be described as 'basal'. For example the environment is not strictly thermoneutral, or patients are anxious or stressed, or they have not been starved before measurement. Therefore RMR includes the BMR, the thermic effect of feeding and a variable degree of activity/thermogenesis. It also includes the energy expended by growing – something that adults shouldn't be doing! As a result it is often more than 15 per cent higher than the BMR.

    An 'activity factor' should be applied when calculating total energy expenditure even when patients are apparently at rest but in fact fidgeting. Activity factors approximate to × 1.2 (bed bound) and × 1.3 (mobile).

RESTING ENERGY EXPENDITURE (REE)

    This is the same thing as the RMR, it is measured in kcal/unit time. It can be estimated as

$$(3.0 \times \dot{V}O_2) + (1.1 \times \dot{V}CO_2)$$

where $\dot{V}O_2$ and $\dot{V}CO_2$ are rates of oxygen consumption and carbon dioxide production respectively measured in litres per unit time. The units kcal day^{-1} can be derived from kcal min^{-1} by multiplying by 1440.

THERMIC EFFECT OF FEEDING (TEF)

An obligatory energy consumption is required to absorb, breakdown and assimilate food; this is associated with the generation of heat; the 'thermic' effect of feeding (TEF). It is normally 8 to 12 per cent of TEE. During starvation, REE is reduced.

ENERGY EXPENDITURE ON ACTIVITY (AEE)

This is usually 20 to 30 per cent of TEE. It varies greatly between individuals depending on their level of activity.

TOTAL ENERGY EXPENDITURE (TEE)

This comprises basal metabolic rate plus the thermic effect of feeding and the energy expenditure from activity. In neonates and infants, it includes the thermogenesis occurring in brown adipose tissue. TEE may be calculated from predictive equations or measured by indirect calorimetry. It is measured in kcal kg^{-1}day^{-1}. In the calculation of TEE the BMR may be weighted by 'stress' factors such as those described on p. 100. The considerable variation in BMR and the errors of estimation in the other parameters used for weighting, mean that calculated TEE is often an overestimate.

TEE = (BMR × correction factor) + TEF + energy requirement of thermoregulation + AEE

A neutral energy balance between intake and TEE will result in a static weight. Energy, over and above that required for TEE is required for growth and for 'catch up' after a period of weight loss or failure to thrive.

INDIRECT CALORIMETRY

This measures oxygen consumption and carbon dioxide production. It requires a sealed breathing system (no leaks) and is inaccurate at high FiO_2s.

BROWN ADIPOSE THERMOGENESIS

Brown adipose thermogenesis is a method of heat generation available to neonates and infants (it is decreased in the preterm) which increases with cooler environments and is normally 2 to 3 per cent of TEE.

RESPIRATORY QUOTIENT (RQ)

The RQ is the ratio of $\dot{V}CO_2$ (carbon dioxide production) to $\dot{V}O_2$ (oxygen consumption). As discussed in Chapter 11, Respiratory System, RQ varies with substrate metabolism. Energy generated purely from carbohydrate produces more carbon dioxide, which leads to increased work of breathing. One effect of a diet incorporating a mixture of fat with carbohydrate is to reduce the work of breathing.

NITROGEN BALANCE

This is the balance between nitrogen intake (protein) and loss.

1 g nitrogen = 6.25 g protein

Nitrogen losses, largely in the urine, increase under conditions of major stress (e.g. burns and sepsis). In addition, when fat and carbohydrate intakes are restricted protein is used as an energy source (catabolism), 1g protein generates 4 kcal, thereby increasing nitrogen losses. A negative nitrogen balance is the best way of defining catabolism. It leads to further muscle wasting, delayed wound healing, increased risk of sepsis and increased mortality. The concept of minimising catabolism is pivotal to intensive care nutrition.

NUTRITIONAL REQUIREMENTS

To calculate children's nutritional requirements four elements must be taken into account.

- *Maintenance* – maintenance requirements equate to satisfying the REE, i.e. the minimum requirement for a resting child. Provision of the maintenance requirement of calories does not promote or even allow growth and any activity will result in weight loss.
- *Growth* – all children are growing but at different ages they grow at different rates. During the first 6 months of life 40 per cent of TEE is required for growth.
- *Activity* – with increasing age, children sleep less and are more active. At birth activity accounts for only 10% of TEE but increases to 25% by 6 months. On average, activity accounts for 20% to 30% of TEE after 6 months of age. The additional energy requirement

is a consequence of increased levels of activity and the fact that the associated physical work is harder as the child is heavier.

- *Catch up* – once a child has fallen behind, as judged by growth or growth velocity charts, additional feeding will be required irrespective of the cause. In addition to calories, fat, carbohydrate and protein, additional vitamins and minerals may be required before satisfactory catch-up growth is seen. A common clinical shorthand is to feed to the expected weight, i.e. that which would apply if the appropriate weight gain had been observed or if weight had not been lost. This attempts to avoid underestimating the calorie requirement.

Water and energy

Normal water requirement is closely linked to energy requirements. For babies an enteral food source is available which balances the two perfectly. A breast-fed term newborn baby drinks approximately 150 ml kg^{-1}day^{-1}. This gives the baby 100 kcal kg^{-1}day^{-1} of energy, (the creamatocrit of breast milk increases during a feed but on average it is 67 kcal per 100 ml or 20 kcal per ounce). This ratio of water to energy promotes optimum growth.

A low glomerular filtration rate restricts babies' ability to excrete a water load and tubular immaturity manifests as an obligatory urinary salt loss with accompanying water loss. Babies produce comparatively dilute urine and their ability to concentrate urine is limited to approximately 600 mosmol L^{-1}. A large osmotic load, for example incorrectly prepared infant formula, leads to loss of additional water and hypernatraemic dehydration.

The amount of room for calorie provision may be restricted by the fluid requirements of infusions and drugs within the routine fluid restriction of PIC patients. Attempts to compensate by increasing the calorie content of the feed with supplements (either glucose polymers or medium chain triglycerides) have upper limits. The final calorie content for neonates should not exceed 1 kcal ml^{-1} and older children 1.5 kcal ml^{-1} (the latter can excrete a more concentrated urine but above 1.5 kcal ml^{-1} diarrhoea is common).

As a guide energy requirements (in kcal) equal fluid requirements (in ml), see Table 8.2.

Table 8.2 Energy requirements by age/size.	
Age/Size	**Energy requirement**
Premature neonates	150 kcal kg^{-1} day^{-1}
Neonates	100–120 kcal kg^{-1} day^{-1}
< 10 kg	100 kcal kg^{-1} day^{-1}
10–20 kg	1000 kcal + 50 kcal kg^{-1} over 10 kg day^{-1}
> 20 kg	1500 kcal + 20 kcal kg^{-1} over 20 kg day^{-1}

These figures will achieve adequate growth assuming normal activity. They do not take into account 'catch up' or extra activity.

Protein

Nitrogen (largely as protein) is necessary for maintenance, to replace losses (urinary, faecal and surface) and for growth. In the absence of adequate calories from fat or carbohydrate, protein is catabolised for gluconeogenesis. Normal 'essential' amino acids are those that cannot be synthesised. In addition, other amino acids become *conditionally* essential, in neonates and in older children when nutritionally stressed. These include taurine, tyrosine, cysteine and histidine, glycine, arginine and glutamine.

The quality of protein varies with its source. Egg or milk protein is the gold standard as it is over 95 per cent absorbed and has optimal quantity and diversity of essential amino

Table 8.3 Guidelines for protein requirements by age (milk or egg-quality protein).

Age/Size	Protein requirement
Premature neonates	2.5–4 g kg^{-1} day^{-1}
Neonates	2–2.5 g kg^{-1} day^{-1}
< 10 kg	1.2–1.6 g kg^{-1} day^{-1}
10–20 kg	1–1.2 g kg^{-1} day^{-1}
> 20 kg	1 g kg^{-1} day^{-1}

acids. Vegetable-derived protein may be less well absorbed and is often lacking in one or more essential amino acids. This means that relatively more must be eaten to achieve the same effect, while increasing the renal osmotic load.

Protein is broken down in the gut by luminal and brush-border enzymes into amino acids and di- and tripeptides, which are more easily absorbed. Non-branched chain amino acids and short peptides are absorbed into the portal vein and transferred to the liver for metabolism. Branched chain amino acids enter the systemic circulation and are taken up by skeletal muscle. The optimal protein content of the diet contains the correct amount of amino acids in an easily digestible form, for example breast milk. With a protein intake in excess of requirements, the surplus amino acids are metabolised to glucose and fat with attendant increases in urinary nitrogen excretion. Protein deficiency, even despite adequate calories, produces a starvation-like picture, with wasting and weight loss.

Guidelines for protein requirements are given in Table 8.3. The table assumes normal growth without the need for catch up. It also assumes an adequate calorie intake to minimise protein catabolism for gluconeogenesis (1 g protein generates 4 kcal).

Carbohydrate

The principal ingested forms of carbohydrate are

- the disaccharides – lactose (galactose + glucose) and sucrose (glucose + fructose)
- and starch (glucose polysaccharide).

Amylase breaks up starch into maltose (glucose disaccharide). Disaccharidases (maltase, sucrase and lactase) are brush-border enzymes and cleave disaccharides into their constituent sugars. As lactase is present in the smallest quantity, lactose intolerance is common after enteritic illnesses, whereas the absorption of starch, and short glucose polymers (maltodextrins), is usually unaffected. It is difficult to achieve an adequate calorie intake using enteral glucose alone as the osmotic effect tends to cause diarrhoea. Disaccharides and starches allow greater delivery of glucose with less osmotic effect.

Carbohydrate contributes approximately 50 per cent of calories at birth, ideally rising to over 70% with increasing age, thereby reducing fat calories to below 30% (1 g of carbohydrate generates 4 kcal).

Fat

Dietary fat is a high-density energy source (1 g of fat generates approximately 10 kcal). It reduces reliance on carbohydrate and minimises protein catabolism. If one attempts to satisfy calorie requirements intravenously without fats, the excessive glucose intake leads to hyperglycaemia, osmotic diuresis and fatty liver. Fatty acids are the molecular building blocks for cell membranes (phospholipids) and the precursors of thromboxanes, prostaglandins and leukotrienes. Essential fatty acids (usually those with a C=C below C10) cannot be synthesised and include linoleic (ω–6) and linolenic (ω–3) fatty acids. Fats also include the fat-soluble vitamins (A, D, E and K).

Ingested fat is hydrolysed in the gut by pancreatic and brush-border lipases to monoglycerides which are absorbed and then reform as triglycerides within chylomicrons. Chylomicrons are transported in the lymphatics, via the thoracic duct, into the venous system. Medium chain triglycerides (MCT) behave differently to other fats when ingested; they are hydrolysed and absorbed directly into the portal vein. The associated reduction in lymph flow via the thoracic duct explains its use in chylothorax. MCTs are more soluble than long chain triglycerides (LCT) and do not require bile salts for their absorption. MCTs are transported intact across the mitochondrial membrane, probably without the need for carnitine. This may be of benefit in severely energy-stressed individuals. Disadvantages of using MCTs include

- lower energy density than LCTs
- lower essential fatty acid content
- greater osmotic activity
- unpalatability.

Vitamins

Vitamins A, D, E and K are fat-soluble and require bile salts for absorption. The water-soluble vitamins are ascorbic acid (C), thiamin, riboflavin, pyridoxine, niacin, pantothenate, biotin, folate and B_{12}. Adequate vitamin intake is essential for normal function, repair and growth. Vitamin supplements are only necessary when intake is inadequate. This is particularly true during total parenteral nutrition, during catch-up growth or in the presence of malabsorption. Excessive vitamin intake may be toxic, particularly vitamins A, D and pyridoxine.

Trace elements

Trace elements include iron, iodine, zinc, copper, selenium, molybdenum, manganese, chromium, fluorine and cobalt. Trace element deficiency may occur with prematurity, protein energy malnutrition and prolonged intravenous feeding. Supplementation is necessary when prescribing the nutrition of 'at risk' groups.

INADEQUATE NUTRITION AND MALNUTRITION

Inadequate nutrition will lead to malnutrition if it is not detected early and treated. Small children are at particular risk compared to older children and adults because of limited energy reserves, higher metabolic rate and rapid growth. Their customary positive energy balance (the excess energy above TEE) is used, together with protein and other nutrients, for growth. An even or negative energy balance from reduced input or increased TEE (usually a combination of both) leads to growth cessation, weight loss and eventually severe malnutrition. Furthermore, of particular relevance to premature babies, there is evidence that brain growth occurs in critical phases, which if missed cannot be compensated for later. Neonates that have managed to preserve brain growth in the face of foetal malnourishment (usually late placental insufficiency) display asymmetric growth retardation with preservation of the head circumference.

In extra-uterine life there are three patterns of inadequate nutrition that are discussed here; these are

- starvation and 'catch-up'
- critical illness
- increased activity.

Starvation and 'catch up'

Children periodically receive inadequate nutrition as a consequence of illness. The normal response to relative starvation is first to use up glycogen stores, which are rapidly depleted over hours. Gluconeogenesis then occurs from amino acid oxidation and the metabolism of triglycerides increases. In premature neonates, inadequate gluconeogenesis leads to early hypoglycaemia unless a source of exogenous carbohydrate is provided. In addition, their limited fat stores lead to early protein catabolism. During catch up, normal requirements are exceeded to replace the deficits and replenish stores.

Critical illness

Hypermetabolic states with associated rampant catabolism are common in critical illness. Sepsis, extensive burns and the systemic inflammatory response syndrome (SIRS) are common examples. The biochemical pathways involved are driven by inflammatory mediators, including tumour necrosis factor, interleukin 1 and hormones such as cortisol, growth hormone, glucagon and catecholamines. Gluconeogenesis and triglyceride metabolism are increased and 'insulin antagonistic' effects may occasionally result in hyperglycaemia and even (rarely) ketosis despite high levels of endogenous insulin. Even after the initial period of severe stress, an elevated metabolic rate persists in association with recovery and repair. Diet in this recovery phase must include additional protein nutrition for both catch up and growth.

Such patients are difficult to treat. Catabolism is typically unresponsive to hyperalimentation or even hormonal manipulation. Energy requirements increase proportionally to the degree of stress. Large doses of insulin can reduce hyperglycaemia and prevent skeletal muscle breakdown but not smooth muscle catabolism. Insulin administration inhibits the normal starvation response. It reduces ketone production but can lead to lactic acidosis and hypophosphataemia. In response to exogenous insulin, vital organs remain largely dependent on glucose (and therefore exogenous sources of carbohydrate). Exogenous insulin is therefore usually reserved for situations where hyperglycaemia is of a sufficient degree to raise concerns about its osmotic effects (20 mmol L^{-1}).

The glycerol from triglycerides is rapidly metabolised for gluconeogenesis but the uptake of released free fatty acids for oxidation is more rate limited, leading to increased plasma concentrations. Free fatty acids displace bilirubin from albumin and excessive exogenous lipid (especially phospholipid) administration can exceed lipoprotein lipase activity leading to hypertriglyceridaemia, with lipaemia, fatty liver and ectopic fat deposition. Depending on the circumstances it may not be possible to provide full nutrition during the acute phase of critical illness even using parenteral nutrition and accepting modest hyperglycaemia and hypertriglyceridaemia. Feeding in excess of metabolic requirements confers no additional benefit and increases morbidity.

So how much energy and protein do these children really need during acute stress? Remember that the impact of 'stress factors' increasing the metabolic rate is countered by PIC treatments such as sedation, paralysis and ventilation, which may reduce metabolic rate by up to 45 per cent. Furthermore such factors apply to the metabolic rate, not the TEE. For example a 10 kg child (BMR 55 kcal^{-1}kg^{-1}day^{-1}) with severe septic shock (stress factor 1.6), who is ventilated, paralysed and sedated (correction factor 0.55, AEE = 0) has minimised energy costs of thermoregulation because of paralysis. Thus he/she needs a baseline of

$$(55 \times 0.55 \times 1.6) + 0 = 48.4 \text{ kcal}^{-1} \text{ kg}^{-1} \text{ day}^{-1}$$

On top of this we can be generous and correct for the 10 per cent of the energy supplied used as TEF (correction factor $\times$ 1.11). Furthermore he will only grow if he receives 10 per cent more than he is consuming. Thus he needs approximately

$$48.4 \times 1.11 \times 1.1 \approx 59 \text{ kcal}^{-1} \text{ kg}^{-1} \text{ day}^{-1} \text{ (let's call it 60)}.$$

Further concessions to preventing catabolism include choosing to give this as both fat and carbohydrate in a proportion of 1:2 or 1:3 and, in some institutions, to ignore the protein requirement when determining calorie intake (i.e. to give the protein as extra).

Conversely, a child with severe burns, who is not ventilated and is moving around the bed will need more calories. For children with burns, the burn surface area has a poor correlation with the increase in metabolic rate. A rough guide to TEE under these circumstances is 2.0 × BMR (predicted from the equations). Although the majority of children will get satisfactory calories from 1.55 × BMR, extra calories are still needed for growth.

Increased activity

Normal tidal breathing uses 1 to 3 per cent of the TEE. Respiratory distress may increase this to over 30 per cent of TEE and the additional 27 per cent requires a calorie source, otherwise the energy will be used preferentially at the expense of something else (such as wound healing or growth). Similarly TEE may increase from physiotherapy by up to 30 per cent and from pain by 10 per cent. Depending upon their indication and extent, changes of dressings can cause increases of up to 25 per cent. Conversely, neuromuscular paralysis reduces energy consumption by up to 50 per cent.

NUTRITIONAL ASSESSMENT

Nutritional status can be assessed from

- weight
- height
- weight/height index
- total body fat assessment
- albumin, prealbumin, retinol binding protein, transferrin
- nitrogen balance
- indirect calorimetry.

Nutritional assessment of critically ill patients may be difficult. Patients are often oedematous confounding interpretation of weight and skin-fold thickness. The levels of serum protein markers fall with sepsis, while acute phase proteins rise. Nitrogen balance requires measurement of urine output, which will still not be representative in the oliguric patient. In effect, it may not be possible to accurately assess a child's nutritional state once he is critically ill. It is therefore important that all patients are nutritionally assessed on admission to the PICU, even if this is just a weight and height measurement. Furthermore, nutrition must be commenced as soon as is practicable.

Serum albumin levels are low in cases of malnutrition but the fall in serum albumin frequently seen in critical care patients more often represents a redistribution of albumin to the interstitium rather than malnutrition or catabolism. Hence it will not easily or sustainably respond to repeated albumin infusions. Attempts to supplement serum albumin levels by transfusion in critically ill patients inevitably lead to oedema. Albumin should not be used as an independent source of parenteral nutrition because it is broken down slowly and contains few essential amino acids. These deficiencies lead to catabolism when albumin is the major protein source.

ENTERAL FEEDING

The enteral route for feeding is preferred whenever possible, although it may not be possible where there is a high risk of aspiration or severe breathlessness / respiratory distress. The gut derives much of its own nutrition from the food within the lumen. In addition, enteric hormones, which maintain bowel function and repair, are released in response to the presence of food within the gut. The presence of food in the stomach decreases gastric pH and reduces the level of bacterial colonisation.

Intermittent oral feeding is preferred whenever feasible. Breast-fed babies tend to feed little and often. There are many situations however where the oral approach may not be suitable, including breathlessness, reduced protective oropharyngeal reflexes, coma and the need for endotracheal intubation or extubation. Some of these can be overcome by naso- or orogastric tubes which allow some or all of the feed to remain enteral. Others necessitate interruption of feeding. 'Failure to absorb' as witnessed by gastric aspirates larger than the volume of instilled milk, indicate failure of gastric emptying but not necessarily ileus. In the absence of signs of abdominal distension or pyloric stenosis, persistence with enteral feeding is justified. This may entail the use of a prokinetic agent, or a change to transpyloric feeding, either nasoduodenal or nasojejunal. Nasoduodenal/nasojejunal tubes may be passed under X-ray control, after administration of a prokinetic agent or at endoscopy. Transpyloric feeding is also a potential approach for persistent vomiting/reflux. Bile-stained nasogastric aspirates may represent transpyloric migration of a nasogastric tube or ileus.

Longer term tube feeding requires narrow-bore silk/polyurethane tubes passed over stiffening wires; these must be lubricated before use. Feeding may be continuous or intermittent in which case flush the tube after each feed. Bolus feeds provide satiety but continuous infusions are safer in the context of potential reflux. Transpyloric boluses may cause diarrhoea, malabsorption and the dumping syndrome, and may need to be 'pre-digested' to avoid malabsorption. Alternatively gastrostomy or jejunostomy may be employed. Percutaneous endoscopic gastrostomy (PEG) is a relatively minor procedure but a formal laparotomy is required if a jejunostomy or simultaneous fundoplication is indicated, for example where aspiration is a significant problem. Many patients with reflux can be managed with an antireflux procedure and a gastrostomy or PEG.

There are several types of enteral feed.

1 ORAL SUPPLEMENTS

These are incomplete diets, designed as supplements, they include nitrogen and energy-rich preparations.

2 POLYMERIC DIETS

These diets contain protein, long chain fatty acids and complex carbohydrates with vitamins and minerals. These are for children with normal or near normal gut function and include breast milk, Osmolite®, Pediasure® and Ensure®.

3 'PRE-DIGESTED' DIETS

These diets are for patients with severely impaired gastrointestinal function, such as short gut syndrome. They contain free amino acids, di- and tripeptides, short carbohydrate polymers (e.g. maltodextrin) and fat, usually as MCT, together with vitamins, minerals and essential fatty acids. Preparations include Pregestimil® and Pepdite®.

4 ELEMENTAL DIETS

These diets are reserved for patients with severe gastrointestinal dysfunction, such as Crohn's disease or radiation-induced enteritis, or other conditions where a low residue is necessary such as intestinal fistulae.

5 DISEASE SPECIFIC DIETS

These diets are for specific conditions

- renal failure – emphasis is on essential amino acids and histidine to reduce nitrogen wastage to a minimum
- hepatic encephalopathy – diets high in branch chain amino acids but low levels of methionine and aromatic amino acids (attempts to prove the efficacy of this approach have been inconclusive). Low fat content other than essential fatty acids. Energy source predominately from carbohydrate

- chylothorax –requires a diet based on MCT
- respiratory failure – the diet should have an emphasis on fat as an energy source.

There is limited evidence for the benefit of some of these diets.

6 MODULAR DIETS

There has been a move away from proprietary disease-specific diets to modular diets where individual components can be altered to achieve an optimum diet. Such diets include

- hepatic diets with whole protein, low sodium and MCT (does not need bile salts for absorption)
- renal diets with low potassium and phosphate
- gastroenterological diets where the protein and fat types can be altered depending on their absorption.

Other dietary approaches to modulating the stress response and its effects on the gut include supplements of glutamine, short chain fatty acids, ω 3 fatty acids, arginine and nucleotides. Their use in children is still under investigation.

Choosing between baby feeds

A lot of 'witchcraft' pervades the process of choosing between polymeric feeds for babies. A culture that promotes breast milk should be encouraged but not to the extent that mothers who choose 'formula' are disparaged. There is really no evidence against formula use in affluent western societies and the immunological benefits of breast milk are reduced if it is stored. Enteral breast milk may reduce the risk of developing NEC in preterm babies who otherwise require more sodium, calcium, phosphorous, iron, protein and calories than it contains.

Cows' milk is not appropriate for children under 1 year. It has six times as much casein as human milk resulting in an inappropriate amino acid profile. Human milk protein is 60 per cent whey proteins, largely lactalbumins and lactglobulins. Cows' milk contains too much calcium and phosphate, and insufficient iron and unsaturated fatty acids. These features are adjusted in the manufacture of formula from cows' milk. A variety of cows' milk-derived formulae of similar composition are available including higher calorie milks which generally are significantly stronger osmotically. Goats' milk and soya-based formulae are available for cows' milk protein intolerance which is a rare (< 0.5% of infants) clinical diagnosis.

Many infants on PICU are fluid restricted. To achieve adequate calories from breast milk or infant formula, additional calories must be added. However, this fails to supplement the sodium or protein content of the feed. Therefore it is wise to concentrate the formula feed from the normal 13 per cent to 15 per cent as a first step and then add additional calories, as either fat or glucose polymers (or both). Recently 100 kcal/100 ml infant feeds have been developed that contain correctly adjusted amounts of protein and electrolytes but which have osmolalities in the region of 325 mOsm/kgH$_2$O.

Complications

The commonest complications of enteral feeding are diarrhoea and vomiting/delayed gastric emptying. Most paediatric diseases can present with such symptoms and the feed may not be to blame. Feed-related causes include:

- antibiotic usage
- bacterial contamination of feed
- Candida overgrowth
- excessive calorie density
- other osmotic effects (e.g. sorbitol)
- MCT-based feeds.

Transpyloric bolus feeding causes more cases of diarrhoea than continuous feeding but the reverse is true of gastric feeds. Antibiotic-associated diarrhoea is probably caused by alteration of bowel flora but may be because of Candida overgrowth and can herald pseudomembraneous colitis. Candida overgrowth usually ceases after the course of antibiotics but responds to oral nystatin (if unable to swallow, instil half in the mouth and half down the nasogastric tube). *Clostridium difficile* requires oral vancomycin.

Excessive calorie density applies to carbohydrates and fats. Stools can be tested for reducing substances (sugars) or steatorrhoea. Alternative carbohydrate calorie sources such as maltodextrin or starch may relieve the problem. Long chain triglycerides cause less diarrhoea than medium chain triglycerides.

Hospital diets are frequently protein deficient. Without supplements, progressive development of protein malnutrition will result, depending upon the degree of inadequacy in protein intake and the rate of protein consumption. Catabolism may be measured by the urinary excretion of nitrogen but is reflected by weight loss or growth failure.

Check list for diarrhoea during enteral feeds (see text)

1. check calorie density of feed
2. check mode of administration, bolus versus continuous
3. look for reducing substances in the stool
4. look for lipid in the stool
5. send stool for virology, microscopy (for ova, cysts and parasites) *Clostridium difficile* toxin and culture
6. consider bacterial / candida overgrowth if on or has recently received antibiotics
7. consider sigmoidoscopy.

Check list for vomiting/regurgitation/large aspirates

1. check position of feeding tube
2. check for abdominal pathology distended abdomen, bilious vomiting, bloody diarrhoea, blood stained NG aspirates and treat as appropriate
3. try continuous feeding first, then
4. consider a prokinetic agent
5. consider reducing fat content or calorie density if still no gastric emptying, or
6. establish transpyloric feeding.

PARENTERAL FEEDING

Parenteral nutrition (PN) is not an alternative to enteral nutrition (EN) and total PN (TPN) implies that PN is responsible for all the nutrition provided, i.e. there is no EN. PN should be considered when all attempts at EN are contraindicated or have been tried and still result in inadequate input or absorption. Parenteral nutrition may be given via peripheral or central veins but the prescription must reflect the route of administration. A prescription for peripheral PN must limit maximum glucose concentration to 12.5 per cent and so will require greater volumes to provide adequate calories. Central PN gets around these problems but long-term central vascular access is required.

GLUCOSE

Glucose is the commonest source of energy and reduces protein catabolism for gluconeogenesis although glucose and fat are used as the main source of calories. Using glucose as the sole source of energy may cause hyperglycaemia and fatty liver in addition to producing a greater carbon dioxide load. Most patients will tolerate the normal babies' requirement of 4 to 5 mg kg^{-1}min^{-1}. Growth-retarded infants may require up to 12 mg kg^{-1} min^{-1}. The incidence of hyperglycaemia is lower if the glucose load is increased slowly over 2 to 3 days. Patients on high doses of glucose from PN will rapidly become hypoglycaemic if the glucose is stopped suddenly.

FAT

Fat may be given peripherally; it lowers the RQ and provides essential fatty acids. The amount of lipid should be increased over 3 to 4 days to a maximum of 2 to 3 g kg^{-1}day^{-1}. Lipid hydrolysis is reduced with severe stress and hypertriglyceridaemia may occur, necessitating reduction of exogenous lipid prescription. In this context the 20 per cent lipid emulsion is preferable to 10 per cent emulsion in TPN because of its lower phospholipid : triglyceride ratio. A minimum of 0.5 g kg^{-1} day^{-1} will prevent essential fatty acid deficiency (4% calories from linoleic acid).

NITROGEN

Nitrogen is supplied as amino acids. Several different formulations are available. These vary in the total quantity of nitrogen and the relative quantities of individual amino acids. Basic amino acid requirements are 2 to 3 g kg^{-1}day^{-1} for preterm babies, 2 g kg^{-1}day^{-1} for infants and small children and 1 to 2 g kg^{-1} day^{-1} for older children. These doses will only be adequate if there are sufficient non-protein calories. Excessive amino acid delivery produces uraemia and increased energy usage as the protein is catabolised and stored as fat. As a general rule, with severe stress, the calorie : amino acid ratio should not exceed 20 kcal : 1 g amino acid. Under less stressed conditions, this rises to 30 kcal : 1 g amino acid.

Premature babies require increased amounts of conditionally essential amino acids, cysteine and tyrosine. Specialised amino acid solutions have been devised for renal failure (primarily essential amino acids) and liver failure with encephalopathy (higher amounts of branched chain, lower aromatic amino acids) although their usefulness is unclear.

Glutamine is poorly soluble and is not part of standard PN but is believed to be essential for gut function. Glutamine supplementation improves gut morphology. Currently, soluble glutamine-based dipeptides are being developed to add to TPN but phenomena such as this reinforce the desire to maintain some enteral nutrition, if at all possible, while using PN.

Adequate electrolytes, including sodium and potassium, can be added to the PN. Calcium and magnesium, bicarbonate and phosphate, all produce insoluble salts which limit the quantities that can be added and may necessitate additional supplements. Acetate or lactate are the usual sources of bicarbonate (by metabolism) but in conditions of poor liver function (failure or shock), inadequate bicarbonate may be generated.

Both water soluble and lipid soluble vitamins must be added to the PN. Prolonged PN leads to trace element deficiency. The addition of trace elements is essential but all are toxic in excess.

Complications

Parenteral nutrition has a much higher cost in medical and financial terms than enteral nutrition. Catheter-related problems include potential problems with insertion, such as pneumothorax and bleeding, as well as thrombosis and infection. Sepsis is common because of the nature of the access to the body and the nutrient nature of the infusion. The patients are often susceptible for other reasons such as immune compromise. Prevention of infection requires meticulous technique in handling lines and infusions but not all infections in these patients are catheter acquired. Increased gut permeability and translocation can lead to infections that subsequently colonise the catheter.

Potential metabolic problems include hyperglycaemia, hypertriglyceridaemia, uraemia and electrolyte imbalance of which hypokalaemia, hypophosphataemia and hypomagnesaemia are the most commonly missed. When starting PN, glucose should be measured several times a day with electrolytes, urea, liver function tests, calcium, phosphate and magnesium measured on a daily basis. Lipids should be measured twice weekly and also if the serum appears lipaemic. Once established on PN, amino acids and triglycerides can be measured less frequently. Trace elements are expensive to measure and should only be measured if deficiency is suspected.

Hepatic cholestasis is common in small children on long term PN and will be aggravated by recurrent infection, inadequate EN, high levels of aromatic amino acids and excessive glucose-derived calories. It can lead to cirrhosis ultimately requiring liver transplantation.

Potential causes of the nutritional problems seen with parenteral nutrition include a lack of essential nutrients, such as glutamine and the short-chain fatty acids derived from fibre, and an altered enteric hormone response.

Intralipid is associated with its own problems. Some fatty acids (ω 6) may be immunosuppressive while others may be beneficial in that respect. All intravenous lipids can aggravate intrapulmonary shunt and pulmonary hypertension.

CONCLUSION

Adequate nutrition should be instituted early in the ICU stay, even for well-nourished patients and those predicted to have a short stay. Enteral nutrition is preferred whenever possible. The nutritional approach should be disease appropriate and should take account of energy requirements for catch up and growth. Hyperalimentation cannot control the catabolism associated with critical illness and carries its own risks, but the protein energy malnutrition caused by the illness must be addressed during recovery. Paediatric nutritional services should be consulted routinely.

9 Pharmacology

- **Paediatric pharmacology**
- **Drug administration and absorption**
- **Drug distribution**
- **Drug elimination**
- **Drug interaction**

PAEDIATRIC PHARMACOLOGY

Many pharmacological processes are immature in babies and children, who cannot be relied upon to have the same absorption, distribution and elimination of drugs (pharmacokinetics) as older people, hence the dosage and duration of drug action may be specific to paediatrics. Additionally, the mechanism of drug action and the relationship between drug level and the type and magnitude of response (pharmacodynamics) may be different in children to that in adults. There may also be additional side effects or factors that are of more importance to children than adults that need to be taken into consideration. Teratogenic drugs that have adverse effects on the foetus, may likewise affect the young child, and some drugs may have effects on growth that are highly relevant to the developing child (e.g. tetracyclines and steroids) but of little or no concern in adults. The process of maturation is associated with many non-linear and qualitative changes, in both pharmacokinetics and pharmacodynamics independently and in the interplay between them, all of which heavily influence prescribing. The presence of organ system failure in the PIC patient obviously complicates matters further.

A variety of organ-specific drug effects are peculiar to children. Some of these have been explained by pharmacological studies but others represent observational data independently confirmed but not necessarily adequately explained. Market forces compound a misplaced emotional reluctance to repeat drug trials independently on children. The result is that it is not unusual to encounter disclaimers from drug companies about the use, dose, efficacy and contraindications of various agents that nevertheless form an essential part of treatment in paediatrics.

Children have an increased propensity for some adverse drug effects such as dystonic reactions to centrally acting dopamine antagonists, for example metoclopramide, prochlorperazine and chlorpromazine (treatable with procyclidine). Other aspects of organ-specific physiology can make the clinical impact of effects that are recognised outside paediatric practice far more significant in children. For example the reports of sudden death in infants after verapamil administration in cardiac failure may be explained by the infant myocardium's dependence upon serum calcium (as opposed to sarcolemmal calcium) and the rate-dependent cardiac output during bradycardia.

Children are *relatively* immune to *some* toxic drug effects such as theophylline toxicity. The hepatic injury associated with paracetamol poisoning is less severe in children by virtue of a greater sulphonation ability (see p 315), which avoids generation of the toxic intermediate. Children are also less prone to hepatic toxicity from halothane even after repeated exposure. They are relatively protected from, but not immune to, the vestibular and renal toxicity associated with aminoglycosides. To achieve therapeutic levels of digoxin, children require higher weight corrected doses than adults. They tolerate higher digoxin levels but the therapeutic range is the same.

Effects of critical illness

Considerable variations in pharmacokinetics also occur in critically ill patients. Many but not all of these variations are mentioned in this chapter. The cardiovascular compensation (or otherwise) of shock reduces the distribution of drugs by reducing blood supply to muscle and adipose tissue. Fluid retention and oedema, from any cause, have the opposite effect. Acid–base fluctuations are common in intensive care patients affecting ionisation of weak acids and alkalis. Metabolism and excretion are reduced if the hepatic or renal blood supply and function are compromised, leading to prolonged half-lives, higher drug levels and increased activity for a given maintenance dosage.

Enteral drug absorption can be highly variable in intensive care as a result of combined effects on gut blood flow and transit time. Similarly intramuscular injections may achieve reduced systemic levels when perfusion is poor. The preference for intravenous drug administration is partly because it is the least problematic in terms of delayed effect but it is not immune. Even intravenous injections exhibit delayed responses in shock states – the obvious example being an intravenous anaesthetic induction in a shocked patient where a considerable delay may occur between injection and anaesthetic effect.

PICU protocol

Intravenous drug administration also has other attendant problems. Every doctor working with children has a tale to tell about difficulties in obtaining vascular access. Patients who have been chronically unwell, or chubby infants for example, may become your worst vascular access nightmare during intensive care, where difficulties may be compounded by shock or by patients who need minimal handling (remember in emergencies the insurance of intra-osseous access). Furthermore the volume of fluid available for intravenous drug administration is often small because of the size of the child, their age or a therapeutic fluid restriction. This frequently leads to the use of low volume, high concentration intravenous infusions. This approach has a number of implications:

- the resultant concentration may require central intravenous administration when it would not otherwise be required
- the impact of factors such as the dead space in intravenous lines and the dangers of incomplete dosage, underdosing and overdosing are magnified
- dangers of inadvertent drug bolus are introduced, for example those caused by technical problems such as pump runaway and syphonage.

Meticulous care must be taken in the manner in which drugs are administered to the patient. Prescribing and drug preparation should be supervised and double-checked and intravenous access sites properly monitored. Every effort should be made to ensure that drug quality as well as quantity is optimal before it reaches the patient. Chemical interactions and physical processes need to be taken into account. Syringes of drugs for continuous infusion may deteriorate over time or in response to sunlight. Multiple drug infusions may have to travel to the patient through the same lines but not all the resulting mixtures are appropriate. Many are incompatible but not all incompatible solutions precipitate floridly like mixtures of thiopental and vecuronium, or calcium and bicarbonate do. In many instances visual

---

Useful drug calculations for infusions

Adrenaline (epinephrine), noradrenaline (norepinephrine), isoprenaline
0.3 mg/kg in 50 ml solution   1 ml hr^{-1} = 0.1 µg kg^{-1} min^{-1} dose range 0.5–5 ml hr^{-1}

Dopamine, dobutamine
30 mg/kg in 50 ml solution   1 ml hr^{-1} = 10 µg kg^{-1} min^{-1} dose range 0.2–2 ml hr^{-1}

Morphine
body weight (kg) gives the number of mg to add to 50 ml solution, 1 ml hr^{-1} is then 20 µg kg^{-1} hr^{-1}

changes in the solution occur only after most of the drug has been lost. The dangers are not just chemical. Physical effects such as haemolysis of blood when sharing lines with dextrose or mannitol, flocculation of lipid emulsions and adherence of drugs to the plastic syringes and lines must also be considered.

It is often wise to keep a short wide-bore cannula free in a large vein for colloid administration. Blood products should only be allowed to mix with each other (not with other substances) in the lines. Normal crystalloid maintenance can run peripherally but concentrated solutions have to be administered centrally because of the potential for chemical thrombophlebitis and the dangers of tissue burns with extravasation. It is not unusual to need as many as six different points of vascular access in an intensive care patient. Multiple lumen intravenous central lines have therefore been an enormous advance and their use has an etiquette of its own. The end hole (distal lumen) should be used for pressure measurements. If necessary a lumen(s) should be distinguished and protected (sealed) from the time of insertion for later use in administering parenteral nutrition. Catecholamines may be mixed with each other but not with all other vasoactive drugs. Lines used for administration of sedatives, anaesthetic agents or relaxants should be flushed immediately after discontinuing the infusion and lines used for intravenous boluses of drugs must be thoroughly flushed with saline before and afterwards.

DRUG ADMINISTRATION AND ABSORPTION (See Figures 9.1 and 9.2.)

Enteral

The choice between routes of drug administration is made on the basis of clinical convenience and consideration of the absorption 'lag time' and 'bioavailability' associated with enteral preparations.

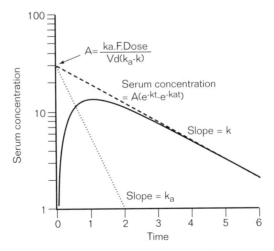

Figure 9.1 Serum concentration *vs* time after oral administration. Serum concentration is graphed against time on semilogarithmic graph paper. The elimination phase (log-linear) is the straight terminal segment of the curve of slope −k where k is the elimination rate constant such that $t_{1/2} = \ln2/k$. The extrapolation of the log-linear phase (heavy dashed straight line) gives the V_d as shown. F is the fraction absorbed (bioavailability) and Ka is the absorption rate constant. Ka is the slope of the fine dashed line which is derived by subtracting concentration during the absorption phase from the extrapolation of the log linear phase. (Adapted from Chernow, B., ed. 1994. The Pharmacological Approach to the Critically III Patient. 3rd edn. Williams and Wilkins, Baltimore.)

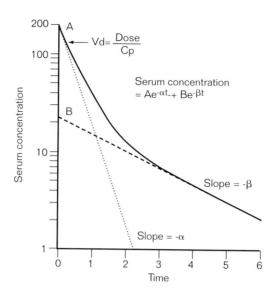

Figure 9.2 Serum concentration vs time after IV administration. Serum concentration is graphed against time on semilogarithmic graph paper. The heavy and light dashed lines are derived as in fig 9.1. α and β are rate constants for the distribution and elimination phases of a two compartment model. V_d is calculated from the extrapolation intercept as shown. See text. (Adapted from Chernow, B., ed. 1994. The Pharmacological Approach to the Critically Ill Patient. 3rd edn. Williams and Wilkins, Baltimore.)

Enterally administered drugs encounter a lag time before they enter the circulation and this is affected by both the preparation and manner of administration. Long lag times do not preclude complete absorption but will affect dosing and steady state drug concentration. A drug that is absorbed from a particular part of the gastrointestinal tract will be dependent upon the transit time to reach that point. Gut transit times vary with age and other factors. Typically they are long in babies but short in children and may be accelerated by metoclopramide. Delayed gastric emptying and other gastrointestinal transit times can result from the administration of drugs such as codeine and other opiates or from electrolyte and acid–base disturbances.

The fraction (F) of the administered dose that is available for absorption by that route is expressed as bioavailability. It can be affected by changes in formulation or by factors such as complexing with milk. For example the concurrent ingestion of tetracyclines with food (i.e. milk, cottage cheese or cheese) and drugs containing multivalent cations (i.e. iron, aluminium, magnesium and calcium) can result in chelation that reduces the bioavailability by up to 90 per cent. A similar dramatic interaction occurs with oral ciprofloxacin. The preparation of a medication can affect bioavailability and absorption, for example highly compressed, poorly soluble tablets or habitually crushing tablets or adding sweeteners.

Changes in gastric pH will affect drugs that are degraded by stomach acid. If the gastric pH rises, the ionised proportion of a weak acid rises and that of a weak base falls. Ionised forms are poorly absorbed since they cannot passively diffuse across lipid membranes. Changes in the ionised proportion of an administered dose greatly affect the pattern of absorption (and distribution). At birth gastric pH is close to neutral but the pH falls rapidly over the first few hours. A functional reserve in terms of gastric acid production develops slowly over the first year but accelerates in the second year.

Rectal administration is used when oral or gastric administration is precluded and intravenous access is not available. This route avoids first-pass metabolism and it is well tolerated by infants and small children. Typical drugs administered rectally include anticonvulsants, sedatives and paracetamol.

Intramuscular

The small muscle bulk, pain, frequent propensity for bleeding and unreliable patterns of absorption lead to a strenuous avoidance of intramuscular injections in babies and children. For many PICU patients additional concerns about absorption in the face of poor peripheral perfusion or paralysis also contribute, for some agents pharmacokinetic concerns add still further to these reservations, for example agents that precipitate when mixed and thence experience delayed and incomplete absorption, such as phenytoin and benzodiazepines.

Intravenous

Intravenous administration gets round many of the problems of absorption and will often entail a marked dose reduction for drugs that were poorly absorbed from other routes. The principal determinants of drug concentration after intravenous administration are those of elimination (see Figure 9.2).

Drug concentration at steady state is as much related to factors governing absorption of the drug as those that describe elimination. The relationship is expressed:

steady state concentration = F × maintenance dose ÷ dose interval × clearance

After oral or rectal administration of the drug, the serum level rises at a rate governed by the absorption rate constant (k_a). Serum levels continue to rise as long as the rate of absorption exceeds that of elimination. The 'therapeutic index' relates the drug concentration required for clinical effect to that associated with toxicity.

DRUG DISTRIBUTION

The serum / plasma concentration of a drug increases with the dose. If the drug sequesters outside the plasma then the concentration is lower and the increases that occur with increasing dose are muted. This phenomenon is described by the volume of distribution (V_d), a contrived parameter relating the dose to the serum concentration that it achieves.

V_d = dose ÷ serum concentration

Volumes of distribution are not physiological parameters. Conceptually the V_d is the answer to the question 'how much plasma/serum would it take to contain this much drug at this concentration?' The V_d can be enormous for drugs that sequester outside the circulation (e.g. lipid soluble agents). Knowledge of the V_d allows the calculation of a loading dose, which as can be seen from the equation below, is independent of 'clearance' and half-life.

Loading dose = (V_d × desired serum concentration) ÷ F

However the loading dose required for a patient already receiving a medication (e.g. theophylline in an asthmatic) *will* be dependent on clearance and half-life since they affect the serum concentration. The relationship is given on p. 119 after a discussion of clearance.

The V_d can be viewed as being divided between compartments, although such compartments are as nebulously defined as the V_d itself. In a 'one-compartment' model, the drug is assumed to instantly distribute homogeneously throughout the distribution volume. The two-compartment model consists of a small volume, rapid, central compartment (that usually corresponds to blood with or without the extracellular fluid of highly vascular organs) and a larger, slower compartment (usually including adipose tissue and intracellular fluid).

The regional distribution of a drug can be a potent influence on its effect. Some, but not all, of these parameters will clearly affect V_d.

BODY SIZE AND COMPOSITION

Changes associated with growth include changes in the relative size of body fluid compartments (see Chapter 7, Fluids, Electrolytes and Blood). The influence that this has on prescribing is most noticeable with drugs that are minimally distributed in the tissues (e.g. muscle relaxants) or are highly water soluble, such as aminoglycosides. A higher dose per kilogram may be needed in infants as compared to older children to produce the same clinical effect, since extracellular fluid in infants makes up a higher proportion of their mass. Critically ill children have a propensity for oedema, exacerbated by capillary leak and MOSF that can wildly elevate total body water. Plasma concentrations of the more lipid soluble drugs tend to be higher in neonates and small infants because fat and muscle proportions are smaller. The proportion of body mass accounted for by fat can increase by a factor of 20 between a preterm infant and a healthy 1-year-old.

ACID–BASE BALANCE

The non-ionised proportion of drug may have greater lipid solubility and therefore tissue affinity than the ionised form. Changes in pH therefore affect the V_d by affecting the pK of drugs that are weak acids. At a high pH, ionisation is encouraged and tissue affinity reduced. Clinical examples include tricyclic poisoning where dysrhythmias can be treated by alkalinisation, and salicylate and barbiturate poisonings, where CNS toxicity is reduced, by the same approach. The normal range for blood pH in neonates (especially preterm) is lower than that in older children.

PROTEIN BINDING

When drugs are highly protein bound, only the free drug is available for its pharmacodynamic action. Changes in the proportion of protein-bound drug (e.g. from pH changes) affect the amount of drug that is available for action as well as elimination, leading to a new steady state that may have different characteristics to that in normal subjects. Drugs that are highly protein bound include penicillins, cephalosporins, sulphonamides, propranolol, phenytoin, bupivocaine, theophylline, morphine, diazepam, phenobarbital and warfarin. These will compete with each other for albumin binding and also with endogenous compounds that are protein bound such as urea, free fatty acids and bilirubin. Total protein and albumin concentrations are low in the neonate and infant and there is also some qualitative impairment of protein-binding capacity. In such relative hypoalbuminaemia, low total drug concentrations of such agents may not be subtherapeutic. For example 70 per cent of the measured theophylline level is free (active) in neonates compared to 40 per cent in adults. The competition of such drugs for protein binding can be of critical importance in jaundiced patients when the drugs compete with bilirubin for albumin. For example phenytoin and caffeine can precipitate kernicterus.

ORGAN SPECIFIC EFFECTS

Poor perfusion of particular organs will reduce the drug effects on them. The most potent example is the development of portal hypertension in liver disease. The dose–response relationship for drugs with an extensive first pass metabolism is very susceptible to changes in liver function. For drugs with a high extraction ratio, hepatic blood flow determines the rate of drug metabolism and the effects of an oral dose will be increased by portal hypertension.

Clearance

Clearance is best thought of as the volume of blood, serum or plasma that is cleared of drug per unit time. In a steady state, the serum concentration obeys the relationship described under absorption. This can be rearranged to clearance = (F × maintenance dose) ÷ (dose interval × serum concentration).

For most drugs, the movement between compartments and out of the body is 'first order'. In first order kinetics a constant proportion of drug is removed per unit time. Thus the amount of drug removed depends upon its serum concentration. The nature of the process of drug elimination is most clearly defined from the decay portion of the absorption–elimination curve but drug elimination is occurring even as the drug is being absorbed. The drug elimination constant (k_e) is measured in units of reciprocal time and is related to the half-life $(t_{1/2})$ by the relationship

$$t_{1/2} = \ln(2) \div k_e$$

Some drugs (e.g. phenytoin) display non-linear or 'zero order' kinetics when in their therapeutic range. For such drugs, clearance decreases and the half-life increases as the dose is increased. This is because elimination pathways become saturated and cannot increase proportionately (hence the term 'saturatable kinetics'). Elimination therefore occurs at a constant rate independent of serum level. The point at which saturation occurs may change in disease states depending upon factors such as liver function and enzyme induction from other drugs. Dose increases must be monitored carefully by measurement of drug levels. Many drugs which display first order kinetics in their normal therapeutic range, display zero order kinetics at higher levels (e.g. phenobarbitone).

When a drug is given intravenously the decay of the serum concentration (Figure 9.2) has two components. The α phase or early, rapid or distribution phase between compartments and the β phase which represents elimination, α and β are both rate constants for first order processes. The points A and B (their intercepts with the y axis (serum concentration)) can be extrapolated from the slope of the decay during those phases. These components allow the following relationships to be determined:

Serum concentration $= Ae^{-\alpha t} + Be^{-\beta t}$

$$\begin{aligned} V_d &= \text{dose} \div \beta AUC \\ &= \text{dose} \div \beta(A/\alpha + B/\beta) \\ &= (\text{dose} \times t_{1/2}) \div (0.693 \times AUC) \end{aligned}$$

$$\begin{aligned} \text{Clearance} &= \text{dose} \div AUC \\ &= \text{dose} \div (A/\alpha + B/\beta) \\ &= (\text{dose} \times 0.693) \div (t_{1/2} \times \text{concentration at } t_0) \end{aligned}$$

$$t_{1/2\alpha} = \ln2/\alpha$$

$$t_{1/2\beta} = \ln2/\beta$$

where AUC = the area under the curve of serum concentration versus time, and t_0 is time zero.

Thus clearance is inversely proportional to half-life and directly proportional to the V_d. Furthermore, even without knowledge of the existing drug level one can calculate a loading dose if required as follows:

$$\begin{aligned} \text{loading dose} &= (\text{maintenance dose} \times t_{1/2}) \div (\text{dose interval (hr)} \times \log_e 2) \\ &= (\text{maintenance dose} \times t_{1/2}) \div (\text{dose interval (hr)} \times 0.693) \end{aligned}$$

A further consideration of exponential processes such as first order kinetics is given in Chapter 18, Physics for the Intensivist.

DRUG ELIMINATION

As absorption and distribution are completed, the rate of change of drug concentration over time is governed by the characteristics of elimination. The β phase of clearance in a two-compartment model represents drug elimination from the body. Elimination is a net effect of two processes – metabolism and excretion.

Metabolism

The liver's role is principally to metabolise the drugs into water-soluble forms that can be excreted in bile or urine. In phase I reactions, lipid solubility is reduced by adding or exposing polar molecule groups such as hydroxyl, carboxyl or amino. In phase II reactions conjugation enhances active tubular excretion. Metabolites may themselves be pharmacologically active and in some cases have enhanced activity. Most of the microsomal enzyme systems required for biotransformation of drugs are present at birth, but their concentration and activity is reduced (to as much as 20% of adult levels in the case of neonatal cytochrome P_{450}). Immaturity has more affect on conjugation than degradation but conjugating ability reaches adult levels by 3 months of age. This is accelerated if enzyme induction has occurred in utero. Normal levels of conjugation do not mean the same pattern as in adulthood. Sulphate conjugation is far more prevalent than glucuronide until puberty. Plasma enzyme activity increases as total plasma proteins increase, reaching adult values at 1 year. The overall result is prolonged elimination half-lives for almost all drugs in neonates. In early childhood there is then a marked increase in metabolic clearance, particularly involving the degradative reactions. Many drugs have shortened half-lives in infants, by factors as high as two and three. This is not fully explained by increases in distribution volume. Additional factors include the fact that the liver is relatively large and that age-related metabolic differences are present in both phase I and phase II reactions giving more options for routes of metabolism.

Children display the same patterns of enzyme induction from drugs such as phenobarbitone and rifampicin, as adults. They are also subject to the same drug interactions that result from inhibition of metabolism, for example the inhibition of cytochrome P_{450} by erythromycin, clarithromycin, ketoconazole and cimetidine that potentiates toxicity of other agents (such as cisapride) using the same pathway.

Excretion

> In general terms, if drug elimination is a clinical problem the same loading dose should be applied but the maintenance dose and frequency should be reduced.

Renal excretion is the major route for excretion of water-soluble metabolites. Term infants handle drugs that depend on the GFR for excretion (like aminoglycosides) better than preterm. For patients receiving renal replacement therapy in the form of peritoneal dialysis or haemofiltration, the GFR equivalence is best judged from the ultrafiltration rate. Renal tubular secretion (an active process) reaches adult levels by 6 months of age, until which time excretion of penicillins and sulphonamides for example, are reduced. Passive tubular reabsorption of weak acids is impeded in babies because the relatively high urine pH leads to increased ionisation. Lipid-soluble drugs may be eliminated via the gastrointestinal tract. Even if not excreted in bile and administered intravenously, their clearance may be enhanced by the nasogastric administration of activated charcoal.

DRUG INTERACTION

The variety of drugs prescribed to intensive care patients introduces a huge potential for interaction. Pharmacokinetic effects are legion but include the actions of H_2 receptor antagonists, proton pump antagonists and antacids on gastric pH, and the use of prokinetic agents or drugs with negative effects upon transit time. Also there are the effects of vasoactive drugs and inotropes on global and regional circulations (particularly renal perfusion and the GFR), competition for protein binding, enzyme induction and drug metabolism, use of diuretics, use of extracorporeal circulation, and many more.

Pharmacodynamic interactions are also relevant whether they involve competition at receptor sites (e.g. aminoglycosides potentiating reversible neuromuscular blockade) or cumulative non-specific interactions. The significance of pharmacodynamic interactions may be specific to, accentuated or attenuated in children.

Antagonism and agonism are properties of drugs that exert their effects via receptors. Receptors are molecular species appearing on cell surfaces or within cells. Binding of receptors with 'ligands' produces specific effects and receptors are defined by their affinities in this regard. Ligands may be agonist or antagonist. Competitive antagonists bind in proportion to the relative concentration of agonist, their effects can therefore be overcome by raised concentrations of agonist. Non-competitive antagonists are immune to agonist concentration. Common mechanisms of non-competitive antagonism are irreversible binding of ligand to receptor or binding to the receptor ligand complex in a manner that blocks the stimulated effect. Specificity of a ligand is a useful property when talking about drugs but ligands may also be hormones, neurotransmitters, toxins, etc. all with varying specificity.

Receptor responses can be modulated naturally or pharmacologically by fast and slow processes. Down and up regulation are slow responses usually mediated by changes in the number of accessible receptors. Down regulation contributes to tachyphylaxis – the phenomenon where increased dosage is required to attain the same effect. Rapid desensitisation of receptors can occur after phosphorylation, which inhibits the effector mechanism of a receptor–ligand complex. These phenomena are typically observed in responses to vasoactive medications such as catecholamines and glyceryl trinitrate.

Non-specific interactions are also common on the intensive care unit. It is not unusual to find oneself trying to balance drugs with different mechanisms of action but opposing effects, for example inotropes and vasodilators on the blood pressure or opiates and prokinetic agents on gastrointestinal function. The net effect is observable but similar results can be achieved with different dose combinations. The correct course of action may not be intuitive for the trainee.

The key lessons to remember from this chapter are:
- that considerable care should be taken with prescribing and administering drugs in the PICU
- it is never a sign of weakness to refer to a paediatric pharmacopoeia
- it is always wise to seek advice from an experienced colleague or a paediatric pharmacist.

10 Metabolic Intensive Care

- **Blood gases**
- **Interpretation of blood gas data**
- **Specific conditions**

Despite its broad title, this chapter concentrates on blood gas analysis, the intensive care approach to inborn errors of metabolism and the treatment of diabetic ketoacidosis.

BLOOD GASES

Acid–base

The normal hydrogen ion concentration ($[H^+]$) is 37 to 48 nmol L^{-1} in babies; this corresponds to a pH in the range of 7.43 to 7.32. The normal pH range in infants and children is 7.34 to 7.43 corresponding to $[H^+]$ of 46 to 37 nmol L^{-1}. Values higher than the upper limit of normal $[H^+]$ (lower pH) are acidotic and values lower than the lower limit (higher pH) are alkalotic.

The principal (but not the only) hydrogen ion buffer in the body is carbonic acid and its relation with bicarbonate. Other buffers include phosphate, haemoglobin, proteins and ammonia. Buffers provide an immediate control over $[H^+]$ by a process of reversible binding. The Henderson–Hasselbach equation

$$CO_{2aq} + H_2O \rightleftharpoons H_2CO_3 \rightleftharpoons H^+ + HCO_3^-$$

expresses the chemical equilibrium between dissolved carbon dioxide and hydrogen and bicarbonate ions. Derangements that are due primarily to fluctuations in $Paco_2$ are termed 'respiratory', all others are 'metabolic'.

These acid–base fluctuations are associated with a variety of effects. Most importantly a level of compensation is achieved by altering levels of carbon dioxide or bicarbonate respectively. The respiratory compensation for metabolic derangements is mediated by changes in respiratory drive and is effected as altered minute ventilation controls the $Paco_2$. Metabolic compensation for respiratory acidosis is much slower and is effected by renal conservation of bicarbonate. In either case, full compensation is unusual but it would bring the pH right back into the normal range if it worked (Figure 10.1). When interpreting blood gas measurements on the intensive care unit remember that the changes invoked by mechanical ventilation can accentuate the respiratory component of the acid–base state to the extent of complete compensation (normal $[H^+]$). That is not to say that such an approach is appropriate or that it would be to therapeutic advantage. It is just to help you interpret the results. In addition to compensation, acid–base derangements have other metabolic consequences.

Acute rises in $[H^+]$ (acidosis) equilibrate across the cell membrane. An efflux of intra-cellular potassium ions (K^+) preserves the transmembrane electrical potential but results in hyperkalaemia. Similarly alkalosis from any cause results in an influx of potassium into the cells causing hypokalaemia. These changes occur without perturbing the whole body potassium. The relationship between acid–base and potassium flux is complicated if insulin is being administered, since insulin promotes potassium movement into cells along with glucose. Alkalosis increases the ratio of bound to unbound (ionised) Ca^{2+} and can lead to tetany. Acidosis increases the P_{50} of the haemoglobin dissociation curve creating potential problems with oxygen delivery, and alkalosis decreases it creating potential problems with oxygen uptake. $[H^+]$ fluctuations (especially those caused by carbon dioxide) affect vascular tone. Hypercapnic acidosis causes cerebral vasodilatation and pulmonary vasoconstriction.

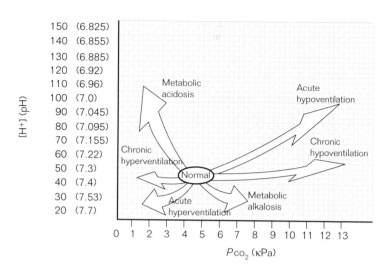

Figure 10.1 Acid–Base Description. Recognisable patterns of change in the bicarbonate buffer system and their interpretation (see text for provisos).

Acid–base disorders

RESPIRATORY ALKALOSIS

Hyperventilation causes a reduction in Pa_{CO_2}, and acute changes in Pa_{CO_2} have a linear effect on $[H^+]$ (1 kPa to 5.5 nmol L^{-1}). Thus $[H^+]$ is low and Pa_{CO_2} is low. Common causes include excessive mechanical ventilation, central hyperventilation associated with encephalopathy, CNS infection, trauma, etc. Acutely hypoxic and acidotic patients can hyperventilate. In the latter case some degree of compensation for the high $[H^+]$ is achieved. One would expect the calculated bicarbonate and base excess to be normal. Treatment is directed at the specific cause.

RESPIRATORY ACIDOSIS

Hypoventilation causes a rise in Pa_{CO_2}. Acute changes in Pa_{CO_2} have a linear effect on $[H^+]$ (1 kPa to 5.5 nmol L^{-1}). Thus $[H^+]$ is high and Pa_{CO_2} is high. Common causes include respiratory depression, obstructive and restrictive respiratory diseases, terminal exhaustion, inadequate mechanical ventilation, etc. Similar derangements may be caused by muscle weakness and increased carbon dioxide production (malignant hyperthermia, seizures, etc.). One would expect the calculated bicarbonate and base excess to be normal (see p. 125–26). Treatment is directed at improving respiratory function and support, and to a lesser extent minimising carbon dioxide load. If it is unsuccessful then compensation occurs over several days through renal conservation of bicarbonate. A compensated respiratory acidosis therefore has a near normal (but high) $[H^+]$ and a high Pa_{CO_2} and one would expect the calculated bicarbonate and base excess to be high.

METABOLIC ALKALOSIS

An acute fall in hydrogen ion concentration without a fall in carbon dioxide may be caused by a rise in bicarbonate concentration or less commonly a loss of H^+ ions. Some compensatory carbon dioxide retention may occur and reduced respiratory drive should be anticipated, for example if one is attempting to wean mechanical ventilation. The calculated base excess would be expected to be high but under most circumstances confusion should not occur with a compensated respiratory acidosis because the $[H^+]$ will be near normal (but *low*).

Chloride depletion is associated with increased sodium reabsorption in the proximal convoluted tubule and excess hydrogen ion and K^+ loss, the former resulting in increased bicarbonate absorption. Chloride depletion is a common consequence of loop diuretic therapy but can also occur from gastrointestinal losses or as a secondary consequence of chronic respiratory acidosis. By contrast to the relation between $[H^+]$ and distribution of K^+ between extracellular fluid and intracellular fluid, genuine hypokalaemia results in compensatory renal excretion of H^+ ions and *causes*, or aggravates, alkalosis. Chloride-sensitive causes of metabolic alkalosis are associated with low urinary chloride (< 20 mmol L^{-1}) and chloride insensitive forms with higher urinary chloride. The former include diuretic therapy, vomiting and chloridorrhoea and the latter include citrate poisoning. Diminished extracellular fluid volume will perpetuate a metabolic alkalosis because it is associated with an obligatory increase in proximal tubular Na^+ reabsorption.

In the rare circumstances where a metabolic alkalosis requires treatment it is important to treat the cause rather than the effect. Treat hypokalaemia with K^+ supplements and hypochloraemia with saline infusion. Acid loads can be delivered, however, in the form of ammonium chloride. Which is to be avoided in cases of liver failure in favour of dilute hydrochloric acid 200 mmol L^{-1} of 85% dextrose. (Dose = BE × Wt × 1.65 to fully correct. Normally half correction is used).

METABOLIC ACIDOSIS

An acute rise in $[H^+]$ with a normal or even reduced $Pa\text{CO}_2$ (attempted compensation) results from an abnormal bicarbonate loss or a non-carbonic source of excess H^+. Metabolic acidosis is considered further in the section on inborn errors of metabolism (see p. 130). The calculated base deficit (negative base excess) would be expected to be high and the calculated bicarbonate would be expected to be low. Treatment must be directed at the cause.

INTERPRETATION OF BLOOD GAS DATA

Acid–base

In general terms *the use of hydrogen ion concentration $[H^+]$ is preferable to pH* because physiological or therapeutic changes are linear (as opposed to inverse logarithmic) and therefore more easily interpreted. The difference that this makes is elaborated below. Tracking the $[H^+]$ is intuitively easier and makes it easier to monitor the effect of therapeutic interventions, which have their effects primarily on the molar $[H^+]$.

[H⁺] or pH?

A pH of 7.4 corresponds to a $[H^+]$ of 40 nmol L^{-1}. An increase of 40 nmol L^{-1} reduces the pH to 7.1 (because the $[H^+]$ has been doubled and the $Log_{10}2$ is 0.3). A similar numerical change in pH towards alkalosis (pH 7.7) involves a reduction in $[H^+]$ of only 20 nmol L^{-1} (to halve the concentration). A drop in pH from 7.4 to 6.8 involves a sixfold increase in $[H^+]$.

With the exception of pH **it is highly preferable to manage patients on the basis of measured values only**. Blood gas machines measure pH, $P\text{CO}_2$ and $P\text{O}_2$ and by making some fairly coarse assumptions about the Henderson–Hasselbach equilibrium, they then go on to calculate other parameters. It is essential to be familiar with the assumptions made in the algorithms if one is to pay any attention at all to the calculated parameters.

Bicarbonate and base excess

There are two principal sources of error in the estimation of bicarbonate and total carbon dioxide content. These are the erroneous assumptions that the pK of the

Henderson–Hasselbach equation and the solubility coefficient for carbon dioxide are constant. Most blood gas machines assume that the pK of the Henderson–Hasselbach equation is 6.1, when in fact it varies *in vivo* over a much wider range (5.8 to 6.4). The cause of such fluctuation is related to variations in

- the ionic strength of the plasma
- the amount of carbon dioxide in the form of carbamino compounds, and
- protein and urea levels.

The impact of these causes percentage errors in estimation of serum bicarbonate from −50 per cent to +100 per cent.

The term 'base excess' refers to an empirical expression which approximates the amount of acid (or base for a 'base deficit') which would be needed to titrate one litre of blood to a pH of 7.4. The base excess of blood with a pH 7.4, $PaCO_2$ 40 mmHg (5.33 kPa), total haemoglobin concentration 15 g dL^{-1} at 37°C, is zero. The principal sources of error in the calculation of base excess are the use of erroneous estimates of bicarbonate concentration and the use of imprecise or assumed values for haemoglobin concentration. Furthermore different formulae are used to calculate the base excess *in vivo* or *in vitro* or of whole blood and extracellular fluid. The choice made by the programmers may not be easily discernible. The different formulae produce results that disagree even for the same blood gas data and the difference between the results changes the further the result is from zero. They cannot be used interchangeably.

Those clinicians that use calculated parameters, tend to use estimates of the base excess as a shorthand to determine the presence of a metabolic acidosis (negative values) or alkalosis (positive values). This practice is probably reliable once values of greater than or equal to +10 are reached. Normal values actually vary from −4 (or as low as −6 in neonates) to +3. These clinicians also tend to use the base excess of whole blood to calculate the dose of bicarbonate (mmol) required to correct (or half-correct) the acidosis. But this dose is distributed throughout the whole extracellular fluid whereas hydrogen ions are distributed throughout the total body water (the further consequences of which are considered below). Meanwhile the formulae for the dose of bicarbonate contain a 'fudge factor' (usually 0.3) which is an estimate of the fraction of the body weight accounted for by extracellular fluid. The usual formula is

Dose of bicarbonate (mmol) = $0.3 \times BE_{wb} \times wt$ (kg)
divided by two for half correction. (BE_{wb} is whole blood base excess).

In fact extracellular fluid accounts for 50 per cent of the body weight (wt) of neonates and declines to about 27 per cent by the end of the first year. The impact of all these errors on the prescribed dose of bicarbonate is so great as to make the resulting dosage schedule farcical. It is just as effective to use a two-dose regime. For severe acidosis give 2 or 3 mmol kg^{-1} of bicarbonate, and for mild acidosis give 1 mmol kg^{-1}. Nevertheless, routinely treating a metabolic acidosis with bicarbonate is a bit like sticking your head in the sand. If you do not establish and treat the cause, the acidosis will rapidly recur. Bicarbonate therapy is:

- indicated to supplement recognised bicarbonate losses (e.g. urine, ileostomy fluid)
- an important therapy in drug overdose involving weak acids
- a valid emergency therapy if there is associated symptomatic hyperkalaemia
- justified to urgently recruit a response to inotrope therapy in the context of severe acidosis ($[H^+] > 63$, pH < 7.2).

In the latter circumstance, therapy may be of limited effect (although it is still worth trying). Bicarbonate therapy is also used by some doctors to control $[H^+]$ during the early stages of permissive hypercarbia, this approach lessens the extent of renal compensation.

Since bicarbonate does not equilibrate quickly across the cell membrane, intracellular acidosis (including that in the myocardial cell) is not immediately affected by bicarbonate administration. Indeed it may be aggravated since dissolved carbon dioxide, which increases after bicarbonate administration, equilibrates across the cell membrane faster and more effectively than the bicarbonate anions.

Routine investigation of a metabolic acidosis includes measurement of urine pH, anion and osmolar gaps and measurement of the serum lactate and/or $AVDO_2$ (arterial–venous oxygen difference) as markers of the adequacy of tissue perfusion or oxygen delivery. The anion gap is calculated according to the formula

$[Na^+] - ([Cl^-] + [HCO_3^-])$.

An anion gap greater than 12 implies the presence of a 'non-Henderson–Hasselbach' source of acid. The osmolar gap is the difference between measured and calculated osmolality. If the measured osmolality is greater than 15 mosm L^{-1} above the calculated value then this implies the presence of additional osmotically active solutes.

Osmo = 2Na + Gluc + Urea (all in mmol L^{-1})

Inborn errors of metabolism may present with a metabolic acidosis and their investigation is covered on pp.128–132.

Interpretation of the Po_2

The physiology of 'oxygen flux' in the 'macrocirculation' is discussed in Chapter 11, Respiratory System. In that chapter, the concept of comparing arterial and mixed venous oxygen content to assess the adequacy of oxygen delivery (cardiac output) is discussed. However in Chapter 17, Host Defence, one of several physiological states will be described where this approach is confounded, i.e. systemic arteriovenous shunting. An alternative approach to judge the adequacy of oxygenation is to do so from an end-organ perspective. From a cellular perspective one can theoretically distinguish or subdefine hypoxia aetiologically as demonstrated in the following list (although many of these processes may occur simultaneously):

- ischaemic –a fall in cardiac output or regional blood flow leads to a rise in total or regional $AVDO_2$
- shunt (as above)
- hypoxaemia – a low Po_2
- anaemia
- increased affinity of haemoglobin for oxygen caused by a left shift in the oxygen dissociation curve
- low oxygen content because of a right shift in the haemoglobin oxygen dissociation curve
- dysperfusion – an increased diffusion distance for oxygen, for example in the oedema of MOSF (multi-organ system failure)
- cytochrome inhibition which inhibits cellular oxidative reactions, for example cyanide poisoning
- uncoupling between mitochondrial electron transport and adenosine triphosphate (ATP) synthesis
- hypermetabolic – an increased oxygen demand.

These distinctions are also useful if one is to apply the ethic of treating cause rather than effect. Also, from this cellular point of view, blood gases are a very insensitive method of determining oxygenation. Three techniques are worth mentioning that have the potential to detect (if not necessarily aetiologically define) cellular hypoxia. They have been applied to regional circulations and thence used to infer more global derangement. A clear role for each has yet to be defined.

- Near infra-red spectroscopy can discriminate between haemoglobin, myoglobin and intracellular cytochromes in different redox states and has been successfully applied to the brain and liver.
- Gastric tonometry. The 'pHi' is the inferred intracellular pH in the gastric mucosa. It is derived by assuming that the Pco_2 of saline filling a gastric tonometry balloon equili-

brates with that of the gastric mucosa and that the intracellular $P\text{CO}_2$ is buffered against the arterial bicarbonate concentration. A number of assumptions (of dubious reliability) are also made about the pK of the Henderson–Hasselbach equation and the time (t_{eq}) taken for $P\text{CO}_2$ equilibration.

To interpret simultaneous measurements of arterial blood gases and $P\text{CO}_2$ of the saline in the tonometry balloon the following formula is applied

$$pHi = 6.1 + \log_{10} \frac{\text{arterial [HCO}_3^-\text{]}}{P\text{CO}_{2\,(\text{tonometer})} \times t_{eq}}$$

- Lactate is a normal product of carbohydrate metabolism but production is raised in oxygen-depleted cells. Hyperlacticaemia in a venous blood sample therefore implies cellular hypoxia (particularly if the lactate : pyruvate ratio rises above the normal value of 10 : 1). However lactate can be metabolised in the venous circulation or sample bottle by respiring red cells (e.g. if the fluoride oxalate sampling bottle is not adequately shaken) making the positive predictive power of a high lactate more useful than the negative predictive power of a low result. Also when blood pools in the periphery as in sepsis or hypothermic circulatory arrest during cardiac surgery, lactate may not be washed out until later reperfusion. The cellular situation is analogous to that of a limb with a tourniquet applied. Even when lactate is raised in circulatory insufficiency, the initial consequence of resuscitation may be for the lactate to rise further. The further significance of raised lactate levels (in inborn errors of metabolism) is discussed on p. 130.

SPECIFIC CONDITIONS

Inborn errors of metabolism

Those readers of this text who are approaching their PIC training from a non-paediatric background will have had little experience of inborn errors of metabolism, despite the fact that these conditions are not as rare as might be expected when working in a regional PICU. Detailed descriptions of individual conditions are available in textbooks of paediatrics and metabolic disease. In such texts, for clarity, they are usually classified and presented by biochemical pathway. Although such references are essential they are not duplicated here. Instead a pragmatic approach is preferred, focussing more upon the manner of presentation and the intensivist's role in a multidisciplinary team that includes expert paediatric biochemists, paediatricians, dieticians, liaison nurses, social workers, etc. As part of this team the intensivist is required to recognise new cases, even when they present covertly and to **resuscitate, diagnose** and **treat** patients presenting in crisis.

Inborn errors start as a consequence of a genetic mutation in the coding for a specific enzyme in a biochemical pathway. This results in a reduction in the enzyme's activity, not necessarily a complete absence of the enzyme. In any case this has two crucial consequences:

1   levels of precursors to the reaction that the enzyme catalyses build up and may then follow alternative routes of metabolism
2   the normal products of the reaction (which may include ATP production, i.e. energy) are decreased.

These patterns of biochemical derangement are reflected in the clinical presentation. Build-up of precursors and by-products is most evident in amino and organic acidurias, urea cycle defects and the storage diseases. Energy deficiency is more prominent in mitochondrial and fatty acid oxidation disorders. In some disorders both phenomena are prominent since they are by no means mutually exclusive.

The intensive care approach is, as usual, prioritised.

Resuscitate

When a patient presents in a collapsed state as a result of a metabolic crisis, do not get put off if the child's parents hand you a brown envelope with a letter in it stating that the patient has, for example, phosphofructokinase deficiency. Now is not the time for a medline search or a visit to the reference library. You must adopt a prioritised approach to airway, breathing and circulation.

A depressed level of consciousness or seizures will lead to inadequate airway protection and may require intubation. Always give plenty of oxygen but be sure to recognise hypoventilation early (saturation monitors are not sensitive monitors of ventilation for patients receiving supplemental oxygen). A patient with a metabolic acidosis who is not hyperventilating may be in danger of abrupt apnoea. Look for evidence of shock and *always check the blood glucose* during any resuscitation. Treat correctable causes of convulsions such as hypoglycaemia before giving anticonvulsants and remember how few indications there are for intravenous bicarbonate. Also remember to recheck the glucose to be sure that your dose had the desired effect.

Diagnose

The diseases vary in their capacity to produce acute life-threatening crises and hence gravitate to the PICU. Furthermore the presentation may occur in a variety of ways. A high index of suspicion should be applied to children of all ages presenting with:

- near miss sudden infant death syndrome
- postulated septicaemic collapse with sterile cultures (neutropaenia and thrombocytopaenia are common features of organic acidaemias)
- acute neurological disturbance, intractable seizures or hypotonia
- acute liver failure, prolonged neonatal jaundice (see Chapter 6, Neonatology) or hepatosplenomegally
- cardiomyopathy
- haemolysis
- characteristic biochemical derangement (after exposure to a specific agent or during the catabolism associated with an intercurrent illness), for example
  - hypoglycaemia
  - hyperammonaemia
  - metabolic acidosis
- intractable vomiting
- a characteristic odour (often accentuated in the urine)
  - musty   phenylketonuria
  - cabbage   tyrosinaemia
  - maple syrup   maple syrup urine disease
  - sweaty feet   isovaleric acidemia, glutaric acidemia type ii
  - cat urine   carboxylase deficiencies
- hepatosplenomegaly, which in this context implies a storage disorder for which PICU presentation is usually incidental.

Look for a history of parental consanguinity and illness in the extended family (n.b. mitochondrial DNA follows maternal inheritance). Look for a history of previous episodes or of failure to thrive. During the clinical examination look for the features listed above and for evidence of dysmorphism (which is rare in those disorders that present in metabolic crisis but will occur for example in peroxisomal and storage disorders) or virilisation (seen in some forms of congenital adrenal hyperplasia).

Perform appropriate screening tests, starting with electrolytes (including chloride), glucose, acid–base, ammonia, liver function tests and urine amino and organic acids.

ELECTROLYTES

Electrolyte derangements may accompany acid–base abnormalities as described on p. 123. Abnormal hydration or encephalopathy will need to be treated on their merits but do not miss the potential diagnostic significance of an electrolyte derangement. For example, an infant with hyponatraemia (especially a virilised patient or one with ambiguous genitalia) raises the possibility of salt losing congenital adrenal hyperplasia.

GLUCOSE

Stressed sick children may be hyperglycaemic (without ketosis) but more commonly get hypoglycaemic quickly. The more common causes of hypoglycaemia are poor nutritional reserve (e.g. growth retardation in neonates) and sepsis. Hyperinsulinism is rare but recognisable by the sheer quantity of glucose required to correct hypoglycaemia (up to 25 mg kg^{-1}min^{-1}). Hypoglycaemia is a feature of many inborn errors such as galactosaemia, glycogen storage diseases, fructose intolerance, propionic acidaemia and methylmalonic acidaemia. It may also occur in tyrosinaemia, maple syrup urine disease, leucine sensitivity and medium chain acyl CoA dehydrogenase deficiency (MCAD).

ACID–BASE

If a metabolic acidosis is detected then be sure that you have adequately treated any component of shock. Then calculate the anion gap to determine whether the acidosis can be ascribed to the Henderson–Hasselbach equation. If it can (anion gap < 12) then determine the source of bicarbonate wasting (e.g. renal or gastrointestinal tract). Bicarbonate wasting from the gastrointestinal tract is unlikely without a history or evidence of diarrhoea, or the presence of a jejunostomy.

Renal tubular acidosis (RTA)

If the anion gap is low and there is polyuria then suspect a proximal RTA. In this condition urine pH remains alkaline until serum bicarbonate falls to a level that the proximal convoluted tubules can keep pace with (as low as 15 mmol L^{-1}), after which urinary acidification is possible. Hyperchloraemia and hypokalaemia are common sequelae aggravated by secondary hyperaldosteronism. Glycosuria and aminoaciduria imply a more generalised proximal tubular dysfunction (Fanconi's syndrome) which may be associated with severe phosphate depletion. Fanconi's may occur as a primary or secondary phenomenon (cystinosis, Lowe's syndrome, galactosaemia, Wilson's disease, tyrosinaemia, fructose intolerance, medullary cystic disease, heavy metal poisoning, tetracyclines, proteinuric states, interstitial nephritis, or carbonic anhydrase inhibition).

Distal renal tubular acidosis is associated with a lower rate of loss of bicarbonate but urinary acidification below pH 5.8 is impossible and so severe acidosis may still result. An acid load (e.g. from ammonium chloride) can be used to distinguish cases presenting with bicarbonate levels > 15 mmol L^{-1} (proximal RTAs will respond by producing urine with pH < 5.5). Distal RTA can also be primary or secondary (e.g. to obstructive uropathy) and is commonly complicated by hypercalciuria. Hyperkalaemic forms are also recognised.

If the metabolic acidosis cannot be ascribed to the Henderson–Hasselbach relation (anion gap > 12 but often much higher) then set about identifying the additional acid(s) by measuring the following variables.

- Lactic acid level and lactate : pyruvate ratio (if available) to distinguish (1) metabolic derangements from hypoxic/ischaemic causes and (2) between metabolic causes. A low ratio implies pyruvate dehydrogenase deficiency whatever the lactate level. An elevated lactate with a normal ratio can also occur in pyruvate dehydrogenase deficiency or may reflect defects in gluconeogenesis, whereas elevated lactate with an elevated ratio implies anaerobic respiration, a respiratory chain defect, a mitochondrial myopathy or pyruvate carboxylase deficiency.
- Urine ketones.
- Urine amino and organic acids.
- Blood sugar and phosphate.

All samples must be taken during the acute phase, handled appropriately and analysed promptly or frozen. Even with these precautions, a diagnostic test result may still be elusive since these tests are subject to errors of spectrum and bias (e.g. from the effects of coexisting disease such as hepatic disease or renal failure). Mixed pictures are also common. For example, fatty acid oxidation defects cause ketosis, hyperammonaemia, and carnitine depletion. Thus the reliable interpretation of the results of these tests requires a paediatric biochemist. However in basic terms:

- Defects in most pyruvate pathways and mitochondrial energy metabolism cause elevated lactate : pyruvate ratios (as above).
- Ketosis is common in inborn errors (the normal ketones are acetoacetic acid and 3-hydroxybutyrate) but otherwise uncommon in sick neonates. Ketosis with hypoglycaemia implies a glycogen storage disease or defect in gluconeogenesis (ketosis and hyperglycaemia is diabetes mellitus).
- Non-ketotic hypoglycaemia implies a fatty acid oxidation defect, or hyperinsulinism.

AMMONIA

Hyperammonaemia to levels greater than 150 μmol L^{-1} produces encephalopathy. It is therefore particularly important to measure ammonia in patients with neurological abnormalities (including hypotonia or seizures). Hyperammonaemia (most often but not always without ketosis) implies a urea cycle defect, transient hyperammonaemia of the newborn or hepatic failure. Hyperammonaemia with ketosis occurs in organic acidaemias. The timing of the onset of (symptomatic) hyperammonaemia may also be of diagnostic significance. An early onset (first 24 hours of life) is more indicative of an organic acidaemia or transient hyperammonaemia. The severity is also of diagnostic significance. The upper limit of the normal range for the ammonia level is higher in neonates and trivial hyperammonaemia can occur as a secondary phenomenon in sepsis or ischaemic hepatic injury. Fulminant hepatic failure may raise levels as high as 400 μmol L^{-1} and transient hyperammonaemia of the newborn regularly produces levels above 1000 μmol L^{-1}.

LIVER FUNCTION TESTS

Inborn errors that cause severe acute hepatic failure tend to present in early life. Unconjugated hyperbilirubinaemia in the neonatal period may be due to defects of erythrocyte metabolism such as glucose-6-phosphate dehydrogenase deficiency and pyruvate kinase deficiency as well as the usual causes (physiological jaundice and a range of feto–maternal blood incompatibilities) and rarer defects of conjugation. However prolonged conjugated jaundice, elevated transaminases and hepatic failure may be caused by many inborn errors for example galactosaemia, tyrosinaemia and $\alpha_1$antitrypsin deficiency. Fulminating neonatal liver failure occurs in neonatal haemochromatosis, which is uniformly fatal without transplantation.

URINE (AND PLASMA) AMINO AND ORGANIC ACIDS

Characteristic profiles will often define many of these conditions. Note that you should really request these analyses whether or not a metabolic acidosis is present, and interpret the results with the aid of a paediatric biochemist.

The presence of encephalopathy has a diagnostic significance. Encephalopathy without hyperammonaemia or metabolic acidosis is still compatible with a diagnosis of inborn error of metabolism since it occurs in organic (and some amino) acidaemias such as non-ketotic hyperglycinaemia. It also occurs in molybdenum co-factor deficiency (look for low uric acid levels) and other conditions such as pyridoxine responsive seizures and peroxisomal disorders. It is important to distinguish cases where encephalopathy is caused or complicated by cerebral oedema and/or raised intracranial pressure.

OTHER SCREENING TESTS

Other screening tests that may prove useful are

- urine Clinitest® for reducing substances (fructose, lactose, galactose, pentose, salicylate, homogentisic acid, phenothiazines); the diagnosis of galactosaemia may be delayed if this screen is not performed.
- a glucose oxidase strip (specific for glucose).

Table 10.1 Methods of accelerating the removal of toxic metabolites.

High anion gap acidosis	carnitine (2.5–4 mg kg^{-1} hr^{-1} of 'L-carnitine', max. 125 mg hr^{-1})
Hyperammonaemia (150–500 µmol L^{-1})	sodium benzoate (neonate 250 mg^{-1} kg over 2 hr followed by 10–20 mg kg^{-1} hr^{-1}) or arginine (300 mg kg^{-1} i.v. over 2 hr) or phenylacetate (neonate 250 mg kg^{-1} over 2 hr followed by 10 mg kg^{-1} hr^{-1})
Severe hyperammonaemia (>500 µmol L^{-1} or severely encephalopathic)	haemofiltration / haemodialysis

The presentation, history, physical examination and the results of these screening tests may indicate second-phase investigations such as the need for a tissue diagnosis (liver, muscle or skin biopsy) or sequential tolerance tests to evaluate carbohydrate metabolism.

Treat

After resuscitation and the initial attempts at diagnosis the next priority is to *accelerate toxic metabolite excretion*.

Carnitine enhances the elimination of organic acids as carnitine esters. Furthermore carnitine deficiency can cause non-ketotic hypoglycaemia and can occur as a result of dietary deficiency or as a secondary phenomenon in organic acidaemias. Arginine reacts with ammonia aiding its excretion in urea cycle disorders. Sodium benzoate conjugates with glycine and phenylacetate conjugates with glutamine. Excretion of the conjugates clears circulating ammonia (irrespective of its cause). However extraordinary levels of ammonia such as those that can occur in transient hyperammonaemia of the newborn will additionally require haemofiltration since the quality of the neurological outcome is adversely affected by the duration of hyperammonaemia.

Meanwhile *prevent catabolism*, which otherwise exacerbates and prolongs most crisis presentations. Calories should be provided in the form of intravenous dextrose in quantities sufficient to maintain a high-normal blood glucose. Insulin therapy may further encourage anabolism. Protein and fat should be avoided until a diagnosis has been made and similarly avoid exposure to known precipitants or exacerbants, for example lactose in galactosaemia,

It may also be possible to augment residual enzyme activity (not all symptomatic patients have zero enzyme function) by prescribing cofactors (usually vitamins) for the relevant enzyme(s), for example thiamine, in maple syrup urine disease and Vitamin B$_{12}$ in methylmalonic acidaemia. Some patients with multiple carboxylase deficiency are responsive to biotin and some cases of Leigh's disease may transiently respond to thiamine.

A metabolic acidosis that is due to the ongoing production of acid will not respond adequately to intravenous bicarbonate. Attempts to maintain a normal pH in this way lead to hypernatraemia unless an anabolic state is achieved quickly (acid production stops). THAM (**T**ris-**h**ydroxymethyl-**a**ino**m**ethane) – a low sodium alternative to bicarbonate – is also hyperosmolar and under the same circumstances will still have to be given indefinitely (until anabolic) in similarly huge quantities with comparably short-lived effect. Severe symptomatic acidosis is best treated by dialysis or reasonably 'high volume' haemofiltration (up to 50 ml kg^{-1} hr^{-1}) with replacement using a fluid containing 35–40 mmol L^{-1} of bicarbonate.

Diabetic ketoacidosis (DKA)

Most cases of DKA do not require PICU admission. PICU admission should be reserved for patients with one or more of the following four criteria:

- young (< 2 years), depending upon local arrangements
- severely acidotic
- shocked (implying moderate (6%) dehydration) – remember low blood pressure is a late sign of shock by the definitions used in this book
- a level of coma that compromises airway protection reflexes.

These cases require a straightforward ABC approach to resuscitation and standard levels of intensive care monitoring ECG, CVP, arterial line, etc. The vast majority of patients with an altered state or depressed level of consciousness can still maintain an airway and should not be sedated as this confounds subsequent neurological assessment. However if the patient is delirious, agitated or confused then monitoring may be difficult to maintain and you will be thrown back on your clinical abilities. Deteriorating level of consciousness is covered under 'Troubleshooting' on p. 134, but beware the agitated patient who becomes easier to handle without becoming lucid. Even airway-competent individuals will require pre-emptive naso-gastric tube drainage because of the high incidence of gastric dilatation and vomiting.

Treat shock

Restoration of the circulating blood volume is a priority and should be achieved relatively rapidly, certainly within 2 hours. If colloids are used, like albumin, then it makes little sense to deduct their volume from the later calculation of fluid replacement regime since your choice was to use fluid that would not distribute outside the vascular space. However if your choice was to use saline for initial resuscitation then it will have required a greater volume and will have distributed more widely so it makes sense to include this volume in the calculation of the subsequent rehydration regime.

Rehydrate

Fluid deficit is estimated – see Chapter 7, Fluids, Electrolytes and Blood (3%, 6% or 9%) – but usually can only be determined retrospectively by the weight change associated with rehydration. Weigh the patient accurately. Remember that hyperosmolal dehydration may have a deceptively reduced effect on urea levels. Rapid rehydration is unnecessary once shock has been treated and carries a significant risk of aggravating cerebral oedema. Use saline (usually with 40 mmol/L of potassium added) for the initial fluid replacement.

fluid requirement = normal maintenance fluid + water deficit + ongoing losses

Replace water deficit over 48 hours. Continuing losses (remember the osmotic diuresis that is occurring) may be corrected hour by hour and can be given as intravenous additional normal (0.9%) saline or half-normal (0.45%) saline. The aim is to preserve osmolality as the serum glucose falls, which will entail a rise in serum sodium. Some people find a concept of sodium equivalence useful to predict the likely peak sodium level during rehydration. Sodium equivalence is the answer to the question 'What would the serum sodium be if all the hyperosmolarity was due to hypernatraemic dehydration?'

1 mmol L^{-1} of glucose and 1 mmol L^{-1} of sodium both = 1 mosmol L^{-1}

A fall in serum sodium should not occur with this regime but is almost inevitable with hypona-traemic resuscitation fluids. If it does occur despite the correct choice of resuscitation fluid then it is a worrying sign of sick cell syndrome or SIADH associated with cerebral oedema.

The sodium content of the rehydration fluid can usually be reduced to 0.45% 12 to 24 hours into rehydration (depending on the progress of the serum glucose in response to insulin replacement) and subsequently lower. Glucose can be introduced into the mainte-nance fluid once the serum glucose is below 15 mmol L^{-1}.

Treat biochemical derangement

Insulin replacement should be given by intravenous infusion – no other route will do. The starting rate is 0.1 units $kg^{-1}hr^{-1}$ of soluble insulin. Only rarely will it need to be higher. Rising glucose levels are more likely to be caused by an inadequate fluid replacement regime, for example one which does not take account of ongoing losses. If the fall in serum glucose is excessive (> 5 mmol L^{-1} hr^{-1}) then halve the infusion rate. Once serum glucose has fallen to below 12 mmol L^{-1} then adjust the rate according to a sliding scale, however do not discontinue the infusion until the acidosis has resolved, as it is insulin infusion that inhibits ketone production. If the serum glucose is low and the intravenous insulin infusion rate is already low (0.02 units $kg^{-1}hr^{-1}$) then it may be preferable to increase the dextrose supply. After 48 hours once haemodynamics and fluid flux have stabilised and the patient is well perfused, a change to subcutaneous insulin is made.

Serum potassium levels may be low, normal or high but there is always total body depletion of potassium. Hyperkalaemia responds to volume resuscitation and disappearance of the acidosis. Potassium should be added to initial replacement fluids (40 mmol L^{-1}) even if there is modest hyperkalaemia. Hyperkalaemic ECG changes and acute renal failure are legitimate reasons for deviation from this protocol. The former usually resolve with restoration of intravascular volume and potassium replacement can then be commenced after a delay of 1 to 2 hours. If acute renal failure has commenced (which is very rare) then management is difficult without continuous venovenous haemofiltration or dialysis. Sugar can easily be removed by dialysis and even these patients end up receiving some carefully titrated potassium supplement usually as a trim in the dialysate.

The rules relating to bicarbonate therapy (outlined above) show that it is clearly **NOT** indicated in the vast majority of cases of DKA.

Troubleshooting
DETERIORATING CONSCIOUS LEVEL

This raises the urgent need to treat or exclude cerebral oedema (but dont miss hypoglycaemia). This complication of DKA is far more common in children than adults and the peak time of presentation is 6 to 12 hours into the resuscitation. Prevention of cerebral oedema would be easy if it were just caused by over enthusiastic volume of fluid replacement or an inappropriate choice of fluid, but whilst these may aggravate it, the true cause is more complex and elusive. Subclinical cerebral oedema is common and may even precede resuscitation. A number of factors probably contribute independently and collectively to its exacerbation including the following.

- The presence of so-called 'idiogenic osmoles' formed within brain cells exposed to a hyperosmolar ECF. The ICF does not just get water depleted, these new osmotically active particles are formed. They appear to dissipate slowly and their quantity and/or osmotic activity may actually increase early in resuscitation. The water content of fluid replacement is consequently rapidly drawn into the cell leading to swelling.
- The speed with which glucose falls.
- The speed with which acidosis corrects.

The latter two factors are also related to the dose of insulin and its effects on membrane ion exchange as well as the fluid regime. Rapid reduction in glucose through dialysis is said to carry less risk of cerebral oedema than a rapid fall due to insulin.

Deteriorating conscious level should be assumed to be due to cerebral oedema and treated aggressively long before a Cushing's response occurs. Deterioration can be very rapid. Stop the rehydration regime, give a large dose of mannitol (1 g kg^{-1}) and initiate neuroprotective intensive care: an appropriate anaesthetic induction, intubation, ventilate to a low-normal $PaCO_2$ under sedation and paralysis, and restrict fluids. Then consider a cranial CT to confirm the diagnosis and exclude haemorrhage, etc. CT does not measure intracranial pressure and it is wise to assume that cerebrovascular autoregulation is deranged so it is likely that intracranial pressure monitoring and jugular venous bulb oximetry will be required if the diagnosis is confirmed. If cerebral oedema is not present then CT may detect other causes such as thrombosis, infarction or haemorrhage.

PERSISTENT ACIDOSIS

This is usually explicable by persistent ketosis and hyperglycaemia and requires either more insulin or more time. Other exacerbating factors may be hyperchloraemia or hypophosphataemia. When phosphate depletion persists after correction of acidosis, 2,3-diphosphoglyceric acid depletion causes a left shift in the haemoglobin dissociation curve and relative hypoxaemia predisposing to lactic acidosis. The phenomenon is correctable with phosphate supplementation. The routine administration of phosphate in DKA may cause hypocalcaemia.

11 Respiratory System

- **Differences between babies, children and adults**
- **Clinical picture of generic 'respiratory failure'**
- **Kinetics of respiratory gases**
- **Ventilation**
- **Non-invasive monitoring**
- **Respiratory support**
- **Extracorporeal membrane oxygenation (ECMO)**
- **High frequency ventilation**
- **Novel approaches to ventilation**
- **Short notes on specific conditions**

Infants and children have less respiratory reserve than adults, leading to a relatively high incidence of respiratory failure during severe illness. This is true even when the patient's primary pathology is in another organ system. Indeed, in both physiological and therapeutic terms, the pulmonary component of intensive care is difficult to separate from other factors such as the cardiovascular, nutritional and metabolic states. Respiratory support for children includes the provision of a secure upper airway and may be indicated:

- for the exercise implications of the work of breathing
- to supplement gas exchange
- for desirable haemodynamic effects
- during sedation or anaesthesia
- in neurological disease

DIFFERENCES BETWEEN BABIES, CHILDREN AND ADULTS

Neonates breathe predominantly through their noses. The position of the larynx is high (C4) and anterior, and the trachea bifurcates at the level of T2. During infancy the larynx and carina gradually descend to assume the adult positions (C6 and T4, respectively). The large, soft epiglottis in infants tends to obscure the laryngeal inlet and throughout childhood the larynx has a gradually tapering shape. The narrowest part of the child's airway is at the level of the cricoid cartilage which corresponds to the subglottic region (Figure 11.1) and any degree of oedema or narrowing exerts a more profound effect on airways resistance in smaller patients. Beyond puberty the vocal cords are the narrowest part of the airway. Uncuffed endotracheal tubes are considered mandatory for children under twelve to minimise the risks of sub-glottic stenosis.

In early life the rib cage is cartilaginous rather than bony, and its elasticity gives the chest wall a tendency to collapse. The ribs are aligned horizontally so that there is less movement in the anterior–posterior direction. Breathing is primarily diaphragmatic and can be seriously impaired by abdominal distension. As children grow, they assume more adult proportions and an upright posture. As part of this process intercostal muscles and 'bucket handle' rib movements become more significant in breathing.

The elastic recoil of the lung is low in infants and the intra-pleural pressure is therefore less negative. This is accompanied by relatively poor total chest compliance (1/20th adult values) because of low lung compliance and high airways resistance (15 × adult values). Thus the neonatal time constant is less than an adult (as low as 0.3 seconds in premature neonates with restrictive lung disease). Babies have a high closing volume, which is especially noticeable when it is expressed as a proportion of their functional residual capacity. However their metabolic rate is much higher than in older children and adults. This is part of the reason why

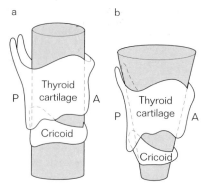

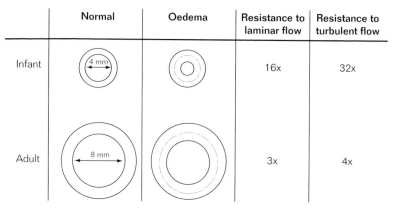

Figure 11.1 Shape and size of the airway. The adult larynx (a) showing its cylindrical nature; the narrowest part is at the vocal cords. The infant larynx (b) showing its cone shaped structure. The transition from the use of an uncuffed to a cuffed endotracheal tube is usually made after puberty. The proportionately greater impact of the same degree of oedema (1 mm) in a smaller airway is calculated in terms of airways resistance, showing why croup is a childhood disease. (With permission from Bion J. (ed.) *Intensive Care Medicine* BMJ Books).

respiratory rate and therefore alveolar ventilation are higher. The high level of alveolar ventilation reduces the effectiveness of the functional residual capacity (FRC) as a buffer between inspired gases and the pulmonary circulation. These terms and their physiology are explained in more detail later in this chapter but it is important to realise from the outset that for these reasons **any interruption in ventilation very quickly leads to hypoxaemia**.

CLINICAL PICTURE OF GENERIC 'RESPIRATORY FAILURE'

It is often necessary to intervene early and electively to support respiration in the critically ill child. Any reduction in muscle tone or respiratory drive, whether from residual anaesthetics, muscle relaxants, fatigue, coma etc., causes a reduction of tidal volume and FRC, exacerbating the tendency to hypoxia. Simultaneously, closure of small airways, decreased compliance (at low lung volume), decreased alveolar minute ventilation and atelectasis occur, all of which increase the work of breathing. The spontaneously breathing child may attempt to compensate for this by increasing respiratory rate and neonates may instinctively grunt which induces positive end expiratory pressure (PEEP). But the combination of fatigue, increased physiological deadspace, and perhaps drug-induced depression of the ventilatory response to carbon dioxide, can combine to prevent restoration of alveolar minu̶ tion. The neonate is even more likely to tire because the diaphragm and intercosta contain a lower percentage of type 1 (slow twitch, high oxidative) muscle fibres ᵢ first few months of life. As respiratory arrest approaches through exhaustion or hyp̶ᵤₓᵢₐ, the child becomes flaccid and respiratory effort dwindles as consciousness is lost.

The clinical picture of respiratory failure is that of a pale, quiet child breathing quickly and using accessory muscles, or of babies concurrently grunting in expiration. Intercostal and subcostal recession are early signs of distress in babies. In children over 5 years, who have a less compliant thorax, they are manifestations of very severe difficulty and imply primary respiratory disease.

KINETICS OF RESPIRATORY GASES

Much of the physiology of respiration, that is of importance in the PICU, is a consequence of the chemical properties of oxygen and carbon dioxide. Oxygen is poorly soluble in water (solubility coefficient 0.0031 ml mmHg^{-1}dL^{-1}) and requires a transport molecule (haemoglobin) to facilitate the movement of serviceable quantities to the cells in the periphery. Each gram of (adult) haemoglobin can carry 1.36 ml of oxygen, which first has to dissolve in the aqueous phase and diffuse from the lumen of the alveolus into a red cell. This makes the overall process of oxygen uptake comparatively slow. In contrast carbon dioxide dissolves rapidly and diffuses comparatively easily.

Oxygen uptake

At *any* respiratory membrane the uptake of oxygen is critically determined by the quantity of haemoglobin supplied to areas where oxygen is accessible. Thus the important factors in oxygen exchange are:

- the amount of blood flow (e.g. the cardiac output)
- the haemoglobin concentration
- the *effective* surface area of the respiratory membrane (after the effects of shunt, dead-space and ventilation-perfusion matching)
- the diffusion gradient for oxygen.

Each of these parameters should be optimised in the intensive care setting.

Carbon dioxide removal – *depends on minute ventilation*

Carbon dioxide diffuses easily across respiratory membranes and dissolves quickly in water. A simple consequence of this physical chemistry determines that the principal factor in carbon dioxide exchange across a respiratory membrane is the diffusion gradient for carbon dioxide. However, since equilibration of carbon dioxide across respiratory membranes occurs quickly, the rate-limiting step in clearing carbon dioxide from the body is the rapidity with which equilibrated (alveolar) gas at the respiratory membrane is replaced with fresh gas into which carbon dioxide can diffuse. The expression for this quantity is the minute ventilation (tidal volume × respiratory rate).

Oxygen content

It is helpful to express the oxygen content of blood as:

$$(1.36 \times [Hb] \times \% \text{ saturation}) + (0.0031 \times Pa_{O_2})$$

The significance of the P_{O_2} in terms of blood oxygen content is achieved through the % saturation of haemoglobin. Thus 15 g dL^{-1} of 100% saturated haemoglobin carries:

$$(1.36 \times 15) \text{ ml of } O_2 = 19.4 \text{ ml dL}^{-1}.$$

139

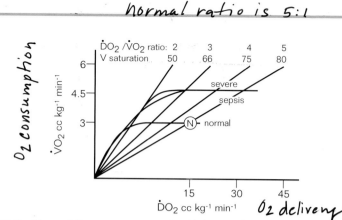

normal ratio is 5:1

O_2 consumption

O_2 delivery

Figure 11.2 Oxygen delivery versus consumption. Under normal circumstances oxygen delivery far exceeds consumption. As delivery falls, extraction increases – hence the superimposed venous saturations. Below a critical point (usually a ratio of 2:1) oxygen consumption becomes dependent upon the rate of delivery. In sepsis this biphasic relation is blunted and rate-dependent consumption occurs earlier e.g. a $\dot{D}O_2:\dot{V}O_2$ ratio of 3:1. NB Do not infer that the relationship between $\dot{D}O_2:\dot{V}O_2$ will always be reflected by the mixed venous oxygen saturation in sepsis. Once peripheral arteriovenous shunts become significant the utility of the mixed venous oxygen saturation is reduced. (With permission from Bartlett RH. Critical Care Physiology Little Brown & Co 1996.)

Add this to the trivial 0.3 ml dL^{-1} of dissolved oxygen and arterial oxygen content is determined at approximately 20 ml dL^{-1}. Repeating this calculation for mixed venous blood (75% saturation) gives an oxygen content of approximately 15 ml dL^{-1} and an arteriovenous oxygen difference ($AVDO_2$) of 5 ml dL^{-1}.

Oxygen delivery

The oxygen delivery ($\dot{D}O_2$) to the tissues, is the product of the oxygen content and the volume of blood being pumped per unit time (cardiac output). The Fick principle, i.e.

blood flow = rate of oxygen consumption ÷ $AVDO_2$

can be paraphrased to the relation that oxygen uptake across the lung is equivalent to oxygen consumption by the tissues. Since the $AVDO_2$ in our example is 5 ml dL^{-1} then oxygen consumption is 5 ml dL^{-1} of blood flow. Typical values for neonates are in fact 7 to 10 ml dL^{-1} and 3 to 4 ml dL^{-1} for adults. Thus knowledge of the cardiac output or index and the $AVDO_2$ quantifies the rate of oxygen consumption ($\dot{V}O_2$) as well as delivery, assuming that blood flow is dispersed to and returned from the tissues appropriately (which may not always be true).

Oxygen consumption

Under normal circumstances oxygen delivery far exceeds oxygen consumption (the oxygen content of venous blood never falls to zero). This physiological reserve is demonstrated in Figure 11.2. Homeostatic mechanisms support these relationships. For example cardiac output increases in the face of acute hypoxia or anaemia to maintain the $\dot{D}O_2$ at its normal 5:1 ratio with $\dot{V}O_2$ (although this response does not occur in premature neonates). In chronic hypoxia the red cell mass increases to levels again sufficient to restore the $\dot{D}O_2$. The exception occurs when cardiac output falls. In the absence of other compensatory mechanisms the tissues extract more oxygen from the supplied blood and the $AVDO_2$ increases – hence the significance of the measurement of mixed venous oxygen content on the ICU.

Oxygen delivery : oxygen consumption relation ($\dot{D}O_2$:$\dot{V}O_2$)

Primary changes in oxygen delivery ($\dot{D}O_2$) do not alter the rate of oxygen consumption ($\dot{V}O_2$) until $\dot{D}O_2$ falls to a ratio of 2 : 1 with $\dot{V}O_2$, whereupon $\dot{V}O_2$ becomes $\dot{D}O_2$ dependant. Why the critical lower limit of this ratio is not 1:1 is not clear. Not all of the oxygen bound to haemoglobin is freely available to the tissues but the haemoglobin dissociation curve only flattens at P_{O_2} values below the physiological range. Microcirculatory perfusion factors such as the inter-capillary distance do contribute and partly explain why the lower limit of the ratio is set even higher in systemic sepsis. Where expansion of the interstitial fluid spaces widens the inter-capillary distances and tissue perfusion is poor due to pre-capillary arteriovenous shunts. In any case, once the critical lower limit of the $\dot{D}O_2$:$\dot{V}O_2$ relation is passed, anaerobic metabolism occurs at a cellular level, acidosis develops and an 'oxygen debt' is incurred.

Haemoglobin dissociation curve

Under most circumstances the intrinsic changes in the affinity of haemoglobin for oxygen have more significance in terms of the behaviour of haemoglobin at different sites within the body than the overall $\dot{V}O_2$:$\dot{D}O_2$ relation, i.e. an increased propensity for binding oxygen in the lung and surrendering it in the tissues. The affinity of haemoglobin for oxygen is decreased (dissociation curve shifted to the right and flattened) by increased [H⁺], temperature, 2,3-DPG and P_{CO_2} (Figure 11.3). Foetal haemoglobin is left shifted compared to adult and is less sensitive to 2,3, DPG.

Shunt   — no amount of hyperventilation will fix this !

Blood returning from non-ventilated alveoli will be hypoxic and no amount of hyperventilation or alteration of the fraction of inspired oxygen (F_iO_2) to ventilated alveoli will compensate for this. This phenomenon is referred to as 'venous admixture' or 'shunt' (Figure 11.4) and is considered in more detail below. In contrast, carbon dioxide excretion is determined by the alveolar minute ventilation. Even if a significant proportion of alveoli are perfused but not ven-

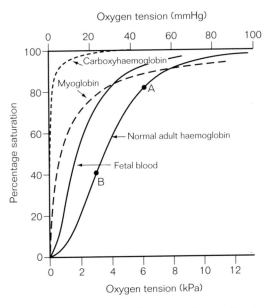

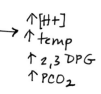

← Fetal Hb

→ ↑[H+]
  ↑ temp
  ↑ 2,3 DPG
  ↑ PCO₂

Figure 11.3 Oxyhaemoglobin dissociation curves. In a normal adult, point A represents serious hypoxia and B the level at which consciousness is lost. The point of note is that A is dangerous because it is on the inflection point of the curve so that a small drop in oxygen tension causes a profound drop in oxygen saturation of haemoglobin and hence oxygen content. (With permission from Nunn JF 1993, *Applied Respiratory Physiology* Heinemann Educational Publishers; p. 273.)

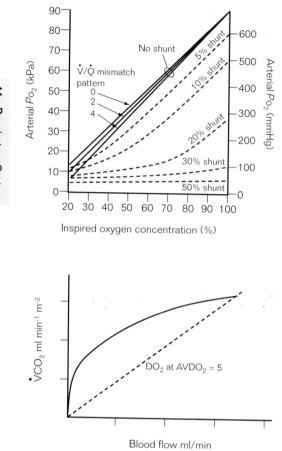

Figure 11.4 Effects of V̇/Q̇ mismatch and shunt upon arterial Po₂. Effect of increasing degrees of V̇/Q̇ mismatch in the absence of shunt (continuous lines) compared to degrees of shunt (dashed lines). A concave downward curve implies that the aetiology is V̇/Q̇ mismatch, a concave upward curve implies shunt. (With permission from Nunn JF 1993, *Applied Respiratory Physiology* Heinemann Educational Publishers; p. 188.)

Figure 11.5 Blood flow versus AVDO₂ and CO₂ clearance. Oxygen delivery (DO₂) is a product of blood oxygen content and cardiac output. Hence for a given arterial–venous oxygen difference (AVDO₂ (= 5 vol% in this instance) there is a linear relation with blood flow (dotted line). The clearance of CO₂ for a typical Pvco₂ is shown (heavy line). At physiological blood flow levels (to the right of the graph) the curve is virtually flat. (Adapted from Chapman RA, Bartlett RH 1991 Extracorporeal Life Support Manual. University of Michigan, Ann Arbor; p. 39.)

tilated, hyperventilation of the remainder can clear sufficient carbon dioxide and equilibration with the rest of the blood occurs during venous admixture. While ventilated alveoli have to receive some blood in order to clear carbon dioxide the flow required is remarkably low compared to that necessary for oxygen uptake (Figure 11.5). Carbon dioxide retention is not a feature of low pulmonary blood flow except in extreme (pre-terminal) situations.

Respiratory exchange ratio (quotient)

Carbon dioxide is produced in quantities determined by the respiratory quotient (RQ or R), which varies according to the principal substrate of chemical respiration.

$$RQ = CO_2 \text{ produced} \div O_2 \text{ consumed}$$

Respiratory Substrate	RQ
Fat	0.7
Protein	0.8
Carbohydrate	1.0

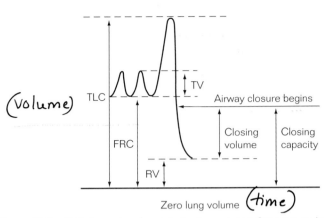

(Volume)

(time)

Figure 11.6 Static lung volumes and closing lung volumes. Spirogram to demonstrate normal static lung volume nomenclature. The y axis is volume and the x axis is time during two normal breaths, a maximum inspiration followed by maximal expiration. The closing volumes are included to help one to visualise how the closing volume to FRC ratio may vary as it does between children and adults. TLC – total lung capacity, FRC – functional residual capacity, RV – residual volume, TV – tidal volume. (With permission from Nunn JF 1993, *Applied Respiratory Physiology* Heinemann Educational Publishers; p. 83.)

Majority of CO_2 in blood is as bicarb.

Factors that affect the VO_2 will therefore have knock-on effects on carbon dioxide production. The majority of carbon dioxide present in the blood is in the form of bicarbonate anions which are in equilibrium with the dissolved/aqueous carbon dioxide. However, it is this latter component that equilibrates with alveolar gas at the respiratory membrane, and bicarbonate levels do not fluctuate quickly. In health, the carbon dioxide production in the periphery and excretion in the lung are in equivalence and the arteriovenous difference for carbon dioxide is (like that for oxygen) approximately 5 ml dL^{-1}.

VENTILATION

Describing respiratory gas exchange

Breathing, whether mechanically assisted or otherwise, establishes a process of gas flow between the outside world and the lung. The gas within the lung is normally described in terms of 'static' lung volumes defined by the actual or potential pattern of gas flow through them (Figure 11.6). In conceptual physiological terms however, a three compartment model is used:

- alveolar ventilation (which achieves perfect gas exchange)
- physiological dead-space (gas which does not participate in gas exchange)
- shunt (blood which does not participate in gas exchange).

Forces impeding gas flow

The forces opposing the gas flow involved in breathing are made up from elastic and non-elastic (frictional) components. The elastic forces are quantified by the 'elastance' (the reciprocal of 'compliance'). The elastance of the lung is greatly decreased by surfactant. On the ICU, the elastance/compliance of the thorax is often added to that of the lung so that as a single unit, total elastance/compliance (C_{LT}) are discussed simultaneously.

The non-elastic forces opposing gas flow are those of airways resistance, the influences of laminar and turbulent flow and the inertia of gas, chest wall, etc. (negligible at normal respiratory frequency). Airways resistance is greater in expiration and at low lung volumes. It may have dynamic components from bronchospasm or flow-related effects. The 'time constant' is the product of compliance and airways resistance. Areas of the lung with reduced compliance and restrictive lung diseases generate short time constants (rapid, small-volume changes) and those with high airway resistance have long time constants (slower, larger volume changes).

Derangements of gas exchange

The four principal respiratory derangements are:

- hypoventilation
- diffusion impairment
- shunt
- ventilation perfusion ($\dot{V}/\dot{Q}$) mismatch

Hypoventilation

Hypoventilation by definition causes carbon dioxide retention because the rate at which alveolar gas is replaced is decreased. However a reduction in alveolar ventilation also causes hypoxia (type II respiratory failure). If an abrupt interruption of ventilation occurs, the fall in Pa_{O_2} is much faster than the rise in Pa_{CO_2}, which is buffered against bicarbonate. The alveolar gas equation links the $P_{A}O_2$ (alveolar P_{O_2}) to the inspired oxygen tension (P_iO_2) and the arterial Pa_{CO_2}.

> ### Alveolar gas equation
>
> $P_{A}O_2 = P_iO_2 - (Pa_{CO_2} \div R) + F$
>
> R = respiratory exchange ratio (or quotient) and F = correction factor. F is required for volume differences between inhaled and exhaled gas. These occur as a secondary effect of the respiratory exchange ratio or changes in inert gas volume, for example inhalational anaesthetic. In normal breathing F is often ignored.

The relation to P_iO_2 is linear, so the hypoxia of hypoventilation can be easily overcome by raising mean airway pressure or preferably FiO_2. An extreme example is apnoeic oxygenation, a technique used in tandem with extracorporeal carbon dioxide removal or without it to allow toleration of apnoeic carbon dioxide retention during the diagnosis of brain stem death.

Diffusion impairment

Diffusion impairment limits the time available for equilibration of alveolar gas and circulating blood. Diffusion capacity is limited in babies but in older children the physiological reserve is large. When disease affects diffusion capacity it causes hypoxia without carbon dioxide retention (type I respiratory failure) and the hypoxia can again be corrected by increasing the inhaled oxygen tension (diffusion gradient for oxygen).

Shunt

Shunt (blood supply without ventilation) is an extreme form of $\dot{V}/\dot{Q}$ mismatch ($\dot{V}/\dot{Q} = 0$) which, as discussed above, causes a form of hypoxia which is characteristically resistant to increases in the inhaled oxygen tension. Carbon dioxide clearance is unaffected (or increased by spontaneous hyperventilation).

> ### Shunt equation
>
> $Q_S \div Q_T = (C_c - C_a) \div (C_c - C_{\bar{v}})$
>
> Q_S = shunt flow, Q_T = total flow (cardiac output), C_c = oxygen content of end capillary pulmonary venous blood (calculated from alveolar P_{O_2} assuming complete equilibration), C_a = oxygen content of arterial blood, $C_{\bar{v}}$ = oxygen content of mixed venous blood.

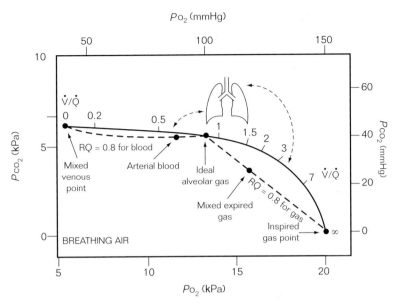

Figure 11.7
Variation in V̇/Q̇. The heavy line indicates all possible values for P_{O_2} and P_{CO_2} when breathing air with V̇/Q̇ varying from 0 (shunt – perfused but not ventilated) to ∞ (ventilated but not perfused). During upright posture the V̇/Q̇ varies within the lung in the manner demonstrated. Note that at P_{O_2} within physiological range within the lung, it will not bear a linear relationship to the % saturation. (With permission from Nunn JF 1993, *Applied Respiratory Physiology* Heinemann Educational Publishers; p. 166.)

Shunt calculations are usually made while breathing an $F_{I_{O_2}}$ of 1. When they are made in lower $F_{I_{O_2}}$ concentrations they attract other names such as 'physiological shunt' or 'venous admixture'. In the presence of low but non-zero V̇/Q̇, shunt calculations performed in an $F_{I_{O_2}}$ of less than 0.5 overestimate the 'true' shunt. They will respond but are relatively resistant to increasing $F_{I_{O_2}}$.

'V̇/Q̇ mismatch'

V̇/Q̇ mismatch can produce disturbances that tend towards shunt (venous admixture) or in the opposite direction (i.e. ventilation without perfusion). It is a common cause of blood gas disturbance in disease. Blood in areas of the lung that are perfused but not ventilated tends to maintain the gas composition of mixed venous blood, and that in areas that are ventilated but not perfused adopts the gas composition of inspired gas (Figure 11.7). In larger (older) children V̇/Q̇ decreases in dependent areas of the lung (less ventilation and more perfusion). Posture-related V̇/Q̇ mismatch contributes to a small physiological alveolar–arterial oxygen difference, which is magnified in disease. In a similar manner to hypoventilation, V̇/Q̇ initiated changes in $P_{a_{O_2}}$ are more rapid than $P_{a_{CO_2}}$. This is because oxygen consumption continues unabated and oxygen stores are small, whereas dissolved carbon dioxide is buffered against bicarbonate. The V̇/Q̇ relationships are described by the V̇/Q̇ equation.

Ventilation perfusion (V̇/Q̇) equation

$$V_A \div Q = 8.63 \times R \times (Ca_{O_2} - C\bar{v}_{O_2}) \div P_{A_{CO_2}}$$

V_A = alveolar ventilation, Q = perfusion, R = respiratory quotient, Ca_{O_2} = arterial oxygen content, $C\bar{v}_{O_2}$ = mixed venous oxygen content and $P_{A_{CO_2}}$ = alveolar P_{CO_2}.

Interpreting hypoxia

Attempts to both quantify and distinguish the cause of hypoxia include tools such as the alveolar–arterial oxygen difference, which is derived from the alveolar gas equation (hypoxia from hypoventilation has a normal alveolar–arterial oxygen difference).

Alveolar–arterial oxygen difference $(A–aDO_2)$:

The ideal alveolar PO_2 (P_AO_2) is that which would pertain if there were no $\dot{V}/\dot{Q}$ mismatch (derived from the alveolar gas equation).

$A–aDO_2 = (P_{bar} – P_{water}) \times FiO_2 – (P_ACO_2 \div R) – PaO_2$

P_{bar} = barometric pressure, P_{water} = saturated water vapour pressure, FiO_2 = fractional inspired oxygen concentration, P_ACO_2 = alveolar PCO_2, R = respiratory quotient, PaO_2 = arterial PO_2.

Assuming that P_ACO_2 is equal to $PaCO_2$, then $A–aDO_2$ is usually

$(716 \times FiO_2) – (PaCO_2 \div 0.8) – PaO_2$ mmHg

$A–aDO_2$ is higher in babies (25 mmHg or 3.3 kPa) than in older children and adults but is lower in children than adults (< 10 mmHg, < 1.33 kPa). Its appeal is that unlike shunt calculations it does not rely on pulmonary arterial blood gas measurements. However the interpretation of a given $A–aDO_2$ depends on the PaO_2 and consequent position on the haemoglobin dissociation curve.

The 'physiological shunt' calculation assumes that shunt is responsible for all hypoxaemia and is expressed as the amount of mixed venous blood that would have to be mixed with ideal blood to give the observed PaO_2.

Physiological shunt

To perform this calculation C_i (the ideal end capillary pulmonary venous oxygen content) is substituted for C_c in the shunt equation given on p.144.

The converse assumption (that all hypoxia is due to the addition of dead-space gas) is used to calculate the 'physiological deadspace'.

Physiological dead space

$V_D \div V_T = (P_i – P_E) \div P_i$

V_D = dead-space, V_T = tidal volume, P_i = PCO_2 in ideal expired gas, P_E = PCO_2 in mixed expiratory gas. The arterial PCO_2 is usually substituted for the P_i.

The **pulmonary vascular resistance**, as with other regional circulations is critically determined by the diameter of the resistance vessels. There are relations therefore with vascular tone, which can be manipulated by drugs and relations with lung volume (Figure 11.8) conferred by stretching out or compressing vessels. Most vasodilators drop pulmonary vascular tone but do so indiscriminately because they are delivered to all perfused areas of the lung. Their administration in the presence of $\dot{V}/\dot{Q}$ mismatch will aggravate the impact of areas of low $\dot{V}/\dot{Q}$ and ameliorate the impact of areas that are ventilated but not perfused. The hope and rationale behind inhaled nitric oxide therapy is that by virtue of its method of administration it will preferentially affect areas of $\dot{V}/\dot{Q} > 1$.

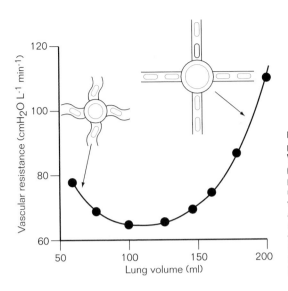

Figure 11.8 Lung volume and pulmonary vascular resistance. When capillary transmural pressure is kept constant, pulmonary vascular resistance rises at both low and high lung volumes, due to compression and stretch of vessels respectively. (With permission from West JB 2000 Respiratory Physiology, *The Essentials.* Lippincott Williams & Wilkins; Baltimore; p. 35.)

NON-INVASIVE MONITORING

Pulse oximetry

The mechanism by which oximetric data can be determined non-invasively is covered in Chapter 18, Physics for the Intensivist. The fundamental appeal of pulse oximetry is due to the far greater significance of haemoglobin saturation compared to the PaO_2 in determining oxygen delivery. The utility of these monitors is impaired by states of altered peripheral perfusion and movement artefact. Reduced perfusion can lead to an underestimation, as can a poorly applied probe in hyperdynamic states when venous pulsation may be detected. If the waveform is poor or the detected pulse rate does not match that of the ECG then the result is unreliable.

Transcutaneous gas electrodes

In mature patients, transcutaneous PO_2 is usually about 80 per cent of the PaO_2. The probes minimise these differences by warming the skin causing local vasodilatation and a right shift in oxyhaemoglobin dissociation. The result is closer agreement and a viable correlation with PaO_2 in premature neonates but in any age group results are still impaired by poor perfusion. Indeed, in older patients these probes are sometimes used as monitors of perfusion rather than oxygenation. Trancutaneous carbon dioxide measurements tend to overestimate $PaCO_2$, a tendency reduced by warming the probe but again aggravated by poor perfusion.

Capnography

Capnometers numerically display the end tidal PCO_2 ($P_{ET}CO_2$). Capnographs show the profile of the expiratory PCO_2 (P_ECO_2) over time. A normal capnograph has four phases (Fig 11.9).

phase I:	dead-space clearance (atmospheric carbon dioxide levels)
phase II:	rapid rise as expiration of alveolar gas starts
phase III:	'alveolar plateau' (slowly rising) culminating in the $P_{ET}CO_2$
phase IV:	fall as inspiration starts.

(a) The capnogram: a continuous trace of CO_2 concentration in expired air

(b) In airway obstruction such as asthma the plateau is lost creating a sawtooth appearance as in the lower of these two traces

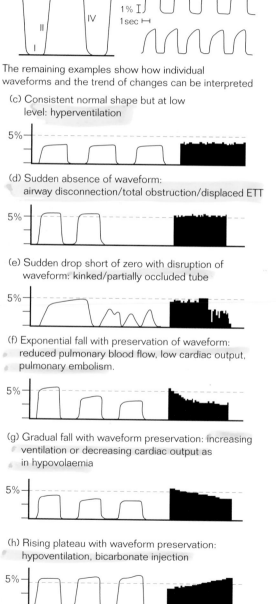

The remaining examples show how individual waveforms and the trend of changes can be interpreted

(c) Consistent normal shape but at low level: hyperventilation

(d) Sudden absence of waveform: airway disconnection/total obstruction/displaced ETT

(e) Sudden drop short of zero with disruption of waveform: kinked/partially occluded tube

(f) Exponential fall with preservation of waveform: reduced pulmonary blood flow, low cardiac output, pulmonary embolism.

(g) Gradual fall with waveform preservation: increasing ventilation or decreasing cardiac output as in hypovolaemia

(h) Rising plateau with waveform preservation: hypoventilation, bicarbonate injection

Figure 11.9 Capnograms.

Table 11.1 Inhaled oxygen concentration equivalents.

Nasopharyngeal catheter		Nasal cannula/face mask		Face mask + reservoir	
$ml\ kg^{-1}\ min^{-1}\ O_2\ flow$	FiO_2	$L\ min^{-1}$	FiO_2	$L\ min^{-1}$	FiO_2
75	0.3	1	0.22	6	0.6
100	0.4	2	0.25	7	0.7
200	0.5	3	0.27	8	0.8
250	0.6	4	0.3	9	0.85
		5	0.35	10 +	0.9
		6	0.4		
		7	0.45		
		8	0.5		

The normal $P_{ET}CO_2$ is close to the $PaCO_2$ and its most frequent use is to track alveolar ventilation and the size of the physiological deadspace. An abnormal $P_{ET}CO_2$ strongly suggests $\dot{V}/\dot{Q}$ derangement which can be confirmed by tracking the $PaCO_2 - P_{ET}CO_2$ difference. Changes in capnograph profile associated with increased $PaCO_2 - P_{ET}CO_2$ suggest changes in dead-space (such as those induced by anaesthesia) whereas changes in $PaCO_2 - P_{ET}CO_2$ with preservation of the profile reflect changes in effective pulmonary blood flow. These monitors can be used to check the integrity of endotracheal intubation. The leak associated with non-cuffed endotracheal tubes flattens the profile of the capnograph, and the use of continuous flow ventilators as well as ventilatory abnormalities (such as dynamic hyperinflation) further reduce the utility of the $P_{ET}CO_2$ as a marker of $PaCO_2$. At high respiratory rates (as in young infants) they lose resolution.

RESPIRATORY SUPPORT

Supplemental oxygen

Supplemental oxygen will usually relieve the hypoxia of hypoventilation and diffusion impairment, but with many methods of supplemental oxygen delivery it is difficult to measure the actual FiO_2 delivered. Table 11.1 gives FiO_2 approximations that are research based but intended as guides only.

Humidification

Humidification is one of the points in PICU clinical practice that proves the maxim that 'good intensive care is about making a big difference by doing simple things well'. Adequate humidification of inspired gases enables prolonged intermittent positive pressure ventilation (IPPV). Poor technique leads to dry and viscous secretions that occlude artificial and anatomical airways, causing respiratory obstruction and atelectasis. Simultaneously cilial motility is ablated and mucosal damage and hyperaemia occur that can predispose to infection.

Water vapour is odourless and colourless. The content of water vapour in a gas is described by the absolute or relative humidity. 'Absolute' humidity is the actual quantity of water vapour in a given volume of gas (expressed in mg L^{-1}). This quantity varies with temperature (Figure 11.10). To raise the absolute humidity of a gas that is already carrying its capacity of water vapour requires a heat source and a water source. The 'relative' humidity

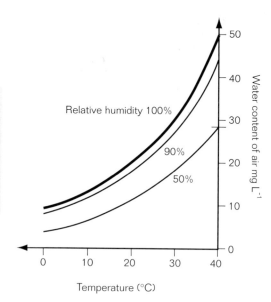

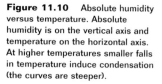

Figure 11.10 Absolute humidity versus temperature. Absolute humidity is on the vertical axis and temperature on the horizontal axis. At higher temperatures smaller falls in temperature induce condensation (the curves are steeper).

is an expression that relates the absolute humidity to the capacity of the gas to carry water vapour at a given temperature. Thus:

relative humidity = (water content ÷ water capacity) × 100

In saturated alveolar air the relative humidity is 100 per cent but the absolute humidity (44 mg L^{-1}) is more than double that of room air of the same relative humidity. The 'dew point' is the point at which saturation and condensation occur respectively during heating and cooling.

The process of raising the absolute humidity of inspired gas is achieved predominantly in the nose and as the temperature of exhaled air falls, an equivalent quantity of water is retrieved from the exhaled gas. Having said this the 'isothermic saturation boundary' (the point at which the inhaled gas reaches body temperature and 100% relative humidity) is frequently below the carina. The magnitude of the water exchange during inspiration and expiration depends on the temperature gradient between the alveolus and the tip of the nose. In a healthy individual this is about 5°C but the gradient is frequently less in a diseased person, in non-humid environments or if the upper respiratory tract is bypassed (e.g. by an endotracheal tube or tracheostomy) resulting in increased water loss. Failure to correct for these effects leads to the morbidity and potential mortality described above.

The more humid a gas the greater its capacity to transfer heat. The loss of humidified gas to the atmosphere can be a very significant heat loss.

When the airway is not intubated, low flow oxygen therapy via a nasal cannula can be delivered, without humidification, up to gas flows of 2 L min^{-1}. At higher flows simple bubble humidifiers (cold-water bath) will add to the humidification, and in warm environments they will achieve absolute humidities as high as 30 mg L^{-1}, but in most circumstances only about 10 mg L^{-1}. Such devices enable oxygen to be delivered at rates of up to 150 ml kg^{-1} min^{-1}. Heated water bath humidifiers are preferable but are difficult to regulate and suffer the drawback of condensation in the inspiratory limb. These humidifiers produce about 25 mg L^{-1} water vapour. Alternatively condensers such as a 'Swedish nose' may be placed in the airway, but small patients will not exhale sufficient water vapour to moisten them and they should therefore be kept wet with added saline. During mechanical ventilation with intubation, the inspired gas must be fully conditioned and a relative humidity of 100 per cent at body temperature achieved before inspiration. This humidity is usually realised using chamber (heated water bath) humidifiers, which heat the inspired gas to 37°C at the humidifier and then to 39°C using a heating wire in the inspiratory limb of the ventilator circuit to prevent 'rainout'. The inspired gas is thus approximately 90 per cent relative humidity at the end of the heating coil and cools to 37°C (100% relative humidity) in the connectors at the top of the endotracheal tube. Both chamber and airway temperatures are regulated by servo mechanisms. The humidification temperature is described as chamber temperature plus the additional temperature imparted in the airway (this is '37 plus 2' as described above). Continuous chamber feed of water avoids temperature fluctuations (and changes in the compressible volume of gas in the circuit). Cooling of the exhaled gases causes condensation and therefore necessitates the use of water traps in the expiratory limb of a ventilator circuit in order to avoid obstruction to gas flow.

Ultrasonic and anvil-type humidifiers increase the water content of gas further by generating nebulised water droplets as well as water vapour. Their use carries a significant risk of water intoxication and increases the density of the gas, thereby increasing turbulence and the work of breathing.

Mechanical ventilation

All mechanically ventilated patients require the close proximity of a full range of airway adjuncts, self-inflating bag, piped oxygen, T-piece, suction, etc. as a back up for equipment failure or compromise of the endotracheal intubation. Mechanical ventilators are only employed when the airway (and intubation where appropriate) are secure. It is customary to use uncuffed endotracheal tubes for pre-pubertal patients and the ideal size is associated with a small leak. The presence of a leak is detected by providing sustained inflation with a T-piece circuit and listening at the mouth, or it is inferred by a drop in expired tidal volume relative to inspired volume. The size of the leak will change with changes in airway diameter (e.g. because of oedema) and with changes in compliance associated with drugs such as relaxants or disease progression or resolution. The degree of leak that can be compensated for by adjusting ventilator settings is lower in non-compliant states. A worsening leak may ultimately require re-intubation with a larger endotracheal tube.

An appreciation of the therapeutics of mechanical ventilation requires an implicit understanding of both respiratory physiology and ICU technology. Despite the variety of ventilators and ventilation techniques the fundamental physical chemistry and physiology of oxygen and carbon dioxide are unchanged, so at one level one can still expect the novice to handle all devices appropriately.

CHOOSING A VENTILATOR

The choice is based upon power source, cycling characteristics, method of flow generation and the provision of gas supply for spontaneous breaths (this may not be the same as that for flow generation). The power source (usually pneumatic or electrical) influences the options for subsequent generation of gas flow (piston, bellows, motor, solenoid-regulated valve, microprocessor-regulated valve or interruption of a high-pressure gas source). Gas flow for spontaneous breaths can be addressed by the provision of continuous flow in the circuit, an inspiratory reservoir (± continuous flow) or a demand valve. The 'cycling' label is attached to the variable (pressure, time, volume or flow) that determines when inspiration stops and expiration starts. Cycling characteristics influence the choice of control modes that each ventilator can offer (e.g. pressure control and volume control). The terms 'support' or 'assist' are applied to modes where the breath is initiated by the patient. 'Mandatory' or 'control' breaths are initiated by the ventilator and may be blended with 'support' (e.g. synchronised intermittent mandatory ventilation with pressure support).

CHOOSING THE MODE OF VENTILATION

The choice of ventilation mode and start settings are made on the basis of :

• clinical examination

- age
- diagnosis
- available respiratory physiological information
- significance of cardiovascular and haemodynamic implications of IPPV
- fluid balance and distribution
- radiographic/CT appearances of the chest.

Once the patient is attached to the ventilator, the adequacy of ventilation is immediately assessed clinically through observation of chest movement, colour, perfusion and auscultation of the chest. A minimum standard of monitoring for typical, acutely ventilated patients includes:

- continuous pulse oximetry
- ECG monitoring
- an alarm that detects failure of cycling (circuit disruption)
- an alarm (integral to the ventilator or otherwise) that detects airway occlusion.

For neonates there is a historical preference for using continuous flow, pressure regulated, time cycled ventilators. They are less susceptible to the fluctuations in tidal volume that are generated by the disparity between tidal volume (V_T) and gas volume in the circuit. Also they do not generate large pressure fluctuations when the patient is uncoordinated with the ventilator and can function in the presence of a modest leak around the endotracheal tube. However when compliance changes (e.g. as muscle relaxants wear off, or disease severity worsens) large changes in delivered V_T occur. Despite being intrinsically sensitive in the detection of circuit disruption, older models may not be capable of detecting absent tidal volume (endotracheal tube blockage). They must therefore be used in combination with an apnoea monitor.

For older patients there is a historical preference for volume controlled ventilation – a mechanical bellows. Nevertheless, improved technology is making it easier and sometimes more appropriate to ventilate smaller patients with such devices. However even with newer models, when compliance changes or airway obstruction develops, airway pressure escalates and effective tidal volume is reduced as gas is compressed in the ventilator tubing.

Thus ventilator control variables must be monitored carefully but when you think about it you will realise that it is actually more important to monitor the effect of ventilator settings upon *non*-control variables. For example tidal volume in pressure-regulated modes

$$(V_T = \Delta P \times C)$$

and airway pressures in volume-controlled modes

$$\Delta P = V_T/C + (R \times F)$$

Table 11.2 summarises some relationships for pure forms of ventilator cycling in high and low compliance states and the legend explains the abbreviations used in this paragraph and in the Table.

In reality relevant safety features are included in ventilator design. Time cycled ventilators are usually pressure regulated or volume controlled and volume cycled ventilators are usually time limited. Ventilation nomenclature can also get confusing e.g. 'time cycled volume limited' is very similar to 'volume cycled', and ventilators designed to deliver one mode (e.g. volume control) can frequently provide others (e.g. pressure support or control).

MONITORING THE MECHANICS OF VENTILATION

The respiratory cycle consists of inspiration and expiration, which both have 'flow' and 'pause' phases. Inspiratory flow occurs at the beginning of inspiration as the result of a pressure gradient between the airway and lung. After a plateau phase, expiration is usually passive. Thus the expiratory pressure time, flow time and pressure volume traces are comparable between most ventilator modes, which is useful since they reflect the compliance and resistance of the system (lung and ventilator).

Table 11.2 Expected behaviour of ventilators in different cycling modes.

	Low compliance / high airways resistance	High compliance / low airways resistance
Volume cycled	V_T becomes a smaller percentage of cycled volume PIP increases	i.t. becomes short PIP falls
Pressure cycled	i.t. and V_T both fall	i.t. becomes very long V_T increases
Flow cycled	i.t. and V_T both fall	i.t. and V_T both rise
Time cycled	No effect	No effect

ΔP = pressure change, V_T = tidal volume, i.t. = inspiratory time, e.t. = expiratory time, C = total compliance, R = total airways resistance, F = flow, PIP = peak inspiratory pressure.

MANAGING VENTILATION: CONTINUOUS FLOW, PRESSURE REGULATED, TIME CYCLED

The start settings that one chooses must be appropriate to the patient and the disease. Premature babies with surfactant deficiency have short time constants and restrictive lung disease. Typical start settings would be peak inspiratory pressure (PIP) 20 to 25 cmH$_2$O, positive end expiratory pressure (PEEP) 3 cmH$_2$O, Fio$_2$ 0.5 and rate 60 with an inspiration : expiration time ratio (I : E) up to 1:1. Older patients (e.g. term babies) with non-restrictive lung disease or healthy lungs have longer time constants. They can be gently ventilated with longer inspiratory times (up to 1 sec) and slower rates. Focal disease such as lobar pneumonia in such patients may create shunt that is not amenable to escalating airway pressure. Babies with cyanotic lung disease and low pulmonary blood flow have normal or increased lung compliance and usually require very gentle ventilation.

With these ventilators the inhaled oxygen tension and the effective surface area of the lung are proportional to the mean airway pressure. Mean airway pressure may be increased by raising; flow rate, PIP, PEEP or inspiratory time (with a constant respiratory rate) (Figure 11.11). Since volumetric data is frequently not available, one has to infer the impact of ventilatory manoeuvres on the Paco$_2$ and check the blood gases for confirmation. The tidal volume is proportional to the difference between the PIP and the PEEP (although this is not a linear

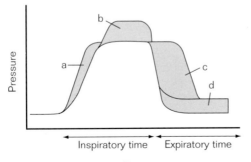

Time

Figure 11.11 Pressure–time curve: pressure control. For a continuous flow, pressure regulated, time cycled ventilator, the effective surface area of the lung is increased by increases in mean airway pressure. These can be achieved by increased flow (a), increased peak pressure (b), increased inspiratory time (keeping rate constant)(c) and increased end expiratory pressure (d). The 'square wave' appearance can be accentuated in inspiration by increased flow but is also accentuated by the short time constant of diseases like respiratory distress syndrome.

relationship). Increases in PIP and decreases in PEEP lower the $PaCO_2$. Additionally increases in respiratory rate will increase minute volume and decrease $PaCO_2$. For many reasons there has been a trend away from elective paralysis for mechanical ventilation in neonates. This requires alternative strategies to achieve coordination with the ventilator. Triggered modes are effective for lower respiratory rates but the more tachypnoeic babies are more likely to come in to phase with a mandatory rate set slightly faster than their intrinsic respiratory rate.

MANAGING VENTILATION: VOLUME CONTROLLED, TIME CYCLED $V_T \approx$

In volume controlled modes, tidal volume is estimated (at approximately 10 ml kg^{-1}), and a rate appropriate to the child's age and *disease* is selected. Minute and tidal volumes can be adjusted directly. To halve the $PaCO_2$ the minute volume is doubled. To increase the $PaCO_2$ by a third, the minute volume is reduced to three quarters of its current value, etc. PaO_2 is again related to the inhaled oxygen tension and the effective surface area of the lung. In essence these are managed by alteration of FiO_2, tidal volume and PEEP. Classic volume controlled ventilation involves delivery of constant flow during the inspiratory flow phase which gives a characteristic pressure–time relation (Figure 11.12). High flow rates give 'squarer' pressure-time curves and higher mean airway pressure.

Decelerating flow (very rapid in early inspiration) is more characteristic of the pressure control modes of volume regulated ventilators (Figure 11.13) but modern devices frequently

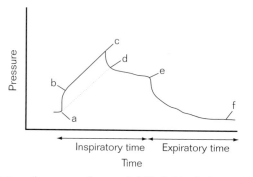

Figure 11.12 Pressure–time curve: volume control. The height ab gives an estimate of the resistance of the system (changes will most likely be due to the patient). The drop cd (due to flow cessation) is equivalent so the gradients of the slopes bc and ad can be used to assess compliance. The plateau de may not be horizontal if there is an air leak or if lung recruitment occurs. Expiration starts at e and a more gradual descent has been depicted reflecting ventilation of a lung with a longer time constant than in Figure 11.11.

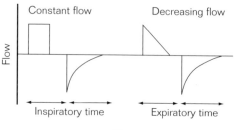

Figure 11.13 Flow time relation in volume control ventilation. This diagram demonstrates the flow and pause phases described in the text. Constant flow produces the classic pressure–time relation shown in Figure 11.12. Decelerating flow produces a squarer wave more like that in Figure 11.11.

incorporate this pattern into volume controlled modes as well to produce a 'squarer' pressure–time relation akin to that in Figure 11.11.

Longer inspired times and inverse I : E ratios may also improve oxygenation by contributing to lung recruitment. The hazards of such approaches include high PIP and intrinsic PEEP (expiratory flow–time curves that do not display a pause (zero flow). Intrinsic PEEP implies gas trapping and can contribute to dynamic hyperinflation. Intrinsic PEEP is not uniformly distributed within the lung and can preferentially affect diseased lung segments.

SUPPORT VENTILATION

In pressure support a predetermined continuous positive pressure is applied above PEEP during spontaneous inspiration. Inspiratory effort from the patient is sensed by a flow or pressure trigger and flow cycling is used to coordinate the duration of the positive pressure support, i.e. the support is withdrawn when inspiratory flow falls to a preset percentage of its peak (e.g. 25%). In volume support a similar decelerating flow velocity is used but the level of pressure applied during inspiration is microprocessor controlled to guarantee a predetermined tidal volume.

BIPHASIC POSITIVE AIRWAY PRESSURE (BIPAP)

Biphasic positive airway pressure is a form of pressure support ventilation (usually flow cycled). It can be administered via an endotracheal tube or by a face or nose mask to make it less invasive. This also makes it well tolerated. Most devices use an electric motor to generate continuous flow. In different settings the BiPAP breaths may be time cycled despite remaining flow triggered. Inspiratory and expiratory pressures can be adjusted independently so that continuous positive airway pressure (CPAP) (inspiration pressure = expiration pressure) can be delivered. Alternatively two levels of CPAP (BIPAP – capital I) can be provided by some devices in which spontaneous respiratory effort is superimposed over the biphasic CPAP each phase of which lasts several breaths. Although triggers ensure the change in pressure is co-ordinated with the respiratory cycle, no support is given per breath.

THE DIFFERENCE BETWEEN CPAP AND PEEP

Children have relatively high closing volumes and commonly require manoeuvres such as CPAP and PEEP to increase or preserve their functional residual capacity. True CPAP delivers positive pressure in inspiration and expiration. PEEP delivers positive pressure at the end of expiration but inspiratory pressure may be negative. The practice of describing both CPAP and PEEP by the end expiratory pressure can blur the difference between them but the work of breathing (represented in Figure 11.14 by the area within a pressure volume loop) is far greater using PEEP than CPAP. Many commonly used methods of generating artificial PEEP will deliver CPAP given sufficient gas flow. As a rule of thumb it requires flow

11 Respiratory System

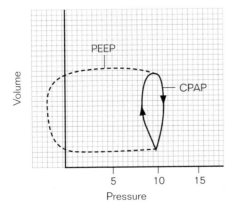

Figure 11.14 The difference between CPAP and PEEP. The solid loop represents CPAP – a positive pressure is maintained throughout the respiratory cycle. In PEEP (dashed line) pressure may drop significantly in inspiration. Patient work is related to the area within the loop (significantly less with CPAP for the same tidal volume). Many support devices generate PEEP and CPAP in the same way (partial occlusion of expiratory circuit) and depend upon the gas flow rate to distinguish the two. Gas flow must exceed peak inspiratory flow rate (estimated as three times the minute volume) to generate CPAP.

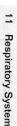

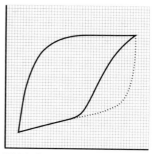

(a) Volume control with constant flow

(b) Modes with decelerating flow

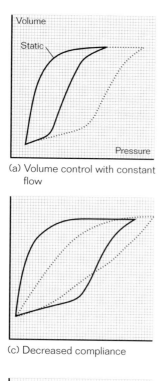

(c) Decreased compliance

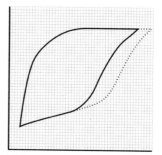

(d) Increased resistance

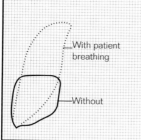

(e) Pressure support

Figure 11.15 Dynamic volume–pressure loops. These differ from static volume–pressure loops because of the additional pressure related to gas flow. They are broadened and the upper inflection point is slurred and may even be lost when the ventilator gas flow decelerates during inspiration (unless there is overdistension). Increased resistance further accentuates these changes whereas decreased compliance slurs the whole loop as shown. Decreased compliance flattens the loop altering the gradient of the inspiratory limb. In pressure support, greater tidal volumes can be achieved if the patient's effort is sustained during the breath rather than just managing to activate the trigger. Hence for a given level of support, the height of the V–P loop changes with the strength of the patient's effort.

greater than the peak inspiratory flow rate (so greater than 3 times the minute volume) to generate CPAP.

TROUBLE SHOOTING VENTILATION USING GRAPHICAL MONITORS

The graphical monitoring provided by many ventilators can be very useful provided that one remembers that it includes effects of both patient and circuit upon each measurement. However non-cuffed endotracheal tubes are associated with a deliberate air leak that can confound the monitors and the graphs are only poor approximations to controlled laboratory pulmonary function tests. For example true pressure–volume loops are assembled from serial static compliance measurements (e.g. via the 'super syringe' method); the dynamic loops generated during ventilator monitoring include errors generated by gas flow against airways resistance, etc. The higher the gas flow, the worse the effect but if gas flow is kept constant then changes in serial pressure–volume loops are more likely to reflect changes in lung compliance than other factors. Figure 11.15 shows the effects of ventilation with constant and decelerating flow upon the displayed pressure–volume relation. Changes in airways resistance and compliance upon the pressure–volume loops are also shown although these may be ablated in modes where flow decelerates during inspiration.

We have already mentioned the use of the flow–time curve in detecting dynamic hyperinflation. Further information can be obtained from the pressure–time relation. The difference in time constants between high airways resistance and decreased compliance are also reflected in the pressure–time relation of classic volume control. Low compliance elevates peak pressure (c in Figure 11.12) and the plateau (de) whereas plateau pressure is unaffected by increased airway resistance.

Diagnostic appearances of flow volume loops usually depend upon cooperation, coordination and active expiratory effort, which are frequently absent in intensive care patients but it is worth remembering the classic patterns of upper and lower airway obstruction.

DETERMINING OPTIMUM PEEP

From pressure–volume loop

If the aim of ventilation is to start inspiration between the inflection points of the inspiratory portion of the pressure–volume loop (given constant flow), then optimum PEEP can be chosen by defining the pressure of the first inflection point and setting PEEP at or above it. This should ventilate the lung within the range of best compliance. The beneficial effects of PEEP persist at lower levels however because of the lower closing pressure of the volume-recruited lung and the fact that the new pressure–volume loop (after PEEP) tracks the expiratory limb of that followed before PEEP.

From pressure–time curve

Further clues as to the probable position on the pressure–volume loop during ventilation can be given from the inspiratory, flow-phase, pressure–time relation (bc in Figure 11.12). If this region is convex then ventilation may be occurring below the first inflection point and if it is concave then the lung may be over distended since the pressure–volume loop in IPPV is steep at its upper right corner.

From estimates of hydrostatic forces

When the water content of the lung is high (pulmonary oedema, ARDS, MOSF) then the hydrostatic forces involved may help determine the optimum PEEP. The height of the water column that needs to be supported is implied by the anterior–posterior diameter of the chest. This leads to PEEP of 5 to 10 cm in a term neonate. PEEP decreases alveolar water but increases total lung water.

From cardiopulmonary interactions

As PEEP is increased, PaO_2 rises but at the point that venous return (and therefore cardiac output) is reduced, peripheral oxygen delivery is reduced proportionately and the mixed venous oxygen content (MvO_2) falls. Thus PEEP can be titrated to choose the level with the highest MvO_2.

HAZARDS OF MECHANICAL VENTILATION

Prolonged hyperventilation causes lung damage. In experiments where spontaneous hyperventilation is induced in animals (e.g. by injection of salicylic acid into the cisterna magna) a progressive fall in PaO_2 occurs within 6 hours and the animals ultimately die a hypoxic death. Laboratory preparations for acute lung injury requiring low FRC and compliance do not have to use lavage to generate disease. High pressure and high tidal volumes generate ultimately fatal lung injury in previously normal lungs within 12 to 36 hours whether positive or negative pressure ventilation is used. Previously injured lungs are more susceptible to ventilator-induced lung injury but it may not be the diseased areas that suffer, since when ventilating a lung with non-homogenous disease the pressures, volumes and flows are preferentially applied to the least diseased segments. Any ventilator settings that induce over-inflation are likely to induce lung injury, although what these settings are will differ between restrictive and obstructive diseases. Two patterns of ventilator induced or aggravated lung injury are seen

- oedema progressing to fibrosis and reduced lung volume (see ARDS, p. 164)
- cyst formation, with or without fibrosis with multiple air leaks.

There is much interest in the relative effects of pressure, volume and shearing forces in the aetiology of ventilator-associated lung damage. It is clear that PIP is far more dangerous than PEEP and that many of the problems previously associated with PIP are as much to do with the associated high end inflation lung volume and V_T as anything else. Furthermore the hazards of mechanical ventilation are not confined to the lung, since the haemodynamic effects of mechanical ventilation and the resultant balance of gas exchange may have profound effects on regional circulations, particularly the cerebral vasculature.

LONG-TERM VENTILATION

Patients may require long-term ventilation for a mixed bag of conditions such as central hypoventilation syndrome, degenerative neuromuscular disorders and high cervical spine injuries. These patients are best managed at home but the support structures and services that this requires are extensive. Supervision of such patients is best allocated to a physician or intensivist with a special interest. Various approaches to the task of mechanical ventilation may be adopted. For example in a recent unpublished survey of the management of North American patients with central hypoventilation syndrome, 80 per cent have tracheostomies and the majority use conventional positive pressure ventilators. However 14 per cent have nasal mask BiPAP, 11 per cent use phrenic nerve pacing and 5 per cent use negative pressure ventilation (cuirasse or box/iron lung).

EXTRACORPOREAL MEMBRANE OXYGENATION (ECMO)

The term 'extracorporeal membrane oxygenation' or ECMO, can be used to describe any extracorporeal circuit incorporating an artificial gas exchange device, whether or not this is specifically a 'membrane' oxygenator and irrespective of the manner in which the blood is propelled. It is a proven therapy in neonatal cardiopulmonary failure. Improvements in technique may have negated the poor results of a randomised controlled trial in adults and there has not yet been a definitive trial for the paediatric age group. In the absence of better evidence, ECMO is used because it can successfully support a patient in the face of complete absence of native heart or lung function. The best results are obtained when ECMO is instituted early before lung damage is aggravated by high FiO_2s and mechanical ventilation.

A classic ECMO circuit is shown in the diagram (Figure 11.16). Blood drains spontaneously from the patient, driven by the central venous pressure and usually assisted by syphonage. This blood is then pumped through the oxygenator and a heat exchanger (to counteract the cooling tendency) before being returned to the patient. In venoarterial (VA) ECMO, blood is returned to the arterial circulation and in venovenous (VV) ECMO it is returned to the veins.

ECMO protocol

The principles of respiratory gas kinetics make ECMO a system that is subject to simple controls. To increase oxygen delivery to the patient, increase blood flow to the oxygenator and to increase carbon dioxide clearance, increase the gas flow (sweep) across it. Carbon dioxide clearance can be achieved at low extracorporeal blood flows. In practice the situation is more complex. Idiosyncrasies of different oxygenators and pumps need to be taken into account as well as the influence of the cannulation upon the performance of gas exchange and circulatory support. Membrane oxygenators are best used at well below their rated flow allowing one to compensate for the fact that the membrane gets wet and its diffusion capacity decreases over time. If one uses high sweep rates to keep the membrane dry, then carbon dioxide must be blended into the sweep gas to avoid hypocarbia. Hollow

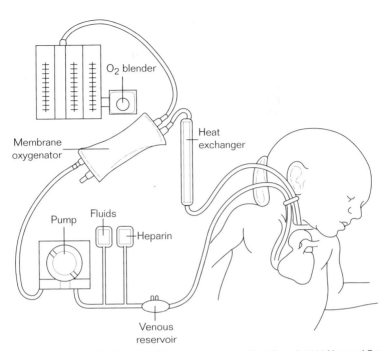

Figure 11.16 Classic ECMO circuit. (With permission from Short B et al. 1986 Neonatal Extra Corporeal Membrane Oxygenation: A Review. J. Intensive Care Medicine 1:47–54.)

fibre oxygenators tend to develop abrupt plasma leaks. Oxygenation of all of the patient's blood requires all of the blood to pass through the circuit. Extracorporeal blood flows of 100 ml kg^{-1} min^{-1} (venoarterial) are usually adequate. This flow rate is just an estimate of the resting cardiac output and is likely to be insufficient during venovenous ECMO and during haemodynamic states of high native cardiac output with low systemic vascular resistance (e.g. septic shock). Tubing must be of sufficient bore to accommodate the desired blood flow but the points of most resistance to blood flow are usually the cannulae. Appropriate cannula size can be judged from the 'm number' although in practice the largest possible cannulae that the vessel can accommodate are usually used. Vascular access for venous drainage should therefore involve the shortest cannula of widest feasible gauge to accommodate the required flow. Venous drainage from the right atrium via the right internal jugular vein is preferred. Return blood flow is under positive pressure allowing smaller cannulae but the smaller the arterial cannula the higher the operating pressure in the circuit and the greater the likelihood of circuit disruption and haemolysis.

Simplicity in ECMO circuit design has distinct advantages such as less risk of component fatigue or failure. Areas of stasis (such as large venous reservoirs) are avoided as they would necessitate prohibitive levels of heparinisation. Typically patients only require an activated clotting time prolonged to about 180 seconds (1.5 times normal). This is achieved by a heparin bolus of 30 to 50 units kg^{-1} during cannulation followed by a continuous infusion of about 20 units kg^{-1} hr^{-1}. Platelets are supplemented to maintain counts above 100×10^9 L^{-1} (higher if there is increased risk of haemorrhage, for example in a post-operative patient).

Unlike VA, the haemodynamics of which are covered in Chapter 12, VV cannulation (double lumen or double venous) has few haemodynamic consequences except for reduction of pulmonary artery pressure (a consequence of improved oxygenation). Two phenomena (recirculation and venous admixture) lead to mild desaturation during VV ECMO, which need not be detrimental to systemic oxygen delivery if cardiac output is maintained. Venous admixture in this context refers to systemic venous return that escapes drainage to the ECMO circuit and continues without oxygen in the native circulation. Recirculation refers to the propensity for oxygenated blood from the circuit to drain back to the circuit without perfusing the patient. This blood cannot take up more oxygen and so limits total oxygen uptake across the oxygenator. Routine blood flow rates are often increased up to 20 per cent to attempt to compensate for this phenomenon during VV ECMO. Recirculation increases with:

- ECMO blood flow rate above the resting cardiac output (giving a descending limb to the graph of oxygen delivery versus ECMO blood flow)
- hypovolaemia
- cardiac arrhythmia
- aberrant cannula position.

VA cannulation offers greater haemodynamic stability but the advantages of VV with respect to coronary and pulmonary perfusion are very persuasive. The relative merits of the different approaches, VV versus VA, in terms of cerebral perfusion during and after cervical cannulation are still debated.

HIGH FREQUENCY VENTILATION

High frequency oscillation (HFO)

HFO is a much more benign form of ventilation than the tidal flow used in spontaneous and most mechanically assisted methods of ventilation. It is associated with lower respiratory morbidity in ventilated neonates and is best suited to homogeneous pulmonary diseases, especially when there are associated air leaks. Its role in larger patients, for example with ARDS, has been less well defined. Some controversy has surrounded the randomised controlled trials associated with its introduction to neonatal ICU. For example the suggestion of increased intraventricular haemorrhage rates in one trial has not been supported by others.

HFO is ventilation using a vibrating CPAP circuit. It relies on laminar gas flow, respiratory rates above 150 breaths per minute and assisted expiration to produce significant ventilation at tidal volumes less than the anatomical deadspace. The oscillating waveform is established around a continuous distending pressure (CDP) applied to the endotracheal tube. This distending pressure is transmitted to the lung fairly efficiently but the oscillations are highly attenuated as they pass down the endotracheal tube. The degree of attenuation is greater with smaller tubes and is marginally reduced by increasing inspiratory time. Thus the effective surface area of the lung (oxygenation) can be manipulated independently of the minute volume (carbon dioxide clearance). The inertial impedance to gas flow increases with respiratory frequency. Therefore increasing frequency (F) disproportionately reduces tidal volume and leads to rising Pa_{CO_2}. Tidal volume itself makes a much greater contribution to minute volume (MV) than in tidal flow ventilation

$$MV = F \times V_T^2$$

A number of devices are available but most clinical papers refer to the use of the Sensormedics 3100A®. To establish a patient on oscillation, first check the oscillator is calibrated and select a bias flow (continuous gas flow rate) appropriate to the size of the patient (10 litres for premature infants, 15 litres for term and over 20 litres for larger patients). Choose an appropriate continuous distending pressure (CDP) (2 to 4 cmH$_2$O higher than MAP for neonates and 4 to 6 cmH$_2$O higher than MAP for older patients). Starting frequency is chosen according to patient weight. Lower frequencies are used for larger patients, they have more power and bigger tidal volumes. Starting frequency is also affected by the type of disease and pathophysiology. The size of the oscillation is expressed by the ΔP, which is usually started at about twice the value of the CDP. Once these parameters have been set the oscillator can be attached to the endotracheal tube and oscillation commenced. Optimal CDP (and hence lung volume) will be that associated with the best Pa_{O_2} for the lowest possible Fio$_2$ and is reached in stages by incremental increases in

CDP. Further increases that lead to overdistension should not be associated with significant rises in PaO_2 and may even cause it to fall. CDP is also the major determinant of the cardiopulmonary interactions of HFO. ΔP controls tidal volume and is adjusted in the light of the effect on $Paco_2$.

High frequency jet ventilation

In this technique an injector is applied to the airway through a side lumen of a special endotracheal tube. Like injectors elsewhere, gas accelerating through a confined nozzle generates a pressure drop at the tip. Additional gas is therefore entrained by a Venturi effect and the sum is delivered to the airway at a regulated driving pressure and respiratory rate of 100 to 150 breaths per minute. The pressure waveform is fairly constant but the percentage time spent in inspiration can be adjusted (usually about 20%). For a given driving pressure the PIP will rise and V_T will fall if compliance or airways conductance fall. Jet ventilation has proved useful in the management of emergency upper airway obstruction after cricothyrotomy, or during instrumentation. In some centres it has recently been used preferentially in the management of neonatal respiratory distress syndrome but this practice has largely been abandoned because of lack of proof of its effectiveness. The hazards of jet ventilation include tracheal mucosal damage (necrotising tracheitis) and the difficulties in countering the drying effects of the jet.

NOVEL APPROACHES TO VENTILATION

Intratracheal pressure release ventilation (ITPV)

In this novel form of ventilation, attempts to minimise deadspace have lead to the use of a specially adapted endotracheal tube with first a Venturi nozzle and more recently a 'reverse thrust' nozzle at its tip. Gas is continuously delivered above the carina via this nozzle and expiration is initiated by pressure release in the circuit. Thus during expiration the Venturi recruits and accelerates the expiratory gases. This allows more efficient use of the tidal volume at lower mean airway pressures than would be generated by other forms of ventilation. Inadvertent PEEP is avoided. Indeed negative pressure is generated at the carina with high gas flows. Promising laboratory models have been followed by case reports of effective ITPV in extreme cases, for example patients with pulmonary hypoplasia who could not be weaned from ECMO.

Liquid ventilation

Perfluorocarbons can dissolve larger quantities of oxygen and carbon dioxide than water, plasma or alveolar fluid. When they are instilled into the lung, the liquid–gas interface has a markedly reduced surface tension, improving lung compliance. Furthermore, because the fluid is non-compressible, the effective surface area of the lung is increased by bulk distension of atelectatic alveoli. Hence deficient gas exchange can be improved. Total liquid ventilation is cumbersome since it requires a method of reoxygenation and CO_2 removal from the liquid before it is recycled and rebreathed. These disadvantages are circumvented by perfluorocarbon assisted gas exchange in which the FRC is replaced with perfluorocarbon and tidal volume ventilation proceeds with a high FiO_2. Promising laboratory studies and early clinical studies in neonates have led to phase three trials. These are likely to be prolonged by the need to recruit high-risk patients.

SHORT NOTES ON SPECIFIC CONDITIONS

Upper airway obstruction

Chronic upper airway obstruction leads to pulmonary hypertension and cor pulmonale. Acute total upper airway obstruction requires immediate resuscitation and is often followed by pulmonary oedema. A degree of palliation can be obtained in subtotal obstruction by breathing helium–oxygen mixtures (see Chapter 18, Physics for the Intensivist). The differential diagnosis depends upon the site of obstruction.

Nasal obstruction is more commonly symptomatic in babies. Symptoms are aggravated by closure of the mouth but the presenting symptom may be recurrent apnoea rather than respiratory distress. Choanal atresia will prevent the passage of nasal tubes, even small nasogastric tubes.

Nasopharyngeal obstruction commonly presents with a long history of sleep disturbance or snoring which may be relieved by a nasopharyngeal airway but can be more acute, for example in association with retropharyngeal abscess formation. Look in the mouth for tonsillar hypertrophy, which is usually associated with adenoidal hypertrophy. Nasal and pharyngeal airway obstruction occurs in a variety of congenital craniofacial anomalies.

Obstruction below the nasopharynx but above the thoracic inlet causes inspiratory stridor. Congenital causes include laryngotracheolmalacia, vocal cord palsy and laryngeal web. Stridor can also result from localised tracheal disease such as a vascular 'ring sling or other thing' within the thorax (diagnosed by barium swallow and angiography, and/or endoscopy).

Stridor with a short history requires the important distinction of epiglottitis from a differential including croup, foreign body and bacterial tracheitis.

Epiglottitis

Epiglottitis presents a toxic patient, drooling with dysphagia and stridor accompanied by a muffled cough. These patients should not be further stressed or examined, unless the individual doing so is capable and prepared to perform advanced airway manoeuvres (including surgical ones). They require expeditious intubation after a gas induction of anaesthesia and then intravenous antibiotics to treat the associated septicaemia and pneumonia (usually caused by *Haemophilus influenzae*). The endotracheal tube can usually be removed within 12 to 24 hours and extubation need not wait for a leak around the tube or resolution of the fever. The disease is rare where Hib vaccine has been introduced.

Croup

Croup or viral laryngotracheobronchitis causes a characteristic barking cough; these patients do not show signs that suggest septicaemia. Treatment is with steroids to treat the inflammation despite the infective aetiology. The need for intubation is judged by the degree of obstruction and the work of breathing. Nebulised adrenaline (epinephrine) may give short-lived symptomatic relief and it delays rather than averts the need for intubation. Frequently acute deterioration has been caused by accumulation of secretions within and below the narrowing necessitating extensive physiotherapy and suction after intubation. The size of endotracheal tube accommodated may be small and it should be left *in situ* until a leak develops. Sputum clearance is enhanced if the patients are nursed awake and coughing. If a leak does not develop after 4 to 5 days then rigid laryngoscopy or bronchoscopy may be indicated to detect and treat granuloma formation.

Foreign bodies

When a patient presents with a foreign body obstruction there is usually a clear clinical history. Toddlers are the worst offenders. Inspiratory and expiratory chest X-ray will help detect obstruction in main and branch bronchi (by far the most common site) but are not helpful in the investigation of stridor. Removal is performed during rigid bronchoscopy under general anaesthesia. When facing acute total airway obstruction from an inaccessible foreign body in the trachea and without access to rigid bronchoscopy it may be possible to advance the foreign body into a main bronchus using a bougie.

Bacterial tracheitis

Bacterial tracheitis causes symptoms like croup but it is a more serious illness with greater severity and toxicity. The usual organisms are *Staphylococcus aureus*, *Haemophilus influenzae* or *Streptococci*.

Inhalation trauma

Inhalation trauma can occur during exposure to hot gases, steam, chemicals or smoke and can cause airway oedema sufficient to obstruct the airway. Early intubation is advisable if the diagnosis is not in doubt since oedema deteriorates in the hours following the trauma.

Post-extubation stridor

This condition results from oedema, inflammation or even granuloma formation at the narrowest part of the airway (subglottic) or below at the site of the tip of the tube. It usually responses to steroids. Nebulised adrenaline (epinephrine) may give symptomatic relief from oedema. Granulomas may be removed during bronchoscopy. Scarring leads to a subglottic stenosis. The degree of obstruction can worsen with time as the child grows and the stenosis does not, or indeed if the stenosis contracts. The diameter of the airway can be increased at this point by a cricoid split procedure which will avoid tracheostomy in about 50 per cent of cases.

Tracheobronchomalacia

Tracheobronchomalacia can (but may not) present with stridor. It may be associated with characteristic cardiac lesions such as a vascular ring or absent pulmonary valve syndrome. Large airway collapse characteristically produces a biphasic expiration which may be ablated by PEEP. The appropriate investigation is a bronchogram which determines the proximal and distal extent of the lesion and, if different amounts of CPAP are applied during the procedure, may also determine its functional severity and the appropriate subsequent ventilatory settings.

Obstruction involving the major bronchi and their branches, the so-called 'conductance airways', causes wheeze provided there is sufficient airflow. Bronchospasm is just one possible cause of wheeze.

Asthma

ICU admission can be avoided if patients respond well to nebulised β_2-agonists and steroids. Nebulised β_2-agonists can be given continuously in severe cases. For patients likely to require ICU admission, intravenous theophylline will reduce the need for ventilation and the required duration of oxygen therapy and therefore ICU stay. For patients already receiving theophylline the loading dose should be reduced to (5.7 × maintenance dose (mg) / dose interval (hr)).

Intravenous salbutamol may also be useful. Occasionally lactic acidosis from salbutamol toxicity causes tachypnoea when otherwise symptoms are improving.

Indications for ventilation include:

- abrupt deterioration
- evidence of exhaustion or a degree of respiratory obstruction likely to cause exhaustion, (patients should be intubated before their respiratory effort dwindles)
- decreasing level of consciousness/somnolence
- a silent chest
- desaturation despite supplemental oxygen ($Fio_2 > 0.5$)
- carbon dioxide retention (if uncompensated and $Paco_2 > 8$ kPa)

A rapid sequence induction is preferred, avoiding histaminergic agents. Ketamine is a useful bronchodilator and both vecuronium and rocuronium will rapidly achieve intubation conditions in place of suxamethonium. Likely difficulties in preoxygenation mean that intubation should be slick. Once intubated, inhalational anaesthetics such as halothane and isoflurane can be used to assist bronchodilatation.

Ventilatory approaches have to take account of severe airflow limitation or they risk exacerbating regional or global hyperinflation, causing air leaks and/or barotrauma. Hyperinflation and high intrathoracic pressures cause haemodynamic compromise by reduction of preload and even cardiac compression. Volume controlled ventilation assures inspiration but risks excessive airway pressures if the patient deteriorates. Pressure limited ventilation (to PIP < 35 cmH$_2$O), preferably time cycled, is safer and carries a lower risk of air leak but tidal volume falls if the patient deteriorates. In reality the morbidity and mortality associated with IPPV are low. Deaths occur principally when access to IPPV is not available in an emergency. With an adequate Fio$_2$, patients can usually be oxygenated and permissive hypercarbia is preferable to a tension pneumothorax. If a hypoxic respiratory arrest has occurred however then one may choose to be more aggressive in removing carbon dioxide for control of cerebral blood flow. Long expiratory times may be necessary to allow for intrinsic PEEP and to prevent further 'dynamic' hyperinflation. Some patients will occasionally demonstrate more effective expiration with PEEP (watch the flow–time curve).

Weaning is appropriate as the ease and effectiveness of ventilation improves, possibly within hours of intubation. This can be judged clinically from peak pressures in volume controlled modes, from oxygen requirement or from cardiovascular parameters such as the degree of pulsus paradoxus during spontaneous respiration.

Bronchiolitis

This infectious winter seasonal malady predominantly affects infants under 1 year. It is usually caused by respiratory syncytial virus, which along with the many other potential viral pathogens may be detected by immunofluoresence of nasopharyngeal aspirate. An elevated oxygen requirement is common among patients who have required hospital admission. However, respiratory failure is rare. In patients with dramatically increased work of breathing the use of pre-emptive nasopharyngeal CPAP decreases the need for IPPV. Formal ventilation is much more likely to be necessary if there is pre-existent lung disease such as bronchopulmonary dysplasia or covert congenital heart disease. Laboratory evidence of response to ribavirin does not translate to clinical benefit and the administration of inhaled ribavirin can be highly problematic during mechanical ventilation.

Adult respiratory distress syndrome (ARDS)

The 'adult' or acquired respiratory distress syndrome (ARDS) is a spectrum of lung disease usually associated with a systemic inflammatory response or non-cardiogenic pulmonary oedema. There is a natural progression which proceeds at different rates in variously affected areas of the lung. The early exudative phase is associated with inflammation with oedema, vascular congestion and hyaline membrane formation associated with preservation of both FRC and compliance, but with $\dot{V}/\dot{Q}$ less than 1. Fibroblast proliferation and hypertrophy of type II pneumocytes then occurs with collagen deposition in the interstitium leading eventually to fibrosis. Hyaline membranes may disappear during this latter phase, which is associated with normal airways resistance but reducing compliance and a fall in FRC (to levels below the normal closing volume of the lung). The rate of progression varies but the degree of eventual fibrosis is aggravated by the necessary therapy with IPPV. The non-uniform distribution of fibrosis is also affected by the ventilatory strategies applied. Asymmetrical atelectasis (affected by the distribution of lung water) gives widespread variation in time constants within the lung and contributes to $\dot{V}/\dot{Q}$ mismatch hypoxia and pulmonary hypertension. The overall prognosis depends upon resolution of the MOSF and hence removal/minimisation of the inflammatory stimulus. Occasionally patients may show improvement with steroid therapy. Such improvement is often temporary and there is no evidence that their use alters outcome. Given a window of opportunity (paradoxically usually from rapid deterioration) survival rates greater than 50 per cent can be achieved with ECMO. After more than 3 or 4 days of high pressure IPPV the results with ECMO are poorer. Ventilatory strategies assume a high V$_D$:V$_T$ and that the normally functioning lung (perhaps 20% of the total) is preferentially ventilated increasing the risk of baro- or volutrauma and oxygen toxicity. Current practice is to limit PIP to less than 35 cmH$_2$O and to use significant PEEP and long inspiratory times to allow one to restrict Fio$_2$. Patients should be moved regularly, rotated or nursed prone to redistribute lung water in order to encourage redistribution of atelectasis. These principles lead to inverse ratio ventilation and can be extended by a policy of permissive hypercarbia in which carbon retention is tolerated allowing low minute volume ventilation. Patients are ventilat pH rather than a PCO_2 and the degree of hypercarbia increases as renal compensation occurs. An alternative approach that allows low tidal volumes is to use a high frequency oscillator.

12 Cardiovascular System

- **Recognising cardiovascular instability**
- **Differences between children and adults**
- **Haemodynamics**
- **The paediatric ECG**
- **Arrhythmias**
- **Non-invasive arterial pressure monitoring**
- **Invasive vascular pressure monitoring**
- **Measurement of cardiac output**
- **Functional echocardiography**
- **Inotropes**
- **Lowering blood pressure**
- **Mechanical circulatory support**

RECOGNISING CARDIOVASCULAR INSTABILITY

The need for cardiovascular monitoring and support is the justification for many PICU admissions. The proficient intensivist must recognise haemodynamic instability or circulatory inadequacy early and intervene before decompensation and collapse occur. The clinical art is the detection of subtle signs of compensation; a sound grasp of age-appropriate normal values is therefore mandatory (Table 12.1).

Shock

Circulatory inadequacy ('shock') is however best defined in terms of end organ function rather than heart rate, function or blood pressure. Shock is therefore present if there is an inadequate supply of oxygen and nutrients to cells, irrespective of the cardiac output. The list in Table 12.2 is an aetiological classification of shock.

Table 12.1 Normal values for cardiovascular vital signs (from Shann 1998 *Drug Doses* Collective Pty Ltd).

Age	Pulse (95% range) (bpm)	Mean blood pressure (95% range) (mmHg)
Term	95–145	40–60
3 months	110–175	45–75
6 months	110–175	50–90
1 year	105–170	50–100
3 years	80–140	50–100
7 years	70–120	60–90
10 years	60–110	60–90
12 years	60–100	65–95
14 years	60–100	65–95
Adult 60 kg	65–115	95–125
Adult 70 kg	65–115	95–125

Table 12.2 Aetiology of shock

Hypovolaemic	Haemorrhage
	Diarrhoea
	Vomiting
	Burns
	Peritonitis
Distributive	Septicaemia
	Anaphylaxis
	Vasodilating drugs
	Spinal cord injury
Cardiogenic	Arrhythmia
	Cardiomyopathy
	Myocardial contusion
	Myocardial infarction
Obstructive	Tension pneumo-/haemothorax
	Flail chest
	Tamponade
	Pulmonary embolism
Dissociative	Anaemia
	Carbon monoxide poisoning
	Methaemoglobinaemia

Compensation for the early stages of shock most reliably, but not always, produces a tachycardia. The detection of tachycardia during clinical examination therefore requires an explanation. Look for corresponding signs of a low cardiac output and for evidence of a pathophysiological diagnosis that could generate shock. A useful algorithm for postoperative cardiac surgical cases is included in Chapter 13, Congenital Heart Disease page 197–98. The most reliable signs of a low cardiac output are a reduction in urine output and an altered level of consciousness or agitation/confusion from inadequate cerebral oxygen delivery. Other signs can help and will not necessarily mislead you, provided you are aware of their possible exceptions. For example a widening differential in core–peripheral temperature may reflect compensatory vasoconstriction of shock or external cooling. If vasodilatation is causal or associated with shock however, then the peripheries may remain warm with full pulses in the early stages and the capillary refill time, which in other circumstances is prolonged, may be preserved. Compensatory vasoconstriction can raise the diastolic and hence mean blood pressure in the early stages of shock. **Systolic blood pressure is normal in compensated shock** hence a fall in systolic blood pressure is the best definition of decompensation.

The definition of decompensated shock is satisfied when the normal physiological lower limit of blood pressure is passed. However one would be foolish to wait for a threshold to pass for intervention if there is a consistent downward trend. Also pre-existing disease can limit the resilience of the patient's circulation to 'stress' making it 'fragile' and allowing decompensation earlier than otherwise expected. Decompensated shock is characterised by hypotension, acidosis (which may produce tachypnoea or other respiratory signs) oligo- or anuria, and syncope or coma. It is generally assumed that a healthy child can compensate for a 25 per cent reduction in intravascular volume. Further loss will be uncompensated and once it exceeds 40 per cent of intravascular volume it will be extreme and 'preterminal' (a retrospective diagnosis).

Heart failure

Children's hearts rarely 'fail' and so the term 'heart failure' is generally best avoided. Failure of the heart *can* occur as a result of cardiomyopathy, anomalous coronary arteries, long-standing arrhythmias or specific congenital heart lesions usually involving systemic outflow tract obstruction. In these instances the mechanical problem is usually related to systolic function. However most children with physical signs that would represent 'heart failure' in an adult are in fact displaying the manifestations of a left to right shunt – high pulmonary blood flow and ventricular volume overload. At the point of presentation, pulmonary oedema and liver enlargement occur at a time when the cardiac output is positively athletic. Indeed the calorie requirement required to sustain this activity is a potential cause of failure to thrive.

DIFFERENCES BETWEEN CHILDREN AND ADULTS

The foetal circulation is discussed in Chapter 6, Neonatology page 71, and cardiac embryology in Chapter 13, Congenital Heart Disease page 191.

The transitional circulation occurs in early neonatal life and is characterised by dwindling foetal connections with changing pressure gradients across them and reducing flow within them. The events of birth are associated with a sudden increase in contractility (compared to foetal levels) that is synchronous with, and related to, surges in catecholamines and thyroid hormone. Sustained changes in ventricular function are also provoked by massive alterations in cardiac-loading conditions. The precipitous fall in pulmonary vascular resistance leads to rising left ventricular preload, corresponding to the increase in pulmonary blood flow and apposition of the atrial septum primum and secundum. With the separation of the systemic circulation from its low-pressure placental sump, systemic vascular resistance and afterload rise correspondingly steeply.

Hence, neonates at birth have little inotropic reserve and the preload reserve of neonatal hearts, paced at fixed rates, is also reduced compared to older children and adults. This all paints the picture of a relatively non-compliant myocardium working vigorously and operating at the upper limits of its function curves (see Fig 12.2). Neonatal myocardium has a greater anaerobic capacity that only partially offsets the limited inotropic reserve. Increases in blood viscosity or arterial pressure (both consequences of hypoxic stress) drop the cardiac output and the heart rate, but the term neonate can mount a tachycardic response to prolonged stress.

The sympathetic innervation of the neonatal heart is less well developed than the parasympathetic and although resting vagal tone is low, a propensity for reflex bradycardia results. The high resting β adrenergic state around the time of birth contributes to a relative resistance to the effects of catecholamines. Increases in heart rate in the newborn achieve limited gain and, if excessive, may even drop the cardiac output. Falls in heart rate are accompanied by less vasoconstriction than in older individuals and are paralleled by disproportionately larger decreases in cardiac output. Similarly, increases in afterload significantly reduce cardiac output whereas output can be preserved but not greatly increased when afterload falls. Aspects of myocardial cellular immaturity make the neonatal heart display muted or accentuated responses to various electrolytes and drugs compared to later life. For example neonates are comparatively resistant to hyperkalaemia but poor calcium uptake by the myocardial sarcolemma makes them more dependent upon serum ionised calcium levels than older patients.

In infancy and childhood the myocardium adapts progressively to its new loading conditions and develops an increased reserve to β adrenergic stimulation. During this period of growth, the morphology of the heart changes. In the foetus and newborn the left ventricle assumes a flattened shape and the interventricular septum is coupled to the right ventricle (RV) rather than the left ventricle (LV). This results in non-concentric LV contraction that can confound functional echocardiographic assessment. In older children the septum is recruited to the LV and the more easily interpreted radial symmetry of the LV develops.

HAEMODYNAMICS

The heart and circulatory system display a high degree of intrinsic autoregulation and are subject to neural, hormonal and local metabolic controls, all of which may be either affected by disease or therapeutically manipulated.

Pump function is described in both volumetric and mechanical terms. Volume-related measures of cardiac function are best standardised by their relation to the child's size, weight or surface area. For example the cardiac output, which is the volume of blood that exits the left ventricle in a minute (stroke volume × heart rate) is best expressed in relation to surface area (the cardiac index).

Volumetric indices of cardiac function are used extensively in adult ICU to derive and infer oxygen delivery. However in paediatrics, intra- or extracardiac shunts may change their relevance radically in this respect. When trying to elucidate the flow across a shunt or root out the causes of blood pressure fluctuations, the concept of a calculated global '*vascular resistance*' (e.g. systemic vascular resistance 'SVR' or pulmonary vascular resistance 'PVR') is frequently employed. The resistance to flow exerted by a circulation is conceptually related to the pressure drop across it divided by the flow. Although simplistic, such assumptions can illuminate clinical problems relating to blood pressure and flow in both systemic and pulmonary circulations.

Under normal physiological conditions, the cardiac output is largely a reflection of its loading conditions. The child's heart can adapt acutely to changes but will also compensate over the longer term with patterns of hypertrophy for pressure loading and dilatation for volume loading. Systolic ventricular performance represents the interactions of four mechanical factors

- preload
- afterload
- inotropic state
- chronotropy

on stroke volume. In addition more subtle considerations of regional wall motion, septal recruitment and ventricular geometry may be highly relevant in the clinical setting.

PRELOAD

Preload is the ventricular wall tension at the end of diastole. It can be inferred from the ventricular end diastolic volume or pressure and will be affected by the circulating blood volume, venous capacitance and heart rhythm. Starling's famous observation that stroke volume increases proportionately to the degree of stretch of ventricular muscle fibres, needs to be qualified:

- there exists a 'limit of preload reserve' beyond which stroke volume falls
- ventricular compliance is not linear (Figure 12.1) and a preload judged from pressure measurements alone (e.g. CVP, left atrial pressure, left ventricular end diastolic pressure or pulmonary capillary wedge pressure) never gives a complete picture.
- *in vivo*, the heart may be constrained in the pericardium and even in the absence of pericardial disease, dilatation of one ventricle can cause compression or limitation of its companion.

Changes in ventricular compliance or other aspects of diastolic function can occur as a ventricle adapts to its loading conditions or as changes in heart rhythm occur.

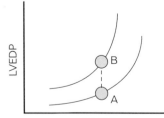

Figure 12.1 End diastolic pressure–volume relation. Ventricular compliance relationship for two different compliance states (A > B). LVEDP = left ventricular end diastolic pressure, LVEDV = left ventricular end diastolic volume. Note that in contrast to the respiratory pressure:volume relation, in graphs of cardiac function, volume is on the *x* axis.

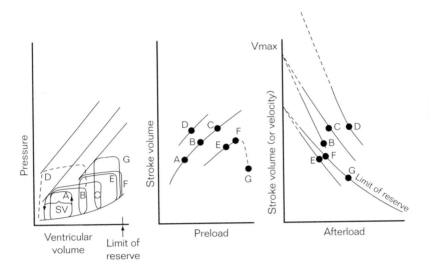

Figure 12.2 Concepts of Myocardial Function. The graph on the left shows Pressure Volume loops for individual cardiac cycles in different functinal states. The stroke volume (SV) is represented by the breadth of each loop. The other two graphs show the Stroke volume: Preload relation (Starling) and the relation between stroke volume and afterload. In these latter two graphs the lines have been derived from multiple beats under the controlled loading conditions/ contractility. Beats A–G represent the same level of function and loading conditions in each graph. A, B, and C represent increasing preload with no change in contractility. A greater stroke volume occurs and the afterload relation shifts to the right (BC) with no change in Vmax (its extrapolation to the y intercept). Beat D occurs at the same loading conditions as B but with enhanced contractility. A greater stroke volume is therefore achieved at modestly increased pressure. Enhanced contractility produces a displaced preload: stroke volume relation and produces a curve with a different Vmax in the stroke volume afterload relation. Beats E and F represent relations in a failing heart. The pressure volume loops move along the relation shown in Fig. 12.1. A reduced stroke volume is achieved for a given preload and the stroke volume afterload relation is flattened. Once the limit of reserve has been reached then increased vascular resistance (infusion of a pressor – Beat G) causes a reduction in stroke volume delivered at a higher pressure. Note how the different contractile states can be characterised by their end systolic pressure volume relations (the three straight trend lines on the pressure volume loops) and by different Vmax. (Adapted with permission from Alexander R et al. 1995 Hurst's the Heart: Companion Handbook. McGraw-Hill, New York; p. 313.)

AFTERLOAD

Afterload is the sum of the forces opposing ventricular ejection, it manifests as the systolic tension in the wall of the ventricle. The most important of these forces is the systolic blood pressure, which is in turn affected by vascular tone – the systemic vascular resistance. Other factors also contribute such as ventricular geometry, aortic input impedance and the inertial properties of blood and other moving components like valves for example.

The heart can produce different stroke volumes and ejection forces for given preload and afterload conditions depending upon its *inotropic state* or contractility. While at one level easy to conceptualise, contractility can be measured or inferred in a number of different ways (see Figure 12.2).

Factors affecting the heart rate are *chronotropic*. Within limits to allow adequate ventricular filling, increases in heart rate have a linear effect on cardiac output and are also associated with an increase in inotropic state. Increases in heart rate are achieved by shortening the amount of time spent in diastole. Rapid rates decrease stroke volume and may impair perfusion of the coronary arteries.

The concept of *stroke work* relates ventricular performance to the afterload. It is the product of the stroke volume and the mean arterial pressure (or mean ventricular systolic pressure). Low levels of stroke work can be caused by a low inotropic state, low vascular resistance or indicate that the limits of reserve have been exceeded (e.g. beat G in Figure 12.2). Increases in stroke work will, like increases in heart rate, increase myocardial oxygen demand. Increased myocardial oxygen demand requires increased coronary blood flow since oxygen extraction from coronary arterial blood is virtually complete even when there is normal perfusion at rest.

There are important distinctions between pressure overload and volume overload so haemodynamic information must always be put into context. The loading conditions of right and left ventricles may be very different from each other. A left to right (L–R) shunt causes pulmonary volume overload and right to left (R-L) shunts cause desaturation or cyanosis. A modest extracardiac R–L shunt is a physiological feature of the pulmonary circulation that can be accentuated by disease.

It is customary to quantify L–R shunts by the relative pulmonary and systemic blood flow ($\dot{Q}p:\dot{Q}s$).

Shunt flow calculations

$\dot{Q}p:\dot{Q}s$ is calculated by manipulation of the Fick equation (see Chapter 18) where blood flow is related to the rate of oxygen consumption ($\dot{V}O_2$) divided by the arteriovenous oxygen difference. These equations can be written for systemic and pulmonary circulations. For Qs the systemic arterial and mixed venous oxygen contents (CaO_2 and $C\bar{v}O_2$) are subtracted.

$$\dot{Q}s = \frac{\dot{V}O_2}{CaO_2 - C_{\bar{v}}O_2}$$

and $$\dot{Q}p = \frac{\dot{V}O_2}{CpvO_2 - CpaO_2}$$

For $\dot{Q}p$ the oxygen uptake (which equals $\dot{V}O_2$) is equivalent to pulmonary vein ($CpvO_2$) minus pulmonary arterial oxygen content ($CpaO_2$). When the ratio between the two is constructed, $\dot{V}O_2$ cancels such that

$$\dot{Q}p:\dot{Q}s = \frac{CaO_2 - C_{\bar{v}}O_2}{CpvO_2 - CpaO_2}$$

it is important to remember that mixed venous oxygen content must be determined in the chamber before the shunt. When necessary this can be calculated from superior vena cava (SVC) and inferior vena cava (IVC) oxygen contents as:

$((3 \times SVC) + IVC) \div 4$. Even this will not work if the pulmonary venous drainage is anomalous (to the systemic veins).

For example, the normal CaO_2 is, say, 20 volumes% and mixed venous ($C\bar{v}O_2 = CpaO_2$) is 15 volumes%. Thus since $CpvO_2$ also equals CaO_2 we have (20–15):(20–15) = 1:1. If a ventricular septal defect is present which raises the $CpaO_2$ to 17.5 volumes%, we have (20–15):(20–17.5) = 5:2.5 = 2:1. An adequate systemic cardiac output in such a situation requires increased cardiac work to compensate for this 'leak'.

$CpvO_2$ is often assumed to equal CaO_2 but provided one is more particular than this, the equation can be inverted to give $\dot{Q}s:\dot{Q}p$ for R–L shunts which is rarely calculated in practice.

DIASTOLIC FUNCTION

The non-linearity of ventricular compliance was discussed under preload (see p. 170). Decreased ventricular compliance gives reduced end diastolic volume for a given end diastolic pressure and this is reflected in the atrial pressures. The classic example of diastolic dysfunction is right ventricular hypertrophy (e.g. in Fallot's). In the face of diastolic dysfunction, higher filling pressure values must be obtained or accepted to give adequate ventricular filling (EDV). Ventricles fill in two phases. Normal early filling associated with ventricular relaxation is rapid and can be assessed by both its rate and extent. Later filling is slow and augmented by atrial contraction (see Figure 12.9). When the ventricle is relatively 'stiff' or non-compliant, for example in normal neonates and infants or in pathological states (e.g. right ventricular hypertrophy) the slow phase predominates. Increases in heart rate and inotropy will both accelerate the rate of relaxation but may also reduce its extent leading to a fall in cardiac output. Ischaemia compromises both the rate and extent of relaxation and, as with systolic function, there may be regional wall motion abnormalities. Extrinsic influences on ventricular diastolic function (the other ventricle, pericardium, etc.) may be profound.

THE PAEDIATRIC ECG

The most important age-related changes of the paediatric ECG are in QRST duration and morphology. Normal values have been reproduced in Table 12.3. The normal neonatal frontal plane QRS axis is right sided, and right ventricular voltages are often of diagnostic significance. For these reasons the recording of right ventricular leads (V3r and V4r) are a routine part of the '12' lead recording in paediatrics.

Neonatal right ventricular dominance is gradually superseded by left dominance during the first year of life. The frontal plane QRS axis shifts from right to left with the initially abrupt neonatal changes, followed by more gradual age-related changes in pulmonary and systemic vascular resistance. These electrical changes lag behind those of blood pressures since they reflect the cardiac adaptation to the changing loading conditions. The behaviour of the ECG as a reflection of loading conditions contributes a diagnostic significance in congenital heart disease. Left axis deviation does not necessarily imply left ventricular hypertrophy and may be a characteristic of the particular congenital lesion (e.g. atrioventricular septal defect). The interpretation of right ventricular hypertrophy is however more specific and it is possible to distinguish pressure overload (dominant R in right ventricular leads with ventricular strain) from volume overload (rSR in the same leads) both of which are usually associated with right axis deviation.

Table 12.3 Normal ECG parameters in paediatric patients (from Moss and Adams 1998 *Heart Disease in Infants, Children and Adolescents* Lippincott Williams and Wilkins).

	0–3 days	3–30 days	1–6 months	6–12 months	1–3 years	3–5 years	5–8 years	8–12 years	12–16 years
PR interval (lead II) (ms)	80–160	70–140	70–160	70–160	80–150	80–160	90–160	90–170	90–180
QRS duration (ms)	25–75	25–80	25–80	25–75	30–75	30–75	30–80	30–85	35–90
QRS axis	60–195	65–185	10–120	10–100	10–100	10–105	10–135	10–120	10–130
Voltages (V1) (mV)									
Q	0	0	0	0	0	0	0	0	0
R	0.5–2.6	0.3–2.3	0.3–2.0	0.2–2.0	0.2–1.8	0.1–1.8	0.1–1.5	0.1–1.2	0.1–1
S	0–2.3	0–1.5	0–1.5	0–1.8	0.1–2.1	0.2–2.1	0.3–2.4	0.3–2.5	0.3–2.2
T	−0.4–0.4	−0.5–0.1	−0.6–0.1	−0.6–0.1	−0.6–0.1	−0.6–0	−0.5–0.2	−0.4–0.3	−0.4–0.3
Voltages (V6) (mV)									
Q	0–0.2	0–0.3	0–0.25	0–0.3	0–0.3	0.02–0.35	0.02–0.45	0.01–0.3	0–0.3
R	0–1.1	0.1–1.3	0.5–2.2	0.5–2.3	0.6–2.3	0.8–2.5	0.8–2.6	0.9–2.5	0.7–2.4
S	0–1.0	0–1.0	0–1.0	0–0.8	0–0.6	0–0.5	0–0.4	0–0.4	0–0.4

Table 12.4 Manifestations of electrolyte derangement in the ECG

Electrolyte abnormality	ECG	Predisposes to
Hypokalaemia	Flattened or inverted T wave Prominent U wave ST depression	Atrial tachyarrhythmias Torsade de pointes Re-entry, VT
Hyperkalaemia	Prolonged P wave Tall peaked T wave	Sinus arrest Varieties of heart block VT or VF (sinusoidal)
Hypocalcaemia	Long QTc (unreliable)	Predominant effect is a negative inotropy
Hypercalcaemia	Short QTc (unreliable)	
Hypomagnesaemia	Prolonged QT	Resistant tachyarrhythmias
Hypermagnaesaemia		Junctional or sinus bradycardia Sinoatrial block AV block Asystole

Continuous ECG monitoring gives an accessible rhythm strip enabling detection of the hallmarks of common electrolyte abnormalities (Table 12.4) or ischaemia in addition to rhythm and conduction abnormalities.

The age-related changes in heart rate (Figure 12.3) are accompanied by increases in P and QRS durations and the PR interval. Rate correction is applied to these intervals by dividing them by the square root of the RR interval.

Determining the heart rhythm

While waiting for your advanced pattern recognition skills to develop, it is best to adopt a structured approach to the interpretation of rhythm from the ECG monitor. The rhythm can be safely determined by answering questions about the presence of a pulse, QRS complexes and shock followed by determination of the rate, regularity and P wave position and morphology.

1 HAS THE PATIENT GOT A PULSE?

If there is no pulse then start cardiopulmonary resuscitation using a structured ABC approach and use the pulseless arrhythmia algorithm (see Chapter 2 page 15).

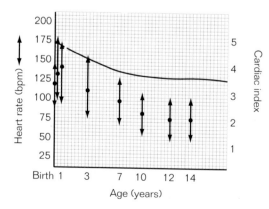

Figure 12.3 Mean cardiac index trend during childhood and mean pulse rate (with 95% range).

2 ARE THERE QRS COMPLEXES?

If there are no QRS complexes but there is a pulse, then there is a technical fault in the ECG monitoring. Check leads, monitor, power supply, etc.

A pulseless rhythm with no QRS complexes is either ventricular fibrillation or asystole and you should have started CPR by now! A pulseless rhythm with QRS complexes is either 'pulseless electrical activity' also known as 'electromechanical dissociation' or pulseless VT and you should still be resuscitating by now!

3 IS THE PATIENT STABLE OR IN SHOCK?

If the patient is in shock then use the arrhythmia resuscitation algorithm on page 18 and worry about the finer details of the rhythm later. Although the route through the algorithm is covered by questions 4–8 below the algorithm includes the appropriate actions to take which are not reproduced here.

4 DETERMINE THE RATE

On a paper trace at 25 mm sec^{-1} the rate is calculated by dividing the RR interval (measured by counting large 5 mm boxes) into 300. Bedside ECG monitors do this for you but may have difficulty registering QRS complexes if their morphology is changing (e.g. some paced beats and some not paced) or if there are tall peaked T waves for example. When in doubt, check the ECG rate against the pulse. This will also allow the detection of pulsus paradoxus and pulsus alternans.

5 IS THE RHYTHM REGULAR OR IRREGULAR?

An irregular rhythm may be sinus (see questions 6 and 7) which speeds up in spontaneous inspiration or may be caused by atrial fibrillation, variable degrees of heart block or intermittent ectopic beats.

6 ARE THERE P WAVES?

P waves represent atrial contraction. They are absent in atrial fibrillation, sawtooth in atrial flutter and hidden in some tachycardias particularly if the QRS is broad. Retrograde P waves can sometimes be seen in nodal and junctional rhythms.

7 ARE THE P WAVES SYNCHRONISED WITH THE QRS COMPLEXES?

Sinus rhythm is indicated by a 1:1 relationship between P waves and QRS complexes.

- First degree block is defined by a prolonged PR interval.
- Second degree block can show a lengthening PR leading to a dropped beat (Wenkebach or Mobitz type I) which implies AV nodal block. Intermittent block with a normal (or constant) PR interval for conducted beats is second degree block of Mobitz type II. It is commonly associated with bundle branch block and implies blockage below the AV node.
- Third degree block is complete AV (P:QRS) dissociation. The idioventricular rate is slow and QRS broad.

8 WHAT IS THE QRS MORPHOLOGY?

Narrow QRS implies normal HIS bundle and ventricular conduction. Thus narrow complex tachycardias are supraventricular, nodal or the lowest junctional. Some degree of differentiation can be provided by the response to vagal manoeuvres or adenosine. Broad complex tachycardias represent, at the very least, bundle branch block (in which case you should still be able to see P waves with each QRS). The broad complex however represents aberrant ventricular conduction and thus likely ventricular tachycardia (in which case there should be no discernible P waves).

Narrow complex bradycardia is usually nodal. (Slow atrial fibrillation is very rare in childhood). A bradycardia with extremely broad complexes is seen as an agonal rhythm (terminal) in all sorts of circumstances. The pulse is usually impalpable and the complexes so broad that your instinct is to call it asystole rather than pulseless electrical activity. This puts you into the correct resuscitation algorithm anyway and it is mentioned here in case the QRS morphology is deteriorating as you watch it.

Pacing and its potential assistance with the differential diagnosis of tachycardia is covered in the section on postoperative care for patients with congenital heart disease in Chapter 13 page 198–201.

ARRHYTHMIAS

At rest, the resting membrane potential of the myocardial cell is maintained or restored by Na^+/K^+ ATPase. Depolarisation follows a 5-phase cycle. Each phase is associated predominantly with the flow of a principal cation. In phase 0 the fast Na^+ channel opens allowing sufficient Na^+ influx to reverse membrane polarity. In phase I the sodium influx slows and it stops in phase II as the slow Ca^+ channel opens. The calcium influx in the plateau of phase II initiates contraction. In phase III potassium efflux continues the repolarisation and the resting membrane potential is restored in phase IV. Arrhythmias may result from abnormal impulse formation (drugs, inflammation, ischaemia, etc.) or abnormal impulse propagation (change in responsiveness or presence of an accessory pathway). In situations of energy depletion, ischaemia or electrolyte imbalance (Na^+, K^+, Ca^{2+}, Mg^{2+}, phosphate) the propensity for dysrhythmia by either mechanism increases.

The most common paediatric tachyarrhythmias are 'supraventricular' and most of these occur in association with the presence of an accessory pathway(s). In their description the terms 're-entrant' and 'reciprocating' tachycardia can be used interchangeably. Pre-excitation can be identified from the resting 12 lead ECG by a short P–R interval and a slurred (delta) onset to the QRS. The appearance results from fusion of propagating ventricular impulses of AV nodal and accessory origin. The overall QRS duration is therefore prolonged and ST and/or T wave changes may be present in leads opposite to the most prominent delta changes. Accessory pathways usually conduct quickly in an antegrade fashion but repolarise slowly giving a longer refractory period. In this way premature atrial contractions can trigger reciprocating tachycardias. They conduct antegrade via the AV node but not via the accessory pathway as it is still refractory from the previous impulse. The accessory pathway can then conduct a ventricular impulse in a retrograde fashion restimulating the atrium. Conduction in this manner is the most common arrangement and is termed 'orthodromic'. Orthodromic reciprocating tachycardias produce classic (narrow QRS) supraventricular tachycardia (SVT) since the ventricular activation is via the AV node. Antidromic reciprocation occurs when antegrade conduction is via the accessory pathway and AV nodal re-entry occurs. Antidromic reciprocation

- is much rarer than orthodromic
- commonly occurs in the absence of structural heart disease
- produces broad QRS complexes during tachycardia because of the abnormal ventricular conduction.

A further minority of patients (< 10%) have multiple accessory pathways; most of these patients also suffer broad complex tachycardias with a variety of conduction patterns. These broad complex tachycardias, when recognisable through the absence of shock, may still respond to adenosine since AV nodal interruption breaks the loop.

The propensity for sinus bradycardia in babies has already been discussed. Bradycardia resulting from sinus node dysfunction may also occur after cardiac surgery though degrees of AV block are more common. The associations of bradyarrhythmia with congenital heart disease are covered in Chapter 13. Complete heart block will usually require pacing eventually but not always precipitously and may certainly resolve spontaneously after cardiac surgery. The surgeon may be able to predict the outcome from the operative history. The idioventricular rate may respond to isoprenaline.

Some common tachyarrhythmias are shown in Figure 12.4.

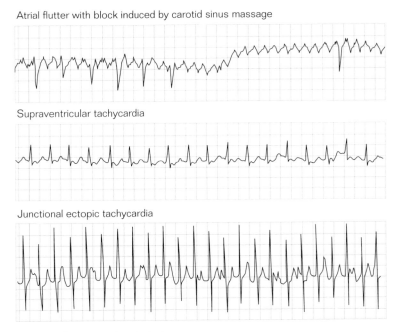

Atrial flutter with block induced by carotid sinus massage

Supraventricular tachycardia

Junctional ectopic tachycardia

Figure 12.4 Common tachyarrhythmias.

Antiarrhythmic drugs

Drug and electrical therapies for arrhythmia are most commonly indicated when there is an associated acute haemodynamic disturbance. Most arrhythmias are however due to hypovolaemia, electrolyte imbalance or other metabolic abnormalities such as acid–base disturbance. Rapid correction of the electrolytes that are more commonly guilty (potassium, magnesium and phosphate) may be more hazardous than the arrhythmia itself, therefore an element of caution is indicated. Arrhythmias presenting as symptoms of myocardial dysfunction from other causes such as ischaemia or the inflammatory effects of cardiopulmonary bypass may respond better if there is a primary problem that can be treated (it is always better to treat causes rather than effects). Reperfusion after ischaemia is a potent cause of aberrant ventricular conduction, dysrhythmia and reflex bradycardia. In vulnerable patients the metabolic stresses of sepsis and pain or agitation may aggravate or predispose to arrhythmia.

All antiarrhythmic drugs should be regarded as potentially proarrhythmic and potentially to have negative inotropic effects (including digoxin). The conventional Vaughan Williams classification of antiarrhythmic agents is based on the effects on the action potential, mediated through blockade of the various associated membrane cation channels. Its use implies incorrectly that the drugs have pure effects and that different agents in the same class have similar mechanisms of action, which is also incorrect. Furthermore the range of antiarrhythmic agents prescribed in paediatric intensive care is limited. Hence the coverage here is restricted to a consideration of haemodynamically robust SVT and a few of the commoner agents use to treat it.

Drug treatment of SVT

The safest way to proceed in the drug treatment of SVT *that is not causing shock* is as follows.

177

- First, prove to yourself that the tachyarrhythmia is persistent, i.e. not self reverting (this may entail a period of observation) and obtain a 12 lead ECG of the tachycardia.
- Second, try vagal stimulation manoeuvres such as unilateral massage of the carotid sinus or attempt to illicit a diving reflex (immerse the face in ice cold water or use a surgical glove filled with crushed ice).
- Third, use drug therapy. Start with incremental doses of adenosine (it is important to make a permanent record of the ECG rhythm strip with each bolus). If these fail, add in amiodarone. Avoid calcium channel and β-blockers during arrhythmia control in infants. Under normal circumstances digitalis is reserved for prophylaxis against recurrence of the tachycardia since it complicates subsequent cardioversion and rapid digitalisation can induce VF during VT.

The sequence of drug administration should be modified in line with the preferences of the local paediatric cardiologists. If shock develops at any stage then conservative efforts should be abandoned in favour of synchronised DC cardioversion under sedation or anaesthesia. Additional agents are available for use if amiodarone infusion fails, but by that time the child should be in a paediatric cardiac centre with access to a full electrophysiological work-up. If the rhythm reverts to sinus or a slower form then get a 12 lead ECG promptly before it recurs.

ADENOSINE

Adenosine must be given as a rapid bolus injection (50 µg kg^{-1} increasing by 50 µg kg^{-1} increments to 300 µg kg^{-1} in successive boluses) and causes brief immediate AV nodal blockade which may interrupt reciprocating and ectopic SVTs. It may also aid the differential diagnosis of both broad and narrow complex tachycardia by slowing the rhythm and revealing the P wave morphology. It will not convert atrial flutter or fibrillation, it may transiently slow a junctional ectopic tachycardia (JET) and has no effect on VT. It naturally aggravates second and third-degree AV block. Indeed the usual ECG manifestation of adenosine's impact is a short-lasting first, second or third-degree AV block, or transient asystole. In the presence of an accessory pathway, antidromic conduction down the accessory pathway may be briefly encouraged. Like the AV nodal block, premature ventricular contractions are usually short-lived effects. Caffeine and theophylline are competitive adenosine antagonists whereas nucleoside transport blockers such as dipyridamole potentiate its effects. It is not blocked by atropine. Its potent vasodilator properties (which do not apply to afferent glomerular arterioles) are not normally observed after bolus injection. Half-life is less than 10 seconds with rapid clearance because of cellular uptake and subsequent metabolism to adenosine monophosphate. It can aggravate bronchospasm.

AMIODARONE

Amiodarone is a useful drug for all recalcitrant tachyarrhythmias. It has mixed effects but basically prolongs the duration of the action potential and the refractory period. Its principal metabolite has a similar profile on fast and slow Na$^+$ channels, K$^+$ channels and Ca^{2+} channels. The conduction depression is more prominent at fast heart rates. It non-competitively antagonises catecholamine receptors and hence has Vaughan Williams class I, II, and IV activity despite being a class III drug by virtue of its potent K$^+$ channel blockade. Oral absorption is slow but not normally associated with negative inotropic effects and the onset of action after intravenous administration may still take several hours. Long-term therapy may be associated with pulmonary infiltrates and respiratory failure, corneal deposits, hypothyroidism (it blocks thyroxine–triiodothyronine conversion) and hepatitis leading rarely to cirrhosis.

DIGOXIN

A summary of digoxin's effects is given in Chapter 19, Ingestion and Poisoning, but in essence it inhibits Na$^+$/K$^+$ ATPase. At the sarcolemmal membrane this increases the availability of sarcolemmal calcium giving a positive inotropic effect which does not demonstrate desensitisation or tachyphylaxis. Antiarrhythmic effects result from augmented effects of vagal tone and decreased sympathetic activity which may counter the positive inotropic effect. The refractory period of the action potential is increased and AV nodal conduction velocity decreased. The resulting rate limitation can limit cardiac output. Routine digoxin therapy in congenital heart disease is out of favour since true heart failure is rare. Oral absorption is so good that intravenous loading is rarely appropriate and paediatric doses are far larger per kilogram than adult.

WORKING OTHER AGENTS

VW class Ic drugs (which slow conduction and prolong refractoriness by a slow onset and offset effect on the fast Na^+ channel) are developing popularity among some paediatric cardiologists. Propafenone has been reported to have greater effect than amiodarone in controlling JET and probably exerts less negative inotropic effect than amiodarone at normal dose (but not high dose). Flecainide has been used to block re-entry and produce exit block from ectopic atrial foci. It also suppresses ventricular tachyarrythmias but has a greater propensity for proarrhythmia than other agents.

NON-INVASIVE ARTERIAL PRESSURE MONITORING

At high arterial pressures, cuffs tend to underestimate blood pressure compared to direct measurement. However small cuffs tend to overestimate blood pressure since a return of pulsation occurs sooner (i.e. at higher pressure) than with larger cuffs. This potential source of error necessitates some standardisation. The width of the bladder in the cuff should be 40 per cent of the mid-circumference of the limb and the length should be twice the width.

The automation of the oscillometric method of blood pressure determination has led to its widespread use in place of the sphygmomanometer. The technique detects pulsation within the cuff caused by the transmitted arterial pulse. As the cuff pressure falls from suprasytemic blood pressure levels, the oscillations abruptly increase in amplitude (systolic), continue to reach a maximum (mean) and then abruptly fall (diastolic) corresponding to the blood pressures. Normal cycles take about 30 seconds to acquire the desired data, which can then be used as a reliable trend. When perfusion is poor the machine struggles to detect a pulse at all and it can be fooled if blood pressure changes quickly during its deflation cycle. Aberrant readings should be rechecked immediately.

INVASIVE VASCULAR PRESSURE MONITORING

The commonly monitored intravascular pressures (arterial and intracardiac) are summarised in Figure 12.5. The process of invasive vascular pressure monitoring involves 'hydraulic coupling' of a remote pressure transducer to a catheter tip via a column of minimally compressible fluid which infuses slowly as a 'flush' to maintain patency. The transducer **must be positioned level with the right atrium and its height altered when the patient's position is changed**. If the tubing making this connection is too compliant then the analogue trace is slurred or damped. Electronic signal processing cannot compensate for this. If the tubing is too stiff then a hyperresonant angular trace with overshoot results which can be electronically damped, hence the preference for non-compliant tubing with signal processing to approximate the physiological appearance. The recorded pressures will also vary depending on the dynamic component of pressure measurement (see Chapter 18 for a more detailed discussion). A preference for distal sites for arterial cannulation minimises the consequences of occlusion or embolism and avoids the errors in pressure recording that can be created by movement or vibration of the catheter. Figure 12.6 shows the different proximal and distal arterial waveforms. Superimposed harmonics reflected from the distal arterioles can lead to overestimation of the systolic pressure and underestimation of the diastolic pressure when using a distal site. Distal arteries also show muted flow-related changes compared to proximal vessels. For these and other reasons the systolic and diastolic values may not precisely mirror the pressure at the catheter tip. Therefore **base most clinical decisions on the mean pressure**. Reliance on the mean pressure minimises error, provided that the mean pressure is being derived by integration of the pulse waveform. If it is approximated (e.g. diastolic + (pulse pressure $\div$ 3)) then estimates will be less accurate from distal sites.

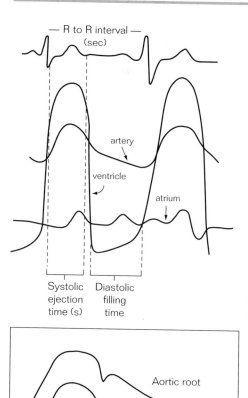

Systolic ejection time (s)   Diastolic filling time

Figure 12.5 Vascular pressure waveforms timed to an ECG rhythm strip.

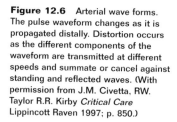

Figure 12.6 Arterial wave forms. The pulse waveform changes as it is propagated distally. Distortion occurs as the different components of the waveform are transmitted at different speeds and summate or cancel against standing and reflected waves. (With permission from J.M. Civetta, RW. Taylor R.R. Kirby *Critical Care* Lippincott Raven 1997; p. 850.)

Arterial lines

Changes in the character of the arterial pressure waveform mirror changes in the flow velocity. Short systolic time intervals occur when systemic vascular resistance (SVR) is high compared to contractility or there is hypovolaemia, which also decreases the total area under the curve. The area under the curve also falls as SVR drops and the diastolic blood pressure falls. The classic sign of poor contractility is a slow systolic upstroke.

Baseline variability of the arterial pressure with respiration occurs if the thoracic pressure excursion is exceptional or if the cardiac function is compromised. Cardiopulmonary interactions frequently entail opposite effects on left and right ventricles because they share

Table 12.5   Normal values of cardiovascular parameters that incorporate flow measurements

Parameter	Derivation	Normal Range
Cardiac index (**CI**)	CO/SA Cardiac Output/Surface area	$3.5–5.5\ \mathrm{Lmin^{-1}m^{-2}}$
Systemic vascular resistance index (**SVRI**)	$79.9 \times$ (MAP–CVP)/CI $79.9 \times$ (Mean arterial – central venous pressure)/cardiac index	$800–1600\ \mathrm{dyne\text{-}sec\ cm^{-5}m^{-2}}$
Pulmonary vascular resistance index (**PVRI**)	$79.9 \times$ (MPAP–LAP)/CI $79.9 \times$ (Mean pulmonary artery pressure – left atrial pressure)/cardiac index	$80–240\ \mathrm{dyne\text{-}sec\ cm^{-5}m^{-2}}$
Stroke index (**SI**)	CI/HR Cardiac index/heart rate	$30–60\ \mathrm{mlm^{-2}}$
Left ventricular stroke work index (**LVSWI**)	$\mathrm{SI} \times \mathrm{MAP} \times 0.0136$ Stroke index $\times$ Mean arterial pressure $\times$ 0.0136	$50–62\ \mathrm{g\text{-}m\ m^{-2}}$
Right ventricular stroke work index (**RVSWI**)	$\mathrm{SI} \times \mathrm{MPAP} \times 0.0136$ Stroke index $\times$ Mean pulmonary artery pressure $\times$ 0.0136	$5.1–6.9\ \mathrm{g\text{-}m\ m^{-2}}$

the pericardial space and have intra- and extra-thoracic sources of venous blood respectively. In spontaneous ventilation excessive inspiratory effort reduces LV preload and causes a downswing of the baseline with reduced pulse volume, the extreme form of which is pulsus paradoxus (the paradox being that a pulse is palpable at the apex but not in the peripheral arteries). In intermittent positive pressure ventilation (IPPV), high intrathoracic pressures can produce a Valsalva effect by reducing RV preload. By contrast, failing left ventricles may demonstrate a baseline upswing during the inspiration phase of IPPV as LV preload is augmented and afterload is reduced.

Central venous pressure (CVP)

Central venous pressure measurements are severely affected by respiratory pressures. The end expiratory value is therefore the most reliable and should be read from the screen in preference to the digital display (which is usually a mean over several respiratory cycles). The pressure alone is not the limit of the utility of the CVP which should also be inspected to interpret the cardiac rhythm and the competence of the right AV valve. In tamponade the CVP rises during spontaneous inspiration (Kussmaul waves), a sign ablated by IPPV.

MEASUREMENT OF CARDIAC OUTPUT

Complex invasive haemodynamic measurement allows informed decision making and is the hallmark of modern intensive care, yet it is not appropriate or available for some children. The first problem is one of size. For example the smallest Swan–Ganz catheter can be difficult to position in children under 18 months. The second problem is one of interpretation because of variable anatomy and shunts. Nevertheless judicious measurement can be inordinately useful if appropriately interpreted.

The limitations of some measurement techniques can sometimes be circumvented by others and there is a whole gamut to choose from. Doppler techniques, bioimpedance, dye dilution and thermodilution are all operator-dependent procedures and the measurements should not be accepted at face value. Accuracy, agreement, consistency, reproducibility,

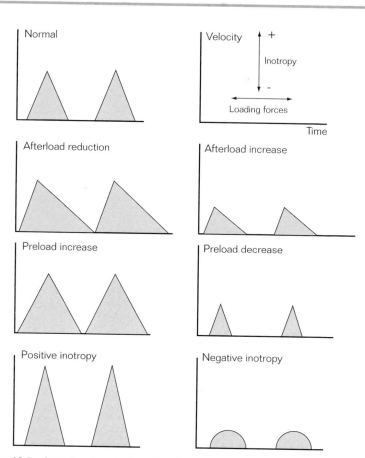

Figure 12.7 Aortic Doppler velocity profiles. Rate corrected flow time varies in proportion to preload and in inverse proportion to afterload. Given a normal profile (top left), the graph at the top right is intended to show which axis will show the biggest (not the only) changes in waveform profile for given changes in mechanics.

sensitivity and specificity should be determined for each operator with each technique before allowing them to influence clinical decision making.

FUNCTIONAL ECHOCARDIOGRAPHY

Where appropriate skills are available and with the provisos mentioned above, functional echocardiography can become indispensable on the PICU. In addition to structural echocardiography it has several uses.

- Estimation of cardiac output from measurements of the cross-sectional area of the aortic root combined with the stroke distance (determined by integration of Doppler waveforms) sampled at the same site.
- The quality of myocardial function and vascular resistances can be inferred from Doppler velocity profiles of the aorta (transthoracic, transoesophageal or trans-tracheal) (Figure 12.7).
- Instantaneous pressure gradients within the circulation can be measured by applying the Bernoulli equation to Doppler measurements (pressure drop = $4V_2^2$ where V_2 is the highest recorded velocity).

i

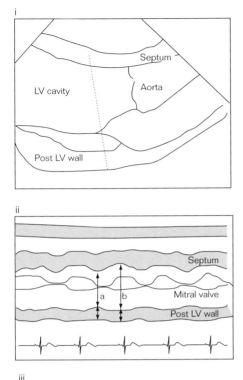

ii

iii

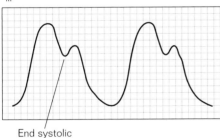

End systolic
blood pressure

Figure 12.8 Indices of systolic
function. Diagrams (i) and (ii) represent
2D and M mode echo appearances. The
fractional shortening (FS) is calculated as
$(b - a) \div b$. The ejection fraction (not
shown) is usually calculated from
changes in the calculated volume of 3D
reconstructions of the LV derived from 2D
measurements in diastole and systole.
Systolic ejection phase indices can be
calibrated to the ejection time (usually
determined from a Doppler trace of the
velocity in the aorta) or to the stress in
the wall of the LV which can be calculated
from its dimension (smaller arrows in (ii))
and the pressure at the time. This is
frequently done at end systole when the
pressure, indicated on (c) the pulse trace,
can be used to infer that of the left
ventricle and the same point in time can
be identified on the echo. Systolic
ejection phase indices calibrated to end-
systolic stress are used as load
independent indices of contractility.

- Indices of left ventricular systolic function (Figure 12.8) with varying sensitivity to loading forces are accessible by combining systolic ejection phase indices with invasive (or calibrated non-invasive) blood pressures. The utility of these indices is limited in smaller or younger patients by the limits of echocardiographic resolution and the LV morphology, which is not conical as many calculations assume but more crescent-shaped in cross section.
- Indices of left ventricular diastolic function (Figure 12.9).
- Contrast echocardiography. Shunts can be delineated by injecting bubbles (peripheral intravenous injection of agitated saline) which are then traced in real time as they pass through the heart.

Pressure gradients determined by Doppler techniques are instantaneous and are a better representation of the physiological gradient than those measured 'peak to peak' in cardiac catheter studies. Such measurements are used creatively to assess stenoses, ventricular outflow tract **183**

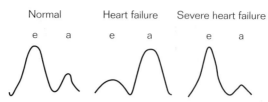

Figure 12.9 Doppler across the AV valve in diastolic dysfunction. One way of assessing diastolic dysfunction is to compare Doppler profiles of left AV valve flow velocity. The normal arrangement where early (e) flow is greater than that produced by atrial contraction (a), reverses in mild to moderate heart failure. A poorly compliant ventricle is more dependent on atrial contraction for filling. In severe heart failure, mitral regurgitation or LV constriction, the pattern becomes 'e' dominant, again with a reduced 'a' component.

obstruction and vascular pressures. The assessment of outflow tract obstruction is also affected by the cardiac output since pressure gradients appear more severe at higher flows.

Continuous cardiovascular monitoring is available from a number of Doppler devices of which the transoesophageal and transtracheal approaches are the most widely used. Its application to paediatrics is complicated by the compliance of the aortic root and variability in the algorithms used to predict its diameter based upon patient surface area. The measurements produced include:

- stroke distance (the integral of the velocity–time curve) that is multiplied by the cross-sectional area of the aorta to give stroke volume and hence cardiac output
- peak velocity and time to peak velocity, which give an indication of contractility but can be affected by afterload. Raised afterload flattens the leading edge of the waveform
- rate-corrected flow time which, if prolonged, implies hypervolemia or reduced SVR, and if reduced implies hypovolemia or raised SVR (see Figure 12.7).

INOTROPES

Inotropes are used to support patients in shock for whom adequate preload augmentation has been assured. There are two principal categories in common usage that have effects on afterload as well as contractility

- sympathomimetics (including the catecholamines)
- phosphodiesterase inhibitors.

Without more detailed measurement or better information the first line inotrope for general use should be dopamine or adrenaline (epinephrine).

CATECHOLAMINES

Catecholamines have a rapid effect, short half-life and undergo peripheral, hepatic and renal metabolism. All stimulate cardiac (β_1) receptors causing membrane adenyl cyclase to raise intracellular cyclic adenosine monophosphate (cAMP) and thence calcium is released from the sarcoplasmic reticulum. Down regulation of receptors leads to tachyphylaxis, which is usually clinically evident within 72 hours of starting a continuous infusion. Stimulation of β_1 receptors has positive inotropic and chronotropic effects but therapeutic agents have different patterns of agonism via the other receptors summarised in Table 12.6. Peripheral α_1 and α_2 receptor agonists cause vasoconstriction, which at physiological levels of noradrenaline (norepinephrine) is predominantly an α_1 effect. Central α_2-agonism causes hypotension and relative bradycardia. The myocardium has α_1 receptors which impart a positive inotropic effect at lower heart rates whereas the positive inotropic effects of β_1 stimulation occur at all heart rates. Vascular β_2 receptors mediate vasodilatation and these receptors are located away from the neuro–effector junction. Thus, even under physiological conditions they rely on circulatory exposure to catecholamines. Agents with any α_1-agonist activity should be

Drug	α_1	α_2	β_1	β_2	Da
Noradrenaline (epinephrine)	✓	✓	✓		
Adrenaline (epinephrine)	✓	✓	✓	✓	
Isoprenaline			✓	✓	
Dopamine	✓		✓		✓
Dobutamine	✓		✓	✓	

Table 12.6 Catecholamine receptor agonism by agent

administered centrally. Dopamine acts at dopamine receptors but has direct and indirect adrenoceptor effects (the latter by causing noradrenaline (norepinehprine) release).

The neonatal myocardium has blunted responses to β_1-agonists. In general the classification of receptor effects of different agents has to be treated with care as effects at different sites and patients' responses at given times may vary. However this is not an excuse for elective polypharmacy. In addition, the evidence to support the use of low-dose dopamine infusions as a routine in intensive care is inadequate and does not, on its own, justify the insertion of a central venous line. The common assertion that dobutamine has predominant selective β_1 activity is also unreliable. In fact vasodilatation, (β_2) is common, it contributes to increased stroke volume and may cause hypotension, although this effect, like its dopamine's chronotropic effect, is weaker than that of isoprenaline.

PHOSPHODIESTERASE INHIBITORS

Phosphodiesterase inhibitors inhibit cAMP breakdown and are much longer acting than catecholamines. Aminophylline has strong chronotropic and weak diuretic properties. The phosphodiesterase inhibition of enoximone and milrinone is more cardiospecific but all three drugs are vasodilators. Enoximone and milrinone have less diuretic action, are predominantly inotropic and may confer increased benefits upon diastolic cardiac function compared to other inotropes.

DOPEXAMINE

Dopexamine inhibits neuronal reuptake of noradrenaline (norepinephrine) and stimulates β_2 and dopaminergic receptors. Experience of its clinical use in children is limited but its actions are likely to mimic those of dobutamine and isoprenaline i.e. chronotropy and vasodilatation being more prominent than inotropy.

GLUCAGON

Glucagon has its own adenyl cyclase receptor enabling it to simulate β_1 activity. This feature is not an unusual property for a hormone. In glucagon's case it has been mostly used to counter excessive or unwanted β blockade but has also been advocated in unusual situations such as tricyclic overdose.

OTHER AGENTS

In addition to the catecholamines other *vasopressor agents* are available although their use is rare and largely confined to septic shock/systemic inflammatory response syndrome or neurogenic shock. Non-catecholamine α-agonists include methoxamine, ephedrine, phenylephrine and metaraminol. Angiotensin II is a potent vasopressor that has a low propensity for arrhythmias and is not susceptible to tachyphylaxis.

LOWERING BLOOD PRESSURE

Hypotensive agents are routinely used in the context of major surgery, cardiac disease and in the treatment of hypertension. Severe hypertension is most frequently due to renal parenchymal disease but other conditions such as endocrine disease (including phaeochromocytoma), renal vascular disease, aortic coarctation, etc., may go so far as to present with encephalopathy.

The choice of hypotensive agent depends upon the context and the desired duration of response. The classes of agent are summarised in Table 12.7.

As with any drug it is important to be familiar with its pharmacology before prescribing or administering it. This is an extensive subject but important notes include:

- no intravenous agent reliably exerts a preferential effect on either pulmonary or systemic circulations
- different degrees and duration of α and β blockade can be achieved by using different agents
- drugs will often display mixed receptor effects, for example α blockade and histaminergic stimulation
- phentolamine produces a competitive α-blockade so its effects can be overcome by sufficient stimulation, for example with noradrenaline (epinephrine) whereas phenoxybenzamine produces a non-competitive block reducing the maximum effect achievable with α-agonists regardless of their dose
- tachyphylaxis is rapid with glyceryl trinitrate and may be partially reversed by sulphydryl-regenerating agents.
- prolonged and high-dose nitroprusside infusions carry a risk of cyanide toxicity.

Hypertensive crisis

Severe hypertension can either be defined by numerical values, which have to be age and context-sensitive, or by the association with organ or system complications, the most critical of which are neurological. When hypertension exceeds the limits of cerebrovascular autoregulation it causes encephalopathy. It is not clear why some patients become encephalopathic and others do not despite equivalent levels of hypertension. Encephalopathy presents with a spectrum of severity from severe headache, vomiting and visual disturbances to paralysis, stupor and coma. Patients presenting with their first seizure must have their blood pressure checked (40% of new hypertensives present this way).

Since the limits of cerebrovascular control are exceeded there is a risk of devastating intracerebral haemorrhage but the most common neuropathology is cerebral oedema. Appreciation of the significance of the associated raised intracranial pressure is important. Control of the blood pressure is usually achieved within 24 hours, therefore many centres do not monitor intracranial pressure and intracranial oxygen consumption. However while the blood pressure is being controlled and cerebral oedema persists, cerebral blood flow will be dependent upon cerebral perfusion pressure. There is no firm evidence that intracranial pressure (ICP) measurement has advantages over supportive measures and control of

Table 12.7 Hypotensive agents	
Class of drug	**Examples**
Centrally acting	clonidine
α-Blockers	phenoxybenzamine, phentolamine
β-Blockers	atenolol, propranolol, labetalol
Ganglion blockers	trimetaphan
Vasodilators	sodium nitroprusside, hydralazine, diazoxide
Calcium channel blockers	nifedipine, diltiazem, nicardipine
ACE Inhibitors	captopril, enalapril

the blood pressure, hence there are wide variations in practice. Management is affected by the degree of depression of consciousness but includes airway support, supplemental oxygen and approaches designed to minimise ICP. The latter include mannitol, fluid restriction and seizure control. In severe cases (GCS < 10) this may progress as far as barbiturate coma with EEG monitoring, paralysis, mechanical ventilation, nursing with the patient's head in the midline and a head-up tilt of 20°. It is important to avoid swings in blood pressure associated with anaesthetic induction. Blood pressure should be controlled gradually (to reduce the risk of ischaemia) over 12 to 24 hours, usually by continuous infusion of a short-acting titratable vasodilator such as sodium nitroprusside. For patients in whom the crisis occurs on a background of recalcitrant hypertension, combination therapy may be necessary, for example with labetalol (α and β adrenergic blockade, dose 1–3 mg kg^{-1} hr^{-1}). Labetalol is longer-acting than sodium nitroprusside and the duration of hypotensive effect can last up to 6 hours, thus labetalol infusion rates cannot be titrated as rapidly.

Infarction of the optic nerve head is a significant risk as blood pressure falls and produces acute blindness without a pupillary light response (treat by raising the mean blood pressure at least 10 per cent depending on the extent of the fall that preceded the pupil change). Transient cortical blindness is also reported.

MECHANICAL CIRCULATORY SUPPORT

Intra-aortic balloon pump (IABP)

The IABP is used to provide diastolic counterpulsation in the aortic arch, improving coronary perfusion. It also reduces systolic left ventricular afterload by deflating during systole and to a lesser extent it enhances diastolic forward flow below the balloon. The balloon is inserted percutaneously by a Seldinger technique and positioned in the descending aorta. Small balloons are available for paediatric patients but the devices are rarely used. The heart rates required make the device impractical for infants despite efforts to maximise the speed of balloon-volume change such as using helium as the standard shuttle gas. When using an IABP it is essential to ensure that balloon inflation (linked to triggers from the ECG or the pulse waveform) is appropriately confined to diastole (which starts at the dichrotic notch). Weaning from IABP can be achieved by delivering counterpulsation on alternate beats or at greater intervals.

Extracorporeal membrane oxygenation (ECMO)

Mechanical circulatory support is most commonly delivered by establishing venoarterial (VA) ECMO. Simpler circuits can be used for left ventricular assist (cannulation of the left atrium and aorta) or right ventricular assist (cannulation of right atrium and pulmonary artery) without using an oxygenator. For a discussion of gas exchange management during ECMO see Chapter 11, Respiratory System (see page 158–160).

The generic indication for mechanical circulatory support is a potentially reversible situation that has proven unresponsive to less invasive approaches. The need is frequently obvious, urgent and irrefutable but its institution is not a 'cure all' or without its drawbacks. Very low survival rates (< 5% in many series) are achieved when failure to wean from peroperative cardiopulmonary bypass is used as an indication for ECMO. Appropriate screening of such patients to exclude residual outflow tract obstruction or septal defects is essential before embarking on mechanical circulatory support. In general the poor historical results for ECMO when used as cardiac support in childhood reflect the lack of reversibility of the primary problem rather than complications of the procedure. Bleeding is more of a concern in postoperative patients necessitating lower levels of heparinisation and more aggressive platelet supplementation. Antifibrinoytic agents such as aprotinin, epsilon aminocaproic acid or tranexamic acid may be helpful.

The haemodynamic effects of ECMO deserve careful consideration. Arterial return from the circuit to the patient increases left ventricular afterload. During VA ECMO, the residual

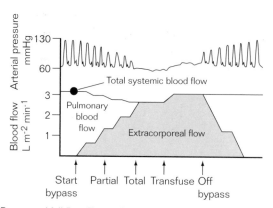

Figure 12.10 Bypass and full flow. The top line is an arterial pressure trace. The lower traces are labelled. The *x* axis is time as venoarterial ECMO is commenced and later weaned. As ECMO flow increases pulmonary blood flow is correspondingly reduced. Full flow is arbitrarily defined as 100 ml kg^{-1} min^{-1} (an estimate of resting cardiac output). At higher levels of ECMO flow total cardiopulmonary bypass may be achieved and the systemic arterial trace is pulseless. This rate of flow should be avoided. Pulsatility returns to the systemic circulation as ECMO flow is weaned and pulmonary blood flow returns. (Extracorporeal Life Support Manual for Adult & Pediatric Patients R.A. Chapman & R.H. Barlett. Uni of Michigan Medical Center 1991.)

left ventricular ejectate contributes disproportionately to the coronary circulation. Myocardial ischaemia and papillary muscle rupture have been reported but the effects of the cannulation cannot be easily distinguished from the severity of the pre-ECMO illness. Rises in left ventricular afterload also have particular significance in the presence of cardiac and extra-cardiac shunts (atrial septal defect, ventricular septal defect or patent ductus arteriosus). Uncontrollable rises in pulmonary blood flow and the risk of pulmonary haemorrhage can necessitate prompt surgical attention to control the shunt. Where necessary, arterial duct ligation on ECMO can be performed in the PICU. VV ECMO provides no circulatory support. However during VV, the pulmonary artery contains the most oxygen-rich blood in the body. Myocardial oxygenation may be optimised if coronary flow is assured. Left ventricular loading forces are unaffected and right ventricular loading is only altered by the fall in pulmonary vascular resistance caused by oxygenation.

The combined effects of reduction in preload and increase in afterload during VA ECMO can lead to cessation of intrinsic cardiac output (Figure 12.10) or 'total cardiopulmonary bypass'. In the total bypass state, the coronary arteries are perfused with oxygenated blood (from the circuit) but the adequacy of this flow is undetermined. 'Myocardial stun' is a separate condition distinguished from total cardiopulmonary bypass. A stunned ventricle does not eject even at low bypass flows. Stun is however by definition, a *potentially reversible* ventricular dysfunction. Distinguishing reversibility frequently requires the passage of time to wait for evidence of recovery (more than 5 days and the prognosis is usually hopeless). In normal ECMO runs, total cardiopulmonary bypass is rarely necessary or desirable and nomenclature distinguishes a different state of 'full flow'. This refers to a bypass flow rate equivalent to the resting cardiac output – usually assumed to be 100 ml kg^{-1} min^{-1} in VA but increased to 120 in VV to make allowances for recirculation.

13 Congenital Heart Disease

- **Incidence**
- **Common associations**
- **Understanding congenital heart disease**
- **Presentation of congenital heart disease**
- **Myocardial diseases**
- **Postoperative care of cardiac surgical patients**
- **Short notes on selected diseases and operations**

In other chapters this book tries to follow a system-based approach to PICU. However in this chapter a more 'disease-specific' primer on congenital heart disease has been included since many people get their first real exposure to these patients on the PICU. As many as 40 per cent of PICU admissions occur in the context of congenital heart disease, so a thorough working knowledge is essential. All children with congenital heart disease should be managed in a specialist centre with on-site access to a PICU.

INCIDENCE

Congenital heart disease has an incidence of about 9 per 1000 live births but the incidence is greater if the abnormalities detected in abortuses and stillbirths are included. The clinical presentation to the PICU may be *de novo* or planned as part of a schedule of palliative or corrective surgery.

The incidence of common conditions and their abbreviations are summarised in Table 13.1. In the subsequent text the common abbreviations are used, for example RA (right atrium), RV (right ventricle), MPA (main pulmonary artery), A° (aorta) and are combined with standard con-

Table 13.1 Types of congenital heart disease, incidence in live born infants, and abbreviation (adapted from Anderson and Yen Ho, 1989).

Lesion	Abbreviation	Average incidence (% of patients with congenital heart disease)	Range (%)
Ventricular septal defect	VSD	30.1	24–34.6
Persistence of arterial duct	PDA	9	5.5–12.6
Atrial septal defect	ASD	7.5	4.3–11.2
Atrioventricular septal defect	AVSD	3.9	2.4–7.4
Pulmonary stenosis	PS	7.2	2.7–10.8
Aortic stenosis	AS	5.2	3.7–8.4
Coarctation of aorta	CoA	6.2	3.4–9.8
Transposition of great arteries	TGA	4.8	2.6–7.8
Tetralogy of Fallot	Fallot's	5.6	3.7–8.6
Common arterial trunk	Truncus	1.2	0–2.5
Hypoplastic right heart	HRHS	2.3	0–4.5

Table 13.1 Types of congenital heart disease, incidence in live born infants, and abbreviation (adapted from Anderson and Yen Ho, 1989).

Hypoplastic left heart	HLHS	2	0.6–3.4
Double inlet ventricle	DILV/DIRV	0.75	0–1.7
Double outlet right ventricle	DORV	0.2	0–1
Totally anomalous pulmonary venous connection	TAPVC	1.1	0–2.8
Miscellaneous		13.7	2.8–21.7

tractions, for example RVH (right ventricular hypertrophy) and LVOTO (left ventricular outflow tract obstruction).

COMMON ASSOCIATIONS

There are well known associations of congenital heart disease with many recognised patterns of congenital deformation and malformation. The associations are not inevitable; not all Downs have AVSDs, but a short list is presented in Table 13.2.

UNDERSTANDING CONGENITAL HEART DISEASE

A sound grasp of the anatomy and physiology of these lesions is a prerequisite to good paediatric intensive care. Many lesions have easy to remember, eponymous titles but their

Table 13.2 Congenital heart defects associated with various syndromes.

Syndrome	Lesion
Apert's	VSD
Crouzon's	PDA, coarctation
DiGeorge	IIIrd arch problems, coarctation, interrupted A° arch, truncus
Down's	Endocardial cushion defects (AVSD), Fallot's
Ehlers–Danlos	Mitral regurgitation
Holt–Oram	ASD, (AVSD)
Kartagener's	Dextrocardia
LEOPARD	Pulmonary stenosis
Marfan's	A° root dilatation, A° regurgitation, mitral prolapse
Maternal hydantoin Rx	PS, AS, coarctation
Maternal rubella	ASD, PS, AS
Noonan's	PS
Osler–Weber–Rendu	Pulmonary AV malformation
Turner's	Coarctation
VACTERAL	VSD
Williams	Supravalvar aortic stenosis, peripheral PS

clear anatomical description requires 'sequential segmental analysis'. This recounts in order; cardiac situs, atrial isomerism, systemic and pulmonary venous drainage, atrioventricular connection, ventriculoarterial connection and the anatomy of associated defects such as those of the septa and valves. Having said this the conceptual key often comes from the embryology (Figure 13.1) followed by a consideration of the loading conditions and shunts, to assess the physiological implications.

> For example, Fallot's tetralogy is *not* just the *random* association of VSD, overriding aorta, pulmonary stenosis and RVH. Rightward deviation of the outlet septum, which can be tracked in the embryology, creates disproportion in the ventricular outflow tracts and accounts for the defect at the top of the ventricular septum where the septum transversum has failed to meet the ventricular septum. Hence the VSD is subaortic. RVH evolves as a simple consequence of the resultant loading conditions – RV outflow obstruction and a VSD. The direction and magnitude of the shunt depend on the balance between the ventricular pressures, the degree of pulmonary stenosis and the beat-by-beat coordination of right ventricular contraction.

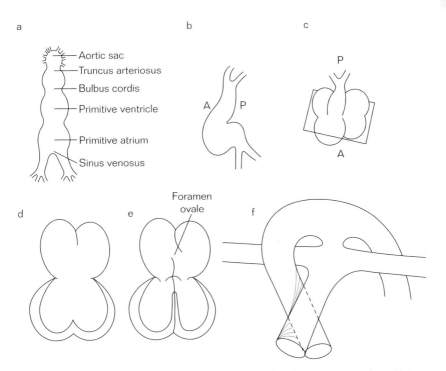

Figure 13.1 Cardiac embryology. (a) The heart forms as a tube, shown in cross section, which twists and bends. This process starts as shown in (b) where A = anterior and P = posterior. (c) is an attempt to show the resultant 3-dimensional relations. A cut in the plane indicated in (c) produces the more recognisable four-chamber views shown in (d) and (e). The atrial septum primum grows and degenerates and with the septum secundum forms the foramen ovale which is kept open by the imbalance between the RA and LA pressures. The endocardial cushions form the AV valves. (f) attempts to show how the spiral septum transversum divides the truncus arteriosus into a pulmonary artery that starts anterior and ends posterior and an aorta which does the reverse. The septum transversum should meet the membranous part of the ventricular septum between the ventricular outflow tracts. In essence transposition results from a straight growth of the septum transversum instead of spiral. Fallot's results from rightward deviation at its lower end and truncus arteriosus from failure of its generation altogether.

Table 13.3 Differentiating congenital heart disease by manner of presentation.

Causes of cardiogenic shock	Lesions associated with a left to right shunt
Preductal coarctation ± VSD	ASD
Interruption of the aorta	VSD
Cardiomyopathies	PDA
HLHS	AP window
Critical AS	AVSD
Anomalous coronary artery	Systemic AV malformation
Arrhythmia	

Lesions associated with a right to left shunt	
With plethoric chest X-ray or pulmonary oedema	TGA ± VSD
	Truncus arteriosus
	TAPVC
	(AVSD)
With oligaemic lung fields on chest X-ray	Pulmonary atresia ± VSD
	Tricuspid atresia ± VSD
	Tetralogy of Fallot
	Critical PS
With atypical vascular markings in the lung fields on chest X-ray	
	Pulmonary AV malformation

The haemodynamics of a heart lesion are conveyed by distinguishing the pressure and/or volume loads on each ventricle. This method is more discriminating than the lists in Table 13.3 (which should not be interpreted too rigidly) since it aids descriptions of heart defects that can demonstrate mixed presentations, for example acyanotic Fallot, Ebstein's anomaly and AVSD, which can otherwise cause confusion.

PRESENTATION OF CONGENITAL HEART DISEASE

Congenital heart disease manifests with one or more of the following:

- pulmonary oedema
- cyanosis
- cardiogenic shock
- arrhythmia
- failure to thrive
- murmur.

These presentations are detected and distinguished by history and physical examination. Chest X-ray, ECG and four limb blood pressures are appropriate discriminatory investigations but echocardiography remains the principal diagnostic tool. In *skilled hands* it frequently provides sufficient anatomical and functional information on its own without further diagnostic investigations such as angiography, catheterisation, nuclear angiography and MRI. To rely on this information one not only has to know the echo result but also who performed the echo.

In presentations to the PICU, pulmonary oedema, cyanosis and cardiogenic shock (including that caused by arrhythmias) are disproportionately common compared to their frequency in the presentation of congenital heart disease *per se*. For these patients **the perceived urgency to establish a diagnosis (by echo) must never supercede the priority for resuscitation.** Although the presentations are discussed separately, they are not mutually exclusive.

Pulmonary oedema

Pulmonary oedema is usually the result of a left to right (L–R) shunt and as such tends not to present with symptoms until several weeks of age when the pulmonary vascular resistance (PVR) has declined to normal levels and the high neonatal haematocrit has fallen. When pulmonary oedema presents in the early neonatal period (higher PVR) it is more ominous since it is far less likely to be due to a L–R shunt. If pulmonary venous drainage is normal then early presentation implies a cardiomyopathy or LVOTO (i.e. true 'heart failure').

Attempts to compensate for pulmonary oedema lead to tachypnoea, which in infants is worse during feeding and may be associated with intercostal recession because of decreased pulmonary compliance. Associated tachycardia with a gallop rhythm and hepatomegally imply ventricular volume overload. Infants with a significant L–R shunt will demonstrate growth failure but in the short term, fluid retention and oedema can manifest as inordinately rapid weight gain. In extreme cases, respiratory failure (initially type I) supervenes. Appropriate treatment is to:

- administer oxygen and consider IPPV early
- minimise orthopnoea
- give loop diuretics
- restrict fluid intake (after treatment of shock)
- correct anaemia (by slow transfusion to a target haemoglobin concentration of at least 12 to 14 gdL^{-1})
- consider inotropic support.

Infants with L–R shunts have dynamic cardiac outputs but at the point of decompensation inotropic support may well be required. If the response to inotropes is muted and there is a severe metabolic acidosis then correction to a pH greater than 7.2 with intravenous bicarbonate may improve the response. The indiscriminate use of digoxin in the treatment of heart failure without arrhythmia is outmoded. Systemic vasodilatation with captopril or shorter-acting intravenous vasodilators can reduce the magnitude of an L–R shunt and offload the heart. This approach requires confidence that the blood pressure is sustainable and that there is not a prohibitive degree of LVOTO.

A primary indication for mechanical ventilation is clinical evidence of a respiratory pattern that will cause fatigue. However IPPV is also a therapeutic modality which can be used electively. Do not wait for evidence of end stage respiratory failure. Increasing oxygen requirement despite therapy and evidence of hypoventilation (carbon dioxide retention) are manifestations of impending collapse and demand urgent intubation. Positive pressure ventilation with paralysis produces immediate effects:

- preload reduced to right ventricle
- preload initially increased to left ventricle
- left ventricle afterload reduced
- variable effects on right ventricle afterload
- decreased work of breathing
- decreased oxygen consumption
- reduced alveolar water

most of which are enhanced by the judicious use of PEEP. Other priorities are to maintain airway pressure without excessive peak pressures or shearing forces (long inspiratory times, inspiratory pauses or reversed inspiration : expiration ratios).

Cyanosis

Hypoxia without carbon dioxide retention in neonates implies cyanotic heart disease and a prostaglandin infusion (2–20 ng kg^{-1} min^{-1}) is mandatory pending echocardiographic diagnosis. In 'duct-dependent' cyanotic lesions, pulmonary blood flow is only via the ductus arteriosus. Prostaglandin infusions inhibit closure of the ductus but may be associated with apnoea. Intubation may be prudent, particularly if the patient needs to be transferred between hospitals. Oxygen will not improve a fixed shunt and these patients are therefore resistant to changes in FiO_2. Furthermore oxygen may cause constriction of the arterial duct so ventilate with FiO_2 0.21 to 0.3 in the first instance. In the absence of pulmonary oedema

193

the lungs are frequently very compliant. Since positive pressure ventilation will further reduce pulmonary blood flow, gentle ventilation is employed. This can mean peak inspiratory pressures as low as 12 cmH$_2$O. Cyanosis in the presence of pulmonary oedema will require higher mean airway pressures and paralysis sometimes with higher FiO$_2$.

The practice of employing a 'nitrogen washout' or 'hyperoxic' test is rarely performed nowadays. Improvements in echocardiography have largely made it superfluous. The procedure involved sampling right radial artery gases after sustained ventilation in an FiO$_2$ of 1, to quantify the right to left (R–L) shunt for diagnostic purposes. Concern has always existed over the potential impact upon duct-dependent lesions.

In long-standing cyanosis, oxygen delivery is usually assured by a high haematocrit and raised cardiac output. However severe hypoxaemia will be accompanied by acidosis and collapse whatever the cause. Cyanotic neonates require urgent assessment at presentation and frequently intervention (e.g. balloon atrial septostomy, Blalock–Taussig shunt or a 'corrective' procedure). Older patients with known cyanotic heart disease and shunt-dependent circulations are at increased risk of complications of hyperviscosity, such as shunt occlusion, if they become dehydrated (whether from intercurrent illness or inappropriate diuretic therapy).

Cardiogenic shock

True heart failure in childhood, particularly infancy, presents with signs of pulmonary oedema, cyanosis and hypotension with weak pulses. In preductal coarctation, right upper limb pulses may be preserved but femoral pulse pressure is reduced. Radiofemoral delay is not discernible in babies because of their faster heart rate. Where there is severe LVOTO or preductal coarctation, systemic blood flow may be duct dependent. In duct-dependent lesions of this type, differential cyanosis (lower limbs only) may be evident but often is not. Treatment consists of:

- prostaglandin infusion for neonates (2–20 ng kg^{-1} min^{-1})
- intubation, ventilation and paralysis
- consider inotropic support.

If the response to inotropes is muted and there is a severe metabolic acidosis then correct to a pH greater than 7.2 with intravenous bicarbonate. These infants require urgent assessment in a specialist centre.

Arrhythmia

There are common associations of cardiac rhythm disturbance in paediatrics. Of these the most well known are the association of Ebstein's anomaly with right-sided re-entrant tachyarrhythmias (Wolff–Parkinson–White type B) and maternal systemic lupus with complete heart block (AntiRo (SS-A) antibody). Complete heart block is also a well-recognised corollary of complex congenital lesions (particularly those with left atrial isomerism). More universal causes of arrhythmias such as pharmacologic effects, ischaemia and trauma are also encountered.

The congenital 'long QT' syndromes Romano–Ward (autosomal dominant) and Lange Nielson (associated sensorineural deafness, autosomal recessive) present with syncopes due to VT or torsade de pointes. The abnormality can be exacerbated by ketoconazoles, erythromycin, some antimalarials and electrolyte imbalances.

Failure to thrive

Failure to thrive in patients with congenital heart disease can be the result of:

- the caloric demands of a L–R shunt and high cardiac output
- poor feeding

- true cardiac failure
- non-cardiac causes.

It should always be aggressively investigated, explained and treated, and should not be dismissed as a feature of the heart disease. Instructive case histories are common where this approach has averted or allowed delayed surgery (with a lower peroperative risk).

Murmur

Classic murmurs abound in paediatric cardiology. They are caused by turbulent blood flow, which is more likely in high-pressure circuits. Murmurs are therefore not typical features of R–L shunts. Since the degree of turbulence is linked more to the velocity of blood flow than its volume, small VSDs make louder noises than large ones. Ventricular leaks (septal defects and AV valve regurgitation) make pansystolic murmurs. Extracardiac L–R shunts tend to make continuous murmurs (the murmur can be heard across the second sound – not necessarily all of the time). Ventricular outflow tract obstructions make ejection systolic murmurs.

Finally and most importantly, heart murmurs can be a normal feature of the paediatric circulation, largely because of its relative dynamism in comparison to the adult. Functional murmurs include soft pulmonary ejection systolic murmurs (made louder by exercise and ablated by a Valsalva manoeuvre), 'venous hums' (which can often be ablated by head position) and so-called 'arterial buzzes' (which can radiate to the neck).

MYOCARDIAL DISEASES

The big difference between childhood and adult heart disease is that in childhood the myocardium is usually healthy. However there are exceptions. Heart disease in childhood is not limited to anatomical derangements. The following diseases still tend to present in comparable ways from a pathophysiological viewpoint.

Ischaemia

Neonatal myocardial ischaemia may occur in association with birth asphyxia and may present with:

- low cardiac output state
- arrhythmia
- thromboembolic phenomena such as stroke.

The differential diagnosis includes cardiomyopathy and the anomalous origin of a coronary artery. Older children can develop myocardial ischaemia as a result of vasculitides such as Kawasaki's disease and coronary artery aneurysms. Some congenital heart diseases associated with high RV pressures may develop coronary AV malformations but in such conditions the RV function is by definition compromised already.

Metabolic disease

A number of inborn errors, endocrine and metabolic diseases may be complicated by 'cardiomyopathy' in terms of the echocardiographic assessment of systolic ventricular function. Primary and secondary carnitine deficiency and Pompe's disease are also associated with cardiomegaly. Myocardial involvement occurs in the muscular dystrophies and Friedreich's ataxia.

Congenital

Dilated, restrictive and obstructive cardiomyopathies have all been described as occurring congenitally. Endocardial fibroelastosis, (which also occurs secondary to ventricular outflow ostruction) and hypertrophic obstructive cardiomyopathy are the two most common. rdial involvement can also occur in more systemic congenital disorders, for example hamartomas in tuberous sclerosis.

Infection

Toxic cardiomyopathy is common in shock associated with septicaemia or toxic-shock syndrome. The presentation of other infective illnesses such as rheumatic fever, botulism and typhoid may be predominantly via cardiac involvement. Viral myocarditis is not just a default diagnosis but has been traced to a variety of agents including coxsackie, echo, rubella, herpes, and influenza viruses.

POSTOPERATIVE CARE OF CARDIAC SURGICAL PATIENTS

Cardiac surgery frequently adopts a staged approach to congenital heart disease. The aim may represent palliation rather than cure and 'normal' anatomy is an unusual end-point. Planning perioperative care requires consideration of:

- the severity of the preoperative presentation
- anaesthetic events
- the nature and quality of the surgery
- the effects of cardiopulmonary bypass (duration, cross clamp time, use and duration of circulatory arrest, etc.).

Procedures not requiring bypass (e.g. PDA ligation, coarctation repair, Blalock–Taussig shunt) may lend themselves to an approach via a thoracotomy in which case perioperative manipulation of the lung, with or without rib resection, will have occurred. Bypass is usually achieved by a direct approach at sternotomy but in unstable situations can be established via extrathoracic cannulation. Bypass involves:

- cannulation of the great vessels
- anticoagulation
- contact of blood with artificial surfaces
- non-pulsatile blood flow
- cooling

and it may also involve

- extensive suction
- direct contact of blood with oxygen
- cardioplegia
- deep hypothermic circulatory arrest.

This cocktail of insults triggers a systemic inflammatory response (SIRS). Patients present postoperatively to the PICU with:

- hypothermia or hyperthermia
- haemodynamic instability
- myocardial dysfunction (and arrhythmias)
- metabolic instability, particularly glucose and electrolyte levels
- bleeding
- renal dysfunction
- capillary leak
- haemolysis
- neurological injury
- susceptibility to infection.

Patients may go on to develop other problems (e.g. chylothorax). A detailed handover from the anaesthetist is essential as the patient returns from theatre but it is also wise to talk to the surgeon (not a messenger) early after the operation as well. Furthermore, liaise with the surgeon early if a patient's condition gives cause for concern. There are many details about an operation that do not make it on to a formal operation note. Only by gleaning some of these details can you be confident about your treatment plan or your interpretation of subsequent progress.

Routine postoperative access, established in theatre, includes central venous and arterial lines and atrial and ventricular epicardial pacing wires. Independent monitoring of left and right-sided pressures (including PA and LA lines) is highly preferable as part of perioperative routine but is crucial when marginal ventricular function, or high or labile PVR are anticipated.

Temperature instability

Patients return from theatre at varying points in their recovery from hypothermia. Although the theatre team should have achieved a normal core temperature before taking the patient off bypass, the temperature may have fallen subsequently and there is frequently a wide toe–core temperature gap. Once hypothermia resolves, fever is a common feature of the SIRS and usually settles within 48 hours. In low output states, therapeutic cooling during pyrexia to normothermia, or even brief (< 24 hours) hypothermia, may be wise to reduce oxygen consumption.

Haemodynamics

The combined effects of hypothermia, vasoactive drugs and diuretics can make many conventional clinical cues about intravascular volume and cardiac output unreliable. Nevertheless try to distinguish the effects of heart rhythm, loading conditions and systolic and diastolic ventricular function. As the normal peripheral circulation is restored during rewarming, a vascular 'space' is regenerated. Without volume replacement this manifests with falling filling pressures (CVP, LA) and hypotension. The former may be disguised if there is AV-valve regurgitation (V waves) or AV dissociation (Cannon waves). Capillary leak (SIRS) also reduces intravascular volume. Volume replacement should be metered to compensate for these effects and any blood loss.

Routine drugs intended to augment the cardiac output include:

- vasodilators to assist rewarming and reduce afterload
- inotropic agents.

Protocols vary between institutions and choices of inotrope are linked to the pattern of vasodilatation. For example the routine use of α-blockers in theatre leads to earlier use of noradrenaline (norepinephrine) in the event of hypotension on the PICU.

> **Key points**
> - Hypovolaemia is common.
> - Hypertension should be avoided since it stresses suture lines and increases the risk of bleeding.
> - Tachycardia is a sensitive but non-specific sign of compensation and should always be adequately explained even if one subsequently elects not to treat it.

Differential diagnosis of tachycardia after cardiac surgery

- Arrhythmia.
- Hypovolaemia.
- Tamponade.
- Poor ventricular function/low output state or hypoxia (older child).
- Other cause of low cardiac output (assuming that there is compensated shock).
- Chronotropic drug effects.

- Pulmonary hypertension.
- Seizures.
- Anaesthetic – inadequate analgesia, paralysed but inadequately sedated, side effect (e.g. histaminergic or vagolytic).
- Fever.
- Sepsis.
- Anaemia (bleeding or haemolysis).

If sudden collapse occurs after cardiac surgery, the resuscitation requires a structured Airway Breathing and Circulation approach, the latter component of which requires the exclusion or treatment of tamponade. '**Tamponade**' means that there is external compression of the heart – particularly the RA. A diseased heart may dilate after surgery and suffer atypical tamponade without the accumulation of much in the way of pericardial fluid/blood. Tamponade causes any combination of high filling pressure (depending on where the measurement is being made), low output, hypotension, tachycardia, dysrhythmia and desaturation. If tamponade is suspected, then while the surgeon is being alerted the skin incision should be opened and the sternal wires should be released (without dislocating the pacing wires) while resuscitation continues.

Myocardial dysfunction

Haemodynamic instability can occur without myocardial dysfunction but contractility is inevitably impaired as part of the SIRS. Additional hazards include coronary air embolism during decannulation. The surgeon may leave the chest or sternum open if the heart is likely to dilate or fail, but this does not provide 100 per cent security against tamponade. Evidence of poor cardiac function should provoke prompt re-evaluation of both the diagnosis and surgical result. Transthoracic or transoesophageal echocardiogram may suffice at first, to exclude residual septal defects or ventricular outflow tract obstruction, but cardiac catheterisation is the definitive investigation. The intensivist should be able to distinguish the effects of heart rhythm, loading conditions and systolic and diastolic ventricular function as they may require opposite therapeutic approaches. Systolic dysfunction requires inotropes, with or without vasodilators, whereas diastolic dysfunction can deteriorate with inotropes and may respond better to volume replacement. 'Myocardial stun' can prove particularly resistant to inotropic support, necessitating ventricular-assist devices, ECMO or a balloon pump (in older patients).

Another manifestation of myocardial dysfunction is a propensity for dysrhythmias, which may be aggravated by electrolyte disturbances. Most dysrhythmias are short lived and asymptomatic. When treatment is required a preference for pacing solutions reflects:

- the opportunity provided by the pacing wires
- the preponderance of bradycardias, usually due to varying degrees of AV dissociation.
- the negative inotropic effects of antiarrhythmic drugs.

Therapeutic cooling can also be used for drug and pacing-resistant tachyarrhythmias (e.g. junctional ectopic tachycardia) if evidence suggests that they are significantly affecting cardiac output. Elective hypothermia requires mandatory paralysis.

Pacing

Convention dictates that perioperative epicardial pacing wires are positioned with atrial wires to the right chest and ventricular wires to the left. Without this access, short-term solutions for bradyarrhythmia may be achieved with transcutaneous or transoesophageal pacing while a transvenous wire is positioned.

The most frequent indication for pacing is bradyarrhythmia. In children the fall in output with bradycardia is precipitate and dramatic. Even in older children and adults the ability to abruptly compensate by increasing stroke volume is limited. The indication for pacing a bradyarrhythmia is clinical evidence of a low cardiac output: altered conscious level, syncope twice low urine output, twice poor peripheral perfusion, twice acidosis or hypotension.

Table 13.4 Pacemaker nomenclature

Chamber paced	Chamber sensed	Response to sensing	Programmability	Tachyarrhythmia functions
O =None	O =None	O =None	O =None	O =None
A =Atrium	A =Atrium	T =Triggered	P =Programme	P =Pace (overdrive)
V =Ventricle	V =Ventricle	I =Inhibited	M =Multiprogramme	S =Shock
D =Dual	D =Dual	D =Dual (T + I)	R =Rate modulation	D =Dual (P + S)

Put another way, if the patient is asymptomatic and the cardiac output appears adequate, then immediate intervention may not be indicated.

Pacing modes are described by a standard nomenclature (Table 13.4) that describes in sequence the chambers; paced, sensed and the mode of pacing. These three nomenclature positions describe modes for bradyarrythmia. The fourth and fifth terms describe programmability and tachyarrhythmia functions.

Other terms in common parlance map to this nomenclature as shown in Table 13.5:

Table 13.5 Mapping pacemaker nomenclature.

Fixed rate pacing	AOO or VOO
Atrial demand pacing	AAI
Ventricular demand pacing	VVI
AV sequential pacing	DVI
AV universal	DDD
AV demand	DDI

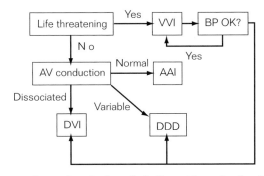

Figure 13.2 The approach to pacing a bradyarrythmia. See text for explanation. With modern devices the popular short cut (dual chamber for all) is usually safe and dual chamber modes are preferable since cardiac output is likely to be greater. Surgeons should be encouraged to site atrial as well as ventricular wires.

A PRAGMATIC APPROACH TO PACING BRADYARRHYTHMIA (Figure 13.2)

1 CONNECT THE PACEMAKER LEADS TO THE PACEMAKER

If there are two atrial wires and two ventricular wires then it is obvious what to do. The two atrial wires connect to the atrial electrodes and the two ventricular wires to the ventricular electrodes. If there is only one ventricular wire then you will need to establish a reference electrode in the skin for a connection to the other ventricular electrode. If you do not have access to purpose-made kit then slide a subcutaneous needle through the skin and connect the reference ventricular electrode to it with a crocodile clip.

2 IF A BRADYARRYTHMIA IS LIFE THREATENING, START VVI AT AN APPROPRIATE RATE.

The native ventricular rhythm will be sensed and there is no danger of inducing a tachyarrhythmia.

3 CHECK THAT THE VENTRICULAR STIMULUS IS CAPTURED AND THAT THE PULSE RATE IS APPROPRIATE

Note to check pulse and not just the ECG. Pacemaker default settings should generate sufficient current to capture but the rate may well be too slow if adult defaults have been programmed. If there is no capture (i.e. no pulse in association with the pacemaker stimulus) then increase the ventricular output.

4 CHECK STIMULATION THRESHOLDS

Once an adequate pulse rate and blood pressure are assured you can check the stimulation thresholds by gradually turning the output down for the ventricular wires until capture is lost. Having noted when this occurs, return the output to 2 mA above this level or twice the threshold depending on your unit protocol.

5 CONSIDER CHANGING TO A DUAL CHAMBER PACING MODE

This will only be possible if there are atrial wires. If you are using atrial wires check their stimulation thresholds in the same manner as above. 'Physiological pacing' describes modes in which the coordination of atrial and ventricular contraction is preserved and the rate is responsive to the SA node (DDD, VDD). These modes have the advantage of being adaptive to meandering native rhythms. Re-entrant tachycardia is a rare, recognised complication of modes like these that involve dual chamber sensing and response. However dual chamber pacing is still frequently preferred because the atrial component to ventricular filling makes a significant (15–30%) contribution to the cardiac output. If a tachyarrhythmogenic effect is observed, the retrograde conduction is likely to be through the AV node and the tachycardia should respond to an increase in the ventricular refractory period.

Successful atrial demand pacing (AAI) requires normal AV conduction, otherwise AV sequential pacing (DVI) will be more effective. If the atria are not being sensed (DVI) and AV synchrony is desired then the paced rate should be set to exceed the intrinsic atrial rate. For some models of pacemaker, dual chamber pacing at physiological rates requires independent adjustment of AV delay and refractory periods.

6 INSTITUTE A REGIME OF DAILY CHECKS OF PACEMAKER FUNCTION

It is important to include pacemaker checks as part of the daily or twice daily routine medical review. However, rule number one is 'if it is not broken don't fix it!' Do not adjust pacemakers unless you are familiar with both the physiology and the technology (i.e. specific knowledge of the model and type of pacemaker being used). Daily checks include:

* determination of the underlying cardiac rhythm by brief interruption of pacemaker output
* checking the stimulation and sensing thresholds by reducing them until capture/sensing ceases then resetting as above.

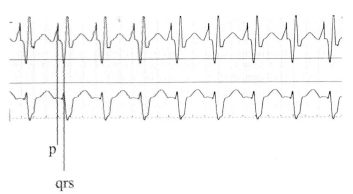

p

qrs

Figure 13.3 Atrial ECG during sinus tachycardia, rate 200 bpm (paper speed 50 mm sec⁻¹). The upper atrial trace clearly distinguishes P waves which can be mapped to the synchronous lead II (lower trace).

This will give early warning of failing wires as the thresholds rise over time before capture is lost. It will also maximise the functional life span of the wires. If the underlying rhythm is absent or inadequate, a backup pacemaker should be kept nearby.

PACEMAKER USE DURING TACHYARRHYTHMIA

FOR DIAGNOSIS

Epicardial pacing wires can facilitate diagnosis by allowing access to an atrial ECG. During a 12 lead ECG, connect the atrial pacing wire to a V lead and produce a rhythm strip that is paired with standard lead II. The atrial ECG helps differentiate different types of narrow complex tachycardias (Figure 13.3).

FOR TREATMENT

Atrial pacing wires also allow the opportunity for pacing solutions to tachyarrhythmias. Pacing is not appropriate for sinus tachycardia or atrial fibrillation but can be useful for paroxysmal atrial tachycardias and flutter. Pacing solutions for tachyarrhythmia should not be attempted without immediate access to DC cardioversion should it be necessary. Pacing approaches for the treatment of VT can speed the dysrhythmia or precipitate VF and are not recommended.

Two pacing techniques are available for supraventricular tachyarrhythmia. The technique of *overdrive atrial pacing* is to commence at a slow rate and increase to a rate 20 per cent higher than the intrinsic atrial rate. This is sustained for 20 to 30 seconds and, if successful, will 'capture' the atrial depolarisation allowing the paced rate to then be slowed to the desired value. If unsuccessful another approach is to try and *induce atrial fibrillation* with very fast atrial pacing (rates > 400 min⁻¹) and then switch the pacemaker off in the hope that the fibrillation will be unstable and decay into sinus rhythm.

Attempts to capture junctional ectopic and nodal tachycardias by overdrive atrial or dual chamber pacing are rarely successful.

Metabolic instability

Metabolic instability is a rather glib phrase, coined here to allow the amalgamation of a series of interrelated electrolyte and biochemical derangements that are commonly seen in postoperative cardiac patients. As in other intensive care situations it is important to treat causes rather than effects and avoid the temptation to treat numbers directly in order to 'buff the charts'. For example at a spinal level a **metabolic acidosis** might prompt a dose of bicarbonate which can aggravate intracellular acidosis. More importantly administering serial doses of bicarbonate to postoperative cardiac patients is like burying your head in the sand. It will mask the nature and extent of the problem and unless the cause is treated, the acidosis will recur. Bicarbonate is a significant sodium load and alternatives like THAM have effects that are just as temporary. There is still a role for rapid correction of pH for example in shocked patients displaying an inadequate response to inotropes but a more appropriate response to isolated acidosis could follow a consideration of the possible causes, for example:

- lactic acid washout from reperfused peripheries
- low cardiac output
- hypovolaemia
- other causes of low oxygen delivery (e.g. anaemia or cyanosis)
- SIRS
- acute renal failure
- bicarbonate losses.

Treat the cause first. If necessary in order to determine the cause measure lactate, oxygen extraction, chloride (to enable calculation of the anion gap) and urinary pH. Where indicated boost the plasma volume, transfuse or increase inotropes, etc. Persistent acidosis (which means the cause has not been resolved) is most effectively treated by dialysis against a bicarbonate-containing dialysate.

Metabolic alkalosis is equally as common as acidosis and results from:

- hypokalaemia (as a result of renal compensation)
- diuresis (hypokalaemia or hypochloraemia)
- chronic respiratory disease (this should have been recognised preoperatively)
- citrated blood products (metabolism of citrate produces bicarbonate).

Serum potassium is closely linked to acid–base status. Acidosis prompts an efflux of intracellular potassium and alkalosis the reverse. In the context of a postoperative patient **hyperkalaemia** may also be a consequence of:

- acute renal failure
- insulin resistance (hyperglycaemia)
- exogenous potassium load (old blood used in the pump prime or a misjudged replacement regime)
- haemolysis (implied by haemoglobinuria or renal failure with a falling haemoglobin).

Treat the cause where possible. Treat the effect if the patient is symptomatic or has ECG changes. Direct treatment options include:

- intravenous insulin and dextrose (0.1 unit kg^{-1} of soluble insulin with 2 ml kg^{-1} of 50% dextrose, and monitor blood sugar).
- nebulised salbutamol (dose is the same as for asthma but the danger of tachyarrythmia is increased).
- intravenous salbutamol 1–5 µg kg^{-1} min^{-1}.
- Rectal administration of an ion exchange resin such as calcium resonium (0.5 g kg^{-1} dose^{-1}) which works more slowly.

Cardiopulmonary bypass, even with a blood prime in the circuit, frequently involves a degree of haemodilution and as a consequence a brisk diuresis is common in the early postoperative period. **Hypokalaemia** is therefore very common and may be exacerbated by:

- diuretic administration
- endogenous or exogenous catecholamines
- metabolic alkalosis
- hyperglycaemia (insulin release).

A culture that demands tight control of serum potassium levels (within limits that are far more stringent than physiological limits) has been inherited from adult cardiac surgery in many centres. It has the advantage of indicating potassium replacement early in circumstances where serum levels may be falling rapidly. However children by and large have a healthy myocardium and are less prone to dysrhythmias from hypokalaemia. Neonates are also remarkably tolerant of hyperkalaemia.

Hyperglycaemia is also common, usually temporary and is not routinely treated since early treatment carries a substantial risk of hypoglycaemia. If it is excessive and persistent then it requires explanation. It is treated if osmotic effects become a concern or if ketoacidosis develops (diabetes mellitus). Exacerbating features may be:

- stress response (circulating insulin antagonists)
- exogenous catecholamines
- hypothermia (reduced consumption of infused carbohydrate)
- dextrose administration (e.g. to treat hyperkalaemia).

Although hyperglycaemia is common, rebound **hypoglycaemia** can even occur without exogenous insulin and calorie input may be deficient as a result of fluid restriction. These factors may be exacerbated by:

- poor nutritional state (this should be recognisable preoperatively)
- insulin therapy for hyperkalaemia
- hepatic failure.

Supplemental dextrose can be administered as a 50% dextrose infusion into a central vein. Normal glucose requirements for babies are 6 mg kg^{-1} min^{-1}. Insulin resistance in postoperative patients can lead to requirements as high as 12 mg kg^{-1} min^{-1} but rarely higher.

Hypocalcaemia can result from alkalosis or diuresis but is a common association of IIIrd branchial arch (aortic arch) anomalies and DiGeorge syndrome. Calcium is a very effective inotrope in children and is antiarrhythmic in the presence of hyperkalaemia.

Haemostasis

Some blood loss is inevitable after cardiac surgery. Hopefully all the blood loss escapes through the surgical drains and the rate of loss can therefore be monitored. However clot occlusion of surgical drains can occur, and if bleeding has not ceased tamponade will result. Persistent bleeding or blood loss at rates equal to or more than 5 ml kg^{-1} hr^{-1} should make one consider surgical re-exploration. Meanwhile, all other parameters should be optimised. Bleeding tendency (not just coagulopathy) can be assessed by the whole blood activated clotting time. More information is potentially available from thromboelastography if available.

Hypothermia inhibits coagulation and many serine proteases in the cascade require calcium as a co-factor during activation. Thus warming the patient to normothermia and supplying a calcium infusion may help. Clotting factors themselves can be supplied by infusion of fresh frozen plasma but fibrinogen depletion can be better supplemented using cryoprecipitate. Unintentional residual heparinisation can be treated with a repeat dose of protamine (always give slowly and be prepared for a marked haemodynamic response, e.g. pulmonary hypertension or systemic hypotension). Platelet counts may be low (sequestered in the bypass circuit or activated and mopped up by the reticuloendothelial system) but platelet dysfunction can contribute to bleeding even if the platelet count is normal. Platelet supplementation is therefore advisable whenever there is bleeding in the early stages after cardiopulmonary bypass.

Drugs that inhibit fibrinolysis may also be useful. Aprotonin is a serine protease inhibitor that prolongs the ACT but has greater effects inhibiting fibrinolysis. Epsilon aminocaproic acid (EACA) and tranexamic acid are antifibrinolytic agents that are less popular because of their theoretical potential for poorly controlled, diffuse thrombogenesis.

Over the longer term, low cardiac output and high venous pressures can cause liver injury, the manifestations of which include a persistent coagulopathy.

Renal dysfunction

In the absence of diuretic administration, urine flow can be a good marker of adequate haemodynamics. The tendency for a capillary leak, myocardial dysfunction and pulmonary oedema make a negative water balance a crucial issue in improving cardiopulmonary function postoperatively. Once adequate intravascular volume is assured postoperatively, it is routine to induce diuresis and implement a simultaneous fluid restriction if the patient received cardiopulmonary bypass. To this end it is often useful to look at colloid and crystalloid balances separately. If hypotension or low cardiac output are precipitating acute renal failure then this will confound attempts to augment the urine output with diuretics alone. In marginal cases, water balance can frequently be controlled with the aid of frusemide infusions, with or without thiazide diuretics such as metolazone. Osmotic diuretics should be avoided in patients with oliguric renal failure. Low dose dopamine causes a natiuresis even when patients are volume depleted. It does not alter the incidence of acute renal failure and should be not be used as a substitute for more direct control of water balance.

There is widespread acceptance (without good evidence) that patients with peritoneal dialysis cannulae, inserted at surgery and allowed to drain freely in the postoperative period, have a smoother course if not a better outcome. Theoretical justification for such an approach is not limited to the ease of institution of peritoneal dialysis but includes potential improved visceral perfusion, which could have ramifications beyond 'kidney' function (gut translocation, etc.). Abdominal pressure can be inferred by transducing the urinary catheter if you are seeking evidence of an abdominal 'tamponade'. Early institution of peritoneal dialysis in low cardiac output states or where there is evidence of capillary leak is also popular and can aid fluid and electrolyte balance even if oliguria is not present. Such an approach could also conceivably shorten or ameliorate the SIRS after bypass. In older patients the surface area of the peritoneum is proportionately smaller and continuous venovenous haemofiltration is preferred.

Capillary leak

The widespread effects of the systemic inflammatory response to bypass and multi-organ system failure are discussed in Chapter 17 (see page 270–277). The key point to reproduce here is the need for resuscitation. Unless fluid replacement keeps pace with the falling intravascular volume during the 'ebb phase' then decompensated shock supervenes. Red cells will not leak as much as colloids which in turn will not leak as much as crystalloids. It is conceivable that in the future elucidation of the mechanisms of SIRS will enable treatment of the cause of this problem, in the meantime a low threshold for peritoneal dialysis pervades.

Haemolysis

Haemolysis may be caused by bypass circuit configuration (e.g. choice of oxygenator) or prolonged bypass even with an optimal configuration. It may be aggravated if venous drainage was difficult or if there was excessive suction, it may persist if prosthetic devices have been introduced (valve replacements or ventricular assist devices) or if VSD regurgitant jets impinge upon valve apparatus. On-going postoperative haemolysis is difficult to control but may be tracked by plasma-free haemoglobin, haemoglobinuria or a fall in red cell haemoglobin. The clear danger is one of acute renal failure. Free haemoglobin precipitates in renal tubules but the free cellular stroma that results from haemolysis can produce a glomerular injury that decreases haemoglobinuria by decreasing the glomerular filtration rate. Haemoglobin levels should be supported by transfusion and renal function supplemented as necessary.

Neurological injury

Generalised hypotonia is a worrying sign of a global hypoxic ischaemic injury, but it may also reflect persistent neuromuscular blockade, sedation or an unusual complication such as critical illness neuropathy. Neurological injury is mercifully rare thanks to meticulous surgical and perfusion techniques. Nevertheless cardiopulmonary bypass accidents are capable of producing catastrophic injuries such as massive cerebral air embolism. Neurological disasters can also result from low perfusion pressures or warm circulatory arrest. Covert preexisting raised intracranial pressure adversely affects cerebral perfusion pressure and can lead to neurological disasters even if bypass perfusion pressures have been normal. Focal deficits as the result of a CNS lesion and focal seizures after surgery imply embolic events which may (depending on the anatomy) have been paradoxical. They usually resolve rapidly in infants because of the plasticity of the developing CNS.

Recognised specific patterns of neurological injury after cardiac surgery include, anterior spinal artery syndrome and occlusion of the artery of Adamkiewicz, both of which cause paraplegia and are most common after prolonged aortic cross clamping, for example in coarctation repair. Controlling a ductus arteriosus is a surgical priority before commencing bypass but can damage the recurrent laryngeal nerve causing vocal cord palsy. The phrenic nerve can be damaged during surgery by direct trauma or by stretching the lateral wall of the mediastinum. Babies rely on diaphragmatic breathing and are more severely affected than older children. Paradoxical movement is more dramatic on the left (non-hepatic) side and is more likely to require plication of the diaphragm to aid weaning from the ventilator. Plication is rarely necessary in children over 2 years old. In the majority of cases the injury is a neuropraxia and recovers eventually, but occasionally a complete neurotmesis has occurred.

Susceptibility to infection

The main concern is the danger of acute staphylococcal endocarditis or septicaemia and the principal problem is the fact that normal reactions to cardiopulmonary bypass produce fever and a left shift in the neutrophil population. Distinguishing septic patients can therefore be difficult, leading to the use of prophylactic antibiotics and a low threshold for re-instituting antibiotic therapy generally. A more discriminant approach is both possible and preferable.

Persistent fever, pericarditis (with effusion) and a raised ESR are signs of the **post-cardiotomy syndrome**; this is an inflammatory condition that arises sporadically after cardiac surgery. It usually responds to NSAIDs.

Chylothorax

Peroperative damage to the thoracic duct is more common after extracardiac procedures such as ligation of a ductus arteriosus, a shunt procedure or repair of a coarctation. Chyle can accumulate without thoracic duct damage if the CVP is high. The lymphatic fluid in a chylothorax is identified by the presence of chylomicrons at microscopy (provided the patient is receiving normal enteral feed). Significant effusions must be drained to avoid respiratory compromise and persistent drainage can prompt further surgical intervention (to repair or over-sew the defect). Medical management involves withholding enteral feeds and providing nutrition from TPN. Alternatively (but less reliably) attempts can be made to feed with calorie-enriched high-protein formulae with a lipid content based on medium chain triglycerides (MCT). Cellular and humoral immune deficiency are potential consequences of prolonged significant drainage and persistent effusions may prompt attempts at pleuradhesis.

SHORT NOTES ON SELECTED DISEASES AND OPERATIONS

Left to right shunts

In general terms delayed surgery and higher pulmonary blood flow carry increased risks of pulmonary vascular disease. A 'pulmonary artery (PA) band' may be used as a palliative procedure to prevent pulmonary hypertension if early surgery is not an option. Preoperative pulmonary oedema may worsen after bypass as a result of the inflammatory insult and an associated decrease in myocardial function.

Right to left shunts

Lesions with a R–L shunt and low pulmonary blood flow (especially those with small pulmonary arteries) may be palliated with a surgically constructed extracardiac shunt. Such temporising procedures buy time before definitive surgery and hopefully promote growth of the PAs. The principal choice is between a modified Blalock–Taussig shunt or a central shunt. The other shunts discussed here, date from the days when definitive surgery for complex lesions was less successful.

Atrial septal defect

The term atrial septal defect (ASD) encompasses stretched persistent foramen ovale, unroofed coronary sinus and three anatomical types of defect defined by their embryological origins. These are primum (low position just above AV valve), secundum (higher position in the fossa ovalis) and sinus venosus (posterior, sub-superior vena cava). ASDs may be associated with many more complex lesions and anomalous pulmonary venous drainage. After ASD repair, patients are more prone to the post-cardiotomy syndrome and pericardial effusion than after other cardiac surgical procedures. Many secundum ASDs are now closed using cardiac catheter techniques.

Ventricular septal defects

Ventricular septal defects (VSD) are also defined by their position:

- muscular
- perimembranous
- subpulmonary
- malaligned outlet, etc.

Size can be measured physically but more usefully functionally, in terms of the magnitude of the L–R shunt. This is expressed by the ratio of pulmonary to systemic flow (Qp:Qs). Depending on the defect's position, the conducting tissue may be closely associated with the rim of the defect and may be damaged during surgery. Small VSDs close spontaneously with an overgrowth of tissue that can cause obstruction or impair right AV valve function. Most surgical repairs are performed through the RA and tricuspid valve without ventriculotomy.

Persistence of the ductus arteriosus

Persistence of the ductus arteriosus is normally avoided by vasoconstriction in response to pulmonary prostaglandin metabolism and oxygenation at birth. Persistence occurs commonly in the premature infant through immaturity, either with or without lung disease, and hypoxia. It also occurs more rarely in mature infants through different mechanisms. Persistence of the ductus arteriosus in older children is a developmental abnormality (as opposed to a feature of immaturity). In these children the ductal tissue may be histologically different from normal. In preterm infants, since persistence of the duct is commonplace, surgery is reserved for symptomatic uncontrolled shunts (left atrial : aortic ratio on M mode echo > 2.5 :1) that otherwise prevent weaning from the ventilator. Pharmacological constriction using cyclooxygenase inhibitors such as indomethacin may be complicated by intraventricular haemorrhage, gastrointestinal bleeding and renal failure. At surgery the duct may be very large, and historically many vessels have been ligated inappropriately through surgical difficulties in identifying the duct (ligated aorta or branch pulmonary artery being the most common). The thoracic duct may also get inadvertently damaged. Non-operative catheter occlusion may be favoured for children who are large enough, and with the appropriate anatomy (short 'hour-glass' shaped duct with open aortic end). Potential complications of catheter occlusion include embolisation of the device or clot, haemolysis, endocarditis and aortic thrombosis.

Atrioventricular septal defects

Atrioventricular septal defects (AVSDs) (Figure 13.4) are defects in the endocardial cushions leading to an abnormal or absent junction with the atrial and ventricular septa. The full

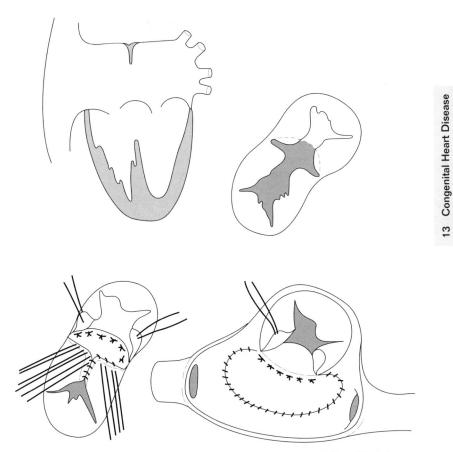

Figure 13.4 Atrioventricular septal defect. Top left: diagrammatic representation of the inflow anatomy. Mid-right and bottom left: superior view of the AV valve. The bridging leaflets are divided and the resulting cleft in the neo-mitral valve sutured. Bottom right: the view from the right atrium at the end of the repair.

anatomical result is a primum ASD continuous with a VSD, which is straddled by a common AV valve (usually 5 leaflet). The surgical approach and the outlook depend on:

- relative ventricular volume – an unbalanced AVSD may only be suitable for univentricular repair
- net shunt – venous mixing gives a fixed R–L shunt but pulmonary blood flow can be raised (risk of pulmonary hypertension) or reduced (aggravating cyanosis)
- the degree of left AV valve regurgitation – a highly regurgitant left AV valve promotes pulmonary hypertension and reduces left ventricular performance.

Total anomalous pulmonary venous connection

Total anomalous pulmonary venous connection (Figure 13.5) is a condition in which the pulmonary veins form a confluence behind the heart that drains anomalously to the heart (e.g. coronary sinus) or via a vertical vein up (to the innominate vein or SVC) or down (below the

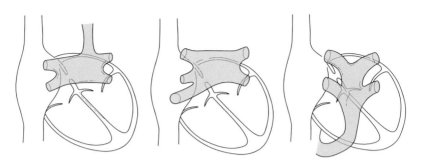

Figure 13.5 Total anomalous pulmonary venous drainage. The pulmonary veins come together in a confluence behind the left atrium that, instead of draining forwards into the LA, drains up, for example to the innominate vein (left), to the heart – usually the coronary sinus (middle) or down below the diaphragm to the hepatic veins / IVC (left).

diaphragm to the IVC or hepatic veins). Infra-diaphragmatic drainage is more likely to be obstructed than the other forms. The anomalous drainage represents a L–R shunt but early presentation due to obstruction is associated with pulmonary oedema, pulmonary hypertension and R–L ductal and atrial shunting. Surgical repair involves ligation of the anomalous channel and anastomosis of the confluence to the LA. The outlook is poor if pulmonary venous drainage is still problematic postoperatively. This occurs when the pulmonary veins are hypoplastic or stenosed, or if the left atrium is small and non-compliant. When pulmonary venous drainage is still impaired there is persistent pulmonary oedema and pulmonary hypertension. Acute rises in pulmonary artery pressure in this context (concurrent rise in LA pressure) may respond to venesection.

Pulmonary hypertension

In normal infants the high foetal PA pressure has dropped to 25 per cent of systemic pressure by 1 month of age (it is always best to compare mean pressures). High flow and high resistance lesions both lead to higher PA pressures and eventually to intrinsic rises in PVR. Pulmonary vascular disease is the result of irreversible muscular hyperplasia in the vessel walls and once established is unaffected by amelioration of the original cardiac defect. Conditions predisposing to pulmonary vascular disease generally involve high flow (e.g. L–R shunts and truncus arteriosus) or impaired venous drainage (e.g. pulmonary venous obstruction or left AV valve disease perhaps in association with AVSD). Alternatively it may arise spontaneously ('primary pulmonary hypertension') or secondary to lung disease such as pulmonary hypoplasia. Finally it may arise from a combination of these causes. Circulations that rely on a passive pulmonary blood flow (after cavo-pulmonary connections) are critically sensitive to the PVR which frequently must be even lower than in normal individuals.

A 'pulmonary hypertensive crisis' refers to an abrupt change where the PVR exceeds the systolic ability of the (right) ventricle. Desaturation and systemic hypotension occur precipitously as the pulmonary blood flow effectively ceases. Patients with an atrial communication (even a patent foramen ovale) may preserve their systemic blood pressure but still become hypoxic. Treatment consists primarily of paralysis and aggressive hand ventilation with oxygen. Intravenous pulmonary vasodilators may be required but all dilate the systemic circulation to some extent and may exacerbate hypotension. Tolazoline was abandoned for these reasons and also because it can precipitate severe gastrointestinal bleeding. Sodium nitroprusside and prostacyclin are more favoured intravenous agents. Ventilation strategies aimed at minimising PVR (see Chapter 11, Respiratory System) include ventilation at optimum lung volume and may include the use of inhaled nitric oxide. Inhaled nitric oxide

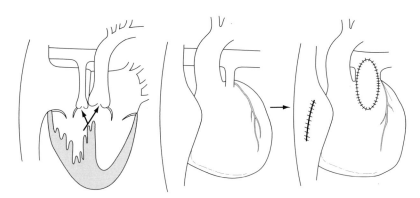

Figure 13.6 Tetralogy of Fallot. The diagrammatic representation (left) represents the internal arrangements (great arteries are drawn side to side for clarity) corresponding to the external appearance (middle). Typically the VSD is closed through the atrium and the RVOT is enlarged from above with minimal ventriculotomy.

improves VQ matching and drops the PA pressure in responsive patients (at most 25% of these cases). Patients rapidly become dependent on inhaled nitric oxide but weaning may be eased by the administration of dipyridamole.

Fallot's tetralogy

'Fallot's tetralogy' (Figure 13.6) was described at the beginning of the chapter as an example of the conceptual advantages of considering anatomy, embryology and physiology to understand a congenital heart lesion. Typically infants with this condition are relatively acyanotic in infancy and the degree of cyanosis increases with age as RVOTO secondary to RVH becomes more significant. Patients with Fallot's syndrome are famous for 'spelling'. A 'spell' is an episode of hypercyanosis resulting from incoordinate RV contraction or a drop in systemic vascular resistance. A child of sufficient age (this is a learned behaviour pattern) will often squat and hyperventilate during the episode. Symptomatic relief results from:

- increasing RV preload
- increasing LV afterload
- decreasing RV afterload

and hence encouraging pulmonary blood flow. The induction of general anaesthesia is notorious for precipitating hypercyanosis usually by dropping the SVR. The secret in dealing with this problem is first to be prepared for it – chance favours the prepared mind – and to use an induction technique likely to preserve the SVR. Therapeutic strategies for dealing with the problem include mimicking the physiology of squatting:

- place the patient's knee to their chest sufficient to cause some abdominal compression
- give supplemental oxygen
- give an intravenous volume bolus, e.g. 10 ml kg^{-1} (to increase RV preload)
- get the patient more deeply anaesthetised or use opiates (with adequate airway protection)
- use β blockade, esmolol (0.5 mg kg^{-1} then 50–200 μg kg^{-1} min^{-1}) provides a short-acting titratable effect.

Persistence of the cyanotic episode longer than a few minutes will necessitate correction of any metabolic acidosis and further therapeutic interventions such as:

- an α-agonist to increase systemic vascular resistance. Methoxamine (0.1–0.2 mg kg^{-1} i.v.) or phenylephrine (2–10 μg kg^{-1} stat and 1–5 μg kg^{-1} min^{-1}) are preferred but noradrenaline by infusion (0.05–0.5 μg kg^{-1} min^{-1}) may be necessary.

The surgical approach is to provide a shunt if the PAs are too small to accommodate a repair. Definitive surgery closes the VSD with a patch and enlarges the RVOT preferably without a ventriculotomy.

Postoperatively, severe RVH can make the RV relatively non-compliant and a ventriculotomy can severely compromise systolic function. Diastolic dysfunction responds poorly to inotropes (with the possible exception of phosphodiesterase inhibitors) and is largely treated by filling the intravascular space (preload augmentation). Beta blockade is of dubious merit for diastolic dysfunction – the stiff RV has a short time constant and filling is not enhanced unless one is treating severe tachycardia. At its worst the RV is little more than a muscular conduit for systemic venous blood.

If the aorta overrides by more than 50 per cent then the description of the lesion is technically one of DORV. Beware of cases that have been redefined as DORV during surgery – this usually means there has been some surgical difficulty. Nevertheless DORV of the Fallot type is treated by a similar surgical approach. An extreme form of Fallot involves pulmonary atresia.

Absent pulmonary valve syndrome

Absent pulmonary valve syndrome (Figure 13.7) is a condition anatomically similar to Fallot. Aortic overide and a subaortic VSD occur in combination with absence of the pulmonary valve in the stenosed RVOT. This leads to severe pulmonary regurgitation and dilatation of the proximal pulmonary arteries. Surgery involves closure of the VSD and plication of the PAs. Severe airway disease is a common corollary of this condition. The main bronchi are extrinsically compressed by the large dilated proximal pulmonary arteries but are often also intrinsically malacial so that airway collapse in expiration persists in the postoperative period, leading to areas of hyperinflation and collapse in the lung. This causes difficulties in weaning ventilation, frequently necessitating high PEEP strategies or long term CPAP.

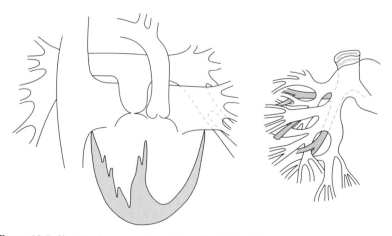

Figure 13.7 Absent pulmonary valve syndrome. The left hand diagram is schematic in the sense that the great arteries are drawn side by side for clarity. The important feature is the stenosed but valveless right ventricular outflow tract with poststenotic dilatation involving the MPA and branch PAs. The right hand diagram attempts to show how these compress the main bronchi from the front. The bronchi appear darker (shaded).

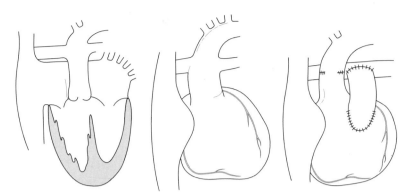

Figure 13.8 Truncus arteriosus. A common arterial trunk gives rise to both pulmonary arteries and aorta. Surgery separates the pulmonary arteries from the trunk and joins them to the RV, usually via a conduit. The back wall of the conduit is used to close the VSD.

Truncus arteriosus

Truncus arteriosus (Figure 13.8) is the persistence of the common arterial trunk. This condition occurs through failure of development of the embryological septum transversum. This defect leads to a single vascular outflow from the heart which fills through an abnormal outlet valve (usually 5 leaflet) overriding a VSD. The anatomical subtypes (1, 2, 3) are defined by the spectrum of PA orifices on the posterior aspect of the trunk (1 MPA, 2 discrete branch PAs in close proximity, 3 discrete branch PAs widely separated). Early presentation and therefore early surgery produces better results principally because pulmonary vascular disease is less likely. Regurgitation of the truncal (neo-aortic) valve is another potential complicating feature.

Coarctations of the aorta

Coarctations of the aorta occur in a number of forms. Coarctation proximal to the ductus arteriosus makes systemic perfusion duct dependent, may present with 'cardiogenic' shock in the neonatal period and requires prostaglandin infusion during resuscitation. The coarctation may be discrete or a tubular hypoplasia of the arch requiring a different surgical approach. Discrete coarctations can be corrected by resection with end to end anastomosis or by a subclavian flap repair which uses the proximal left subclavian artery to augment the arch and avoids a circumferential scar on the aorta. The extreme form of coarctation is a complete aortic interruption. Again sub-types are defined by the position of the interruption in relation to the arch branch vessels. Post-ductal coarctations present late in early adulthood with a murmur and notched ribs on chest X-ray. Surgery may be complicated by bleeding from collateral vessels and postoperatively, patients may demonstrate the 'liberated LV' phenomenon (hypertension). This can demand treatment with hypotensive agents (β-blockers and vasodilators) to preserve the integrity of the anastomosis. Aortic arch abnormalities may be associated with other IIIrd branchial arch abnormalities and other associations include bicuspid A° valve, LVOTO and Schone's complex (tubular hypoplasia of aortic arch, A° stenosis, VSD).

Hypoplastic left heart syndrome

The term 'hypoplastic left heart syndrome' describes a variety of conditions in which the left side of the heart is anatomically insufficient (Figure 13.9). The cardiac outflow is from RV to MPA and its branches, including the descending aorta via the ductus arteriosus. Typically

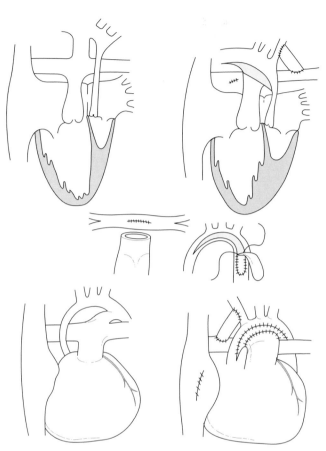

Figure 13.9
Hypoplastic left heart syndrome. The pre- and post-first stage anatomies are shown at the top. The aortic arch is drawn to the right to clarify the connections. The 3D drawings below show the external appearances. The first stage repair excises ductal tissue, disconnects the branch pulmonary arteries and creates a neoaortic arch. The pulmonary arteries are fed by a shunt and the atrial septum is excised to ensure unrestricted pulmonary venous drainage.

the ascending aorta is a diminutive 'main coronary artery' filling retrograde from the ductus arteriosus. The condition typically presents with cardiogenic shock in the neonatal period (for which prostaglandin therapy is mandatory pending definitive diagnosis).

The haemodynamics are a balance between SVR and PVR. Too much pulmonary blood flow manifests as high (i.e. normal) saturations, low diastolic blood pressure and acidosis (beware of a pulmonary 'steal' phenomenon causing myocardial ischaemia). Too little pulmonary blood flow causes severe cyanosis with preservation of systemic perfusion. Ventilation should be accompanied by paralysis and is aimed at maintaining PVR (appropriate lung volume, low pressure, low FiO_2, normal pH hence high normal $PaCO_2$). A peripheral oxygen saturation in the mid-high 70s is acceptable. Preoperative pulmonary oedema may imply a restrictive ASD (needs earlier surgery) or ventricular failure. If the ASD is not severely restrictive, surgery is best delayed until at least 3 to 4 days of age.

The surgical approach is a three-stage palliation:

Stage 1 – 'Norwood' procedure. This stage has the highest mortality (> 25%) of the three stages. It aims to remove ductal tissue and establish permanent arterial connections (MPA to descending A°) and A° to branch PAs (shunt). Unobstructed pulmonary venous drainage is assured by atrial septectomy. Postoperatively the same balance of vascular resistance pertains as preoperatively. Smaller shunts (3 mm) impart more stability but require earlier stage 2 surgery. Some surgeons prefer larger shunts if the ASD was restrictive in fear of high PVR. Any compromise in shunt patency is usually fatal. There may be great variation in the quality of the neo-aorta.

Stage 2 – Glenn procedure (SVC to RPA).

Stage 3 – complete the total cavopulmonary connection (IVC–LPA).

The Damus–Kaye–Stansel procedure is a close variant of the Norwood. When an adaptive approach is adopted to this sort of surgery it is best to establish the postoperative anatomy on a case-by-case basis by asking the surgeon. If there are two functional ventricles then the haemodynamics are likely to be more robust.

Transposition of the great arteries

Transposition of the great arteries involves an embryological failure of rotation of the septum transversum. This leads to an anterior A° attached to the RV and a posterior PA attached to LV (Figure 13.10). The pulmonary and systemic circulations thence run in parallel rather than in series so the neonate presents with severe cyanosis with normal or raised pulmonary blood flow. Oxygenation is achieved by mixing at ductal (give prostaglandin) and atrial (do a balloon septostomy) levels but the mixing is only effective if the balance of pressures across the duct or atrial septal defect favours it.

The operation of choice is a neonatal arterial switch (with re-implantation of coronaries onto the LVOT). There are two surgical strategies:

1   reposition the MPA, the 'French manoeuvre' (more anatomically correct but can stretch and narrow the LPA)
2   use a RVOT homograft (tends to late MPA stenosis/RVOTO).

Switch patients have a high risk of LV dysfunction postoperatively based on the possibility of compromised coronary flow and increased LV afterload, which can manifest as 'failure' or abrupt ventricular dysrhythmias. Abnormalities of coronary anatomy may alter the surgical approach. The coronaries arise from the aortic root (RV), from the sinuses that face the pulmonary artery. The non-coronary sinus is usually anterior.

Late arterial switch is best contemplated after 'training' the LV by positioning a PA band to provide LVOTO, lasting for months before the attempted switch.

The alternative to an arterial switch is an atrial switch, which uses a baffle to divert systemic venous return across the ASD to the LV and consequently pulmonary venous return around the baffle to the RV. Again there are two surgical approaches

1   the Mustard procedure excises the atrial septum and uses a pericardial baffle
2   the Senning procedure constructs the baffle using the right atrial wall and a flap of atrial septal tissue.

Postoperative atrial dysrhythmias are common to both procedures as is the risk of venous obstruction. Pulmonary venous obstruction presents with pulmonary oedema. The Mustard procedure is more prone to late venous obstruction, which commonly affects the SVC channel (where the baffle crosses the ASD) but IVC and pulmonary veins (or all three) may be affected.

Half of patients with TGA have other cardiac anomalies such as VSDs, PS (may allow later surgery without needing to train the LV), or congenital 'correction' (atrial situs solitus with atrioventricular as well as ventriculoarterial discordance) for which surgery, if contemplated, requires atrial and arterial switches. Conversely other conditions such as tricuspid atresia or DORV may be complicated by transposition. In complicated univentricular hearts with associated transposition, the anterior position of the aorta has few functional consequences for the eventual total cavopulmonary connection.

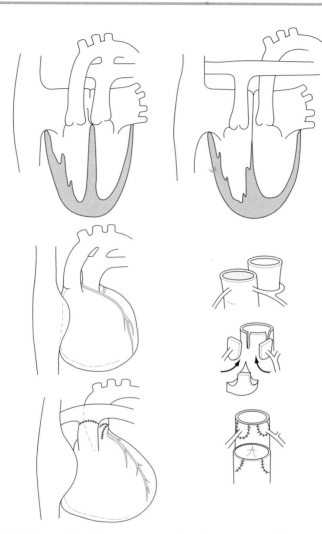

Figure 13.10 Transposition of the great arteries. For clarity the pre- (top left) and post-switch (top right) arrangements are shown with the great arteries side by side. The external appearances below show the true anatomy with the aorta anterior. The surgery involves moving the coronary arteries to the LVOT and switching the arteries above them.

PA band

In the above text a PA band has been mentioned in two contexts – limiting the pulmonary blood flow in a L–R shunt and training the LV in transposition of the great arteries. In the first instance, pulmonary blood flow may still be greater than normal after the procedure but a $\dot{Q}p{:}\dot{Q}s$ of 1.5:1 is a good result compared to 3:1 before the procedure. Therefore do not discount the band just because the patient remains well-saturated in air. Bands can also be measured by their physical dimension (diameter) or by measuring the gradient across them using Doppler ultrasound. A high gradient implies a tight band and can compromise the ventricular function of the ventricle below it. Patients receiving a band for transposition of the great arteries need to be very closely monitored on the ICU. Rising LA pressures and LV dilatation indicate poor tolerance of the LVOTO and impending collapse.

Blalock–Taussig shunt

A Blalock–Taussig shunt (Figure 13.11) is a palliative procedure for low pulmonary blood flow used in duct-dependent cyanotic lesions where primary repair is precluded (e.g. by small PAs). A 'classic' Blalock–Taussig shunt divides the subclavian artery and anastomoses the proximal end to the branch PA. 'Modified' techniques use a Gortex interposition graft, which can leak serous fluid for a time and will not grow (so it may end up kinking the branch PA). Do not site arterial lines in the arm on the side that has recently been or is about to be used for the shunt.

Large shunts allow later definitive repair. The effective size of a shunt relates to the blood flow through it. This is determined by:

- shunt diameter (most significant)
- shunt length
- Pulmonary Vascular Resistance (and size of the PAs)
- Systemic Vascular Resistance
- quality of the anastomosis
- blood viscosity (which may be high because of a high preoperative haematocrit).

Barring catastrophes there are three possible outcome states to shunt surgery:

The shunt is too big:	high saturation (> 90%) with risk of pulmonary oedema (which drops the saturation), low systemic flow (causes acidosis). The patient requires ventilation with PEEP, diuretics, inotropes and/or attempts to raise PVR and reduce SVR and perhaps increase viscosity.
The shunt is too small:	low saturation perhaps no improvement on the preoperative state. Check for shunt murmur and adequate flow by echo or even catheter. If the shunt is blocked redo the surgery. Otherwise promote pulmonary blood flow by weaning from IPPV early. Consider measures to raise the SVR. Do not routinely drop the viscosity/haematocrit as this may compromise tissue oxygen delivery.

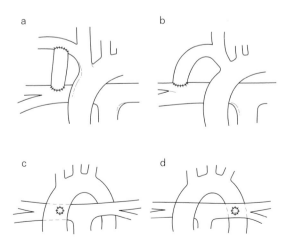

Figure 13.11 Shunts. (a) The most common approach – a modified Blalock–Taussig shunt which is a Gortex interposition between the subclavian and pulmonary arteries. (b) A 'classic' Blalock–Taussig shunt, i.e. using the native subclavian artery. (c) Waterston shunts create an AP window between MPA or bifurcation and ascending aorta.(d) A Potts shunt creates a direct communication between descending aorta and LPA.

The shunt will do: the patient can be weaned from the ventilator and rapidly discharged from the ICU. Growth of the patient will lead to decreasing saturation over time.

Patients are routinely anticoagulated with heparin in the early postoperative phase and later with aspirin, with or without dipyridamole, as prophylaxis against shunt occlusion. Contusion of the upper lobe of the lung on the side of the shunt is common.

Fontan

The eponymous title 'Fontan' loosely includes all total cavopulmonary connections (systemic veins to PAs). These operations are used as palliative procedures in complex heart disease to relieve cyanosis. The modern approach is in two stages:

stage 1 – Glenn (SVC to RPA)
stage 2 – IVC to MPA/LPA sometimes via an extracardiac conduit with variation as to whether continuity of branch PAs is preserved.

In a Fontan circulation (Figure 13.12), pulmonary blood flow becomes the critical determinant of cardiac output and requires a transpulmonary pressure gradient greater than the PVR. If this results in high systemic venous pressures then aggravated oedema includes pleural plus pericardial effusions and ascites. Low cardiac output compounds the effect of high venous pressures on organ perfusion leading to early secondary organ (liver, kidney, brain) failure. Cardiac output may depend on preservation of AV synchrony (sinus rhythm). If a 'fenestration' is left (atrial communication) then cardiac output can be preserved in the face of low pulmonary blood flow but at the expense of a fixed R–L shunt. The surgeon may request postoperative anticoagulation. Postoperative care:

- Nurse the patient with their legs raised or bandaged to decrease venous capacitance.
- Promote pulmonary blood flow (adequate systemic venous pressure, low ventilation pressures, triggered modes and early extubation).
- Adopt an aggressive approach to tachyarrhythmias, particularly atrial fibrillation (more frequent after classic Fontan).
- Preserve oxygen delivery (transfuse patients with [Hb] < 12 g L^{-1} with a target [Hb] of 14–15 g L^{-1}).
- Investigate hypoxia and hypotension promptly. Use the balance of left and right sided filling pressures to distinguish hypovolaemia, high PVR or a left sided problem. Transoesophageal echo is better than transthoracic in reviewing the surgical connections. Both approaches can confirm adequate AV valve function.

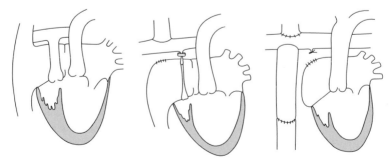

Figure 13.12 Total cavopulmonary connection (Fontan) for tricuspid atresia. The starting anatomy is represented on the (left). Note the atretic tricuspid valve, ASD, VSD and diminutive RV. In this example the great arteries are normally sited. Stage one (middle) closes any arterial connection to the branch pulmonary arteries (usually a shunt rather than the PA) and anastomoses the SVC to the RPA. In stage 2 (right) the IVC is connected to the branch pulmonary arteries either through the atrium or via an extracardiac conduit. A variety of approaches are possible with and without continuity of the pulmonary arteries and with and without a fenestration.

- Catheterise early in failing Fontan circuits to delineate anatomical causes of high PVR, anomalous systemic venous connections (that decompress the right side and cause cyanosis), LVOTO or myocardial dysfunction. This also allows one to locate the position of any R–L shunt within the circuit (e.g. the fenestration or a pulmonary arteriovenous malformation).
- A failing LV may require preload augmentation to what would otherwise be considered high LA pressures. When these patients also have a fluid leak it may be difficult to determine the appropriate or adequate intravascular volume.

Glenn procedure

In a Glenn procedure the SVC is attached to the RPA. If continuity of the branch PAs is preserved then the operation is called 'bidirectional' or 'Kawashima' (this latter eponym is sometimes reserved for when bilateral SVCs have been used). The Glenn forms the first part of a two-stage total cavopulmonary connection and the second stage of a 3-stage approach to hypoplastic left heart syndrome. It frequently includes the taking down of a previously fashioned Blalock–Taussig shunt. The postoperative approach is similar to that for a total cavo-pulmonary connection though one usually anticipates fewer problems.

Konno procedure

The Konno procedure is a surgical solution for a tunnel type LVOTO involving aortic valve replacement and a prosthetic patch to the LVOT.

Potts shunt

In a Potts shunt (Figure 13.11) a window is created between the RPA and the descending aorta to increase pulmonary blood flow. It is a palliative procedure, technically hard to reverse and rarely used.

Rastelli procedure

The Rastelli procedure (Figure 13.13) is a biventricular repair, providing VA concordance when there are transposed great arteries, a VSD and pulmonary stenosis (Taussig–Bing anomaly is defined by the subpulmonary position of the VSD). An intracardiac tunnel connects the LV to the A° through the VSD. The pulmonary artery is disconnected from the LV and attached to the RV via a valved conduit/homograft. Key points are as follows.

- Low cardiac output states require early recognition and diagnosis. For example inadequate ventricular dimensions and/or residual ventricular outflow tract obstruction require revision or change of the surgical approach but the haemodynamic consequences of a large ventriculotomy are not remediable by further surgery.
- Propensity for dysrhythmias, particularly AV dissociation. Permanent conduction defects can occur when the VSD has been enlarged.
- Right ventricular diastolic dysfunction may occur (this is more common when there is right ventricular hypertrophy).

Rev procedure

The Rev procedure is similar to a Rastelli operation but the pulmonary artery is stitched directly onto the RV.

Ross procedure

In a Ross procedure LVOTO is relieved by using the pulmonary valve for the LVOT. The RVOT is then reconstituted with a valved conduit. The postoperative course largely

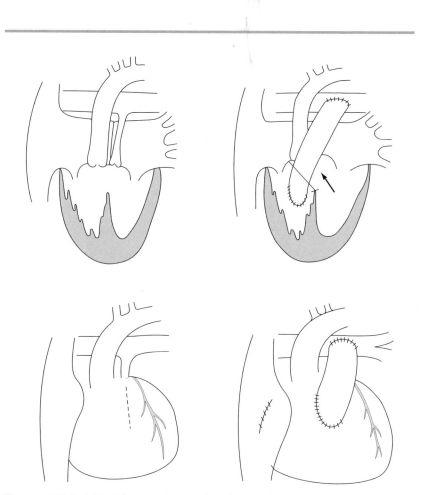

Figure 13.13 Rastelli and Rev procedures. In these diagrams the great arteries are appropriately transposed although they would not necessarily be side by side. There is transposition, VSD and pulmonary stenosis. The RV–PA connection is made with a homograft (Rastelli) or straight to MPA (Rev). The LV outflow is through an intracardiac tunnel involving the VSD. Diagrams on the left are pre-repair and those on the right are post-repair. The upper diagrams reflect internal anatomy and the lower ones external.

depends on LV function. Patients may show a 'liberated LV' response akin to postoperative coarctation repairs.

Takeuchi procedure

The Takeuchi procedure is a creative surgical solution for anomalous coronary artery (usually arising from PA). The condition causes myocardial ischaemia, with or without infarction, and the intention is to prevent extension of an infarct. Tissue that is already infarcted will not recover. An AP window is created and a baffle constructed within the MPA to direct the L–R shunt into the coronary orifice. This operation is still occasionally used when the geometry precludes re-implantation of the coronary. Any preoperative LV dysfunction is likely to persist postoperatively.

Waterston shunt

A Waterston shunt (Figure 13.11) is effectively a surgically created AP window intended to increase pulmonary blood flow in cyanotic lesions. It is difficult for the surgeon to size the connection appropriately and postoperatively patients may have very high pulmonary blood flow (see 'The shunt is too big' under Blalock–Taussig shunt). A more modern approach to cyanotic heart disease where the branch PAs are inaccessible or small is to create a central shunt (Gortex –such as a Blalock–Taussig shunt) onto the bifurcation of the MPA.

14 Central Nervous System

- **Intracranial contents**
- **Cerebral blood flow**
- **Intracranial pressure**
- **The blood–brain barrier**
- **The consequences of cellular injury**
- **Measurement and monitoring**
- **Short notes on multifactorial conditions**

Intensive care routinely involves the manipulation of central and peripheral nervous activity and metabolism. Additionally, patients with specific paediatric 'neurological' diagnoses can visit the ICU for 'neurological' care or for the treatment and support of the respiratory complications of their illness. Encephalopathic patients and those with intractable status epilepticus can arise from any number of parent specialities.

At the risk of using inappropriate teleology, it is fair to say that the ultimate aim of physiological responses to illness or injury is to preserve end organ function and that the body prioritises these relationships with the brain placed at the top of the list. Even if it is inappropriate to apply such 'purpose' to the physiology, the clinical approach to the critically ill child should be the same. Neurological intensive care aims to prevent both the progression of an established neuronal injury and the occurrence of secondary neuronal injury. Much of this is achieved with resuscitation via an ABC approach and subsequent appropriate cardiorespiratory support. However advances in the understanding of neuronal cellular responses to injury raise the prospect of specific therapeutic interventions in this regard. Meanwhile for much of the time we concentrate on structural, mechanical and functional issues and these have therefore been given priority here over diagnostic or diagnosis-specific considerations.

INTRACRANIAL CONTENTS

After the first three months of life the cranium should be regarded as a rigid structure – a closed box. The intracranial cavity contains three minimally compressible compartments, neural tissue, blood and cerebrospinal fluid (CSF) (see Table 14.1).

An increase in the volume of one component of the intracranial space causes a concomitant reduction in one of the other compartments, otherwise raised intracranial pressure (RICP) results. Causes of RICP are shown in Figure 14.1.

Table 14.1 Intracranial compartments.

Compartment	Percentage of total volume	Notes	Examples of expansion
Neural tissue	80%	<10% is extracellular fluid in addition to CSF	Tumour, cerebral oedema
Blood	10%	Mostly in venous sinuses and pial veins	Haemorrhage, aneurysm, arteriovenous malformation
CSF	10%		Hydrocephalus

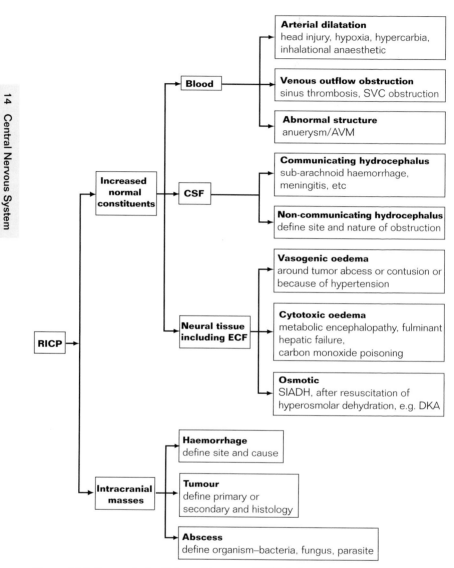

Figure 14.1 Causes of raised intracranial pressure (RICP). Differential of causes of raised intracranial pressure. The most appropriate treatment is usually that which addresses the cause.

CEREBRAL BLOOD FLOW

Increases in the intracranial blood volume can result from the formation of intracranial haematomata or increases in cerebral blood flow (CBF). Since haematomata are extravascular they are best thought of in therapeutic terms as intracranial masses.

Global CBF varies with the age of the patient:

- in infants it is 40 ml 100 g^{-1} min^{-1}
- in children it ranges from 75 to 110 ml 100 g^{-1} min^{-1}
- in adults it is approximately 50 ml 100 g^{-1} min^{-1}.

Changes in CBF are prevented from directly affecting cerebral blood volume (CBV) and intracranial pressure (ICP) by autoregulation of the cerebral vasculature, this maintains cerebral blood flow in the face of fluctuations of:

- cerebral perfusion pressure (CPP)
- $Pa\text{co}_2$
- $Pa\text{o}_2$
- regional metabolic demand
- autonomic activity.

The ability to autoregulate CBF is lost in diffuse brain injury; CBF then develops a linear relationship with CPP. This pressure gradient across the cerebral circulation is derived from the mean arterial pressure (MAP) and the ICP (which, when autoregulation is lost, bears a linear relation to the CVP).

CPP = MAP − ICP

The factors that influence the relationship between CPP and CBF are summarised in Figure 14.2. Normal autoregulation maintains cerebral blood flow across a range of cerebral perfusion pressure and $Pa\text{o}_2$. However even without cerebral injury, if the limits of autoregulation are exceeded, CBF shows a linear relation to CPP. A pathologically low CPP causes cerebral ischaemia and acidosis and conversely, acute sustained hypertension leads to blood–brain barrier disruption and oedema which can then lead to secondary ischaemia.

Over a wide range of perfusion pressure CBF varies directly with the change in $Pa\text{co}_2$. This response occurs rapidly and is related to diffusion of carbon dioxide across the blood–CSF barrier and a consequent change in CSF [H^+]. If this lasts for 6 hours or more, bicarbonate ion shifts return CSF pH to normal. Hypercarbia ($Pa\text{co}_2 > 10$ kPa) is associated with increasing narcosis and there may be a corresponding fall in cerebral metabolic oxygen consumption.

Moderate hypoxia and major hyperoxia do not appreciably affect CBF. Significant hypoxaemia however, ($Pa\text{o}_2$ below threshold values of approximately 6 to 7 kPa) will induce cerebral vasodilatation. This effect seems to be related to the onset of lactic acidosis in brain tissue. In anaemia and polycythaemia where the oxygen-carrying capacity of the blood deviates from normal, CBF is adjusted to maintain oxygen delivery. Normal responses to superimposed changes in $Pa\text{co}_2$ are retained.

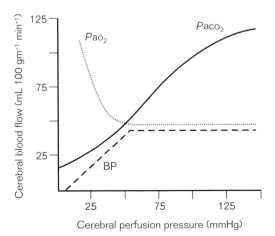

Figure 14.2 Factors influencing the relationship between cerebral blood flow and cerebral perfusion pressure. Cerebral blood flow is normally constant across normal ranges in perfusion pressure but has an almost linear relation to $Pa\text{co}_2$ in the physiological range. Very low perfusion pressure drops cerebral blood flow and very low $Pa\text{o}_2$ (<6 kPa) increases it. (With permission from Rogers MC, Traystman RJ 1985. An overview of the intracranial vault. Physiology and philosophy. Crit Care Clin 1:195–204.)

The cerebral metabolic utilisation of oxygen is between 3.0 and 5.8 mL 100 g^{-1} min^{-1} in adults and does not vary between states of sleep and intense mental activity. CBF is however coupled to cerebral metabolic rate (and hence temperature). Local increases in neuronal activity do cause a concomitant rise in substrate and energy demand, provoking an increase in regional blood flow. Increased cerebral blood flow occurs during epileptic seizures. Barbiturate coma causes a reduction in cerebral blood flow over and above the effects of falling CPP.

Pain and anxiety increase CBF. This forms the rationale for the need to provide adequate sedation and analgesia during the intensive care of patients with decreased intracranial elastance. The sympathetic nerve supply may contribute to the ability of cerebral vessels to autoregulate and influence resting vessel tone. Endogenous catecholamines raise MAP and CPP.

INTRACRANIAL PRESSURE

The relationship between intracranial volume and pressure change is defined by the intracranial elastance (the reciprocal of compliance)

$$elastance = \Delta\ pressure \div \Delta\ volume$$

The relationship follows a typical compliance curve. When the volume of the intracranial contents increases initial pressure changes are minimal, but once a limit is reached the pressure changes are dramatic. The limit shifts when chronic changes occur. The normal ICP in adults and children is below 15 mmHg, while in the infant it is below 8 to 10 mmHg.

ICP waveforms

The following categories of waveform pattern are recognised in the ICP.

1 THE NORMAL WAVEFORM IS SYNCHRONOUS WITH ARTERIAL PULSATION

The waveform is said to have three components, the amplitude of which reflect the factors that contribute to the ICP (Figure 14.3).

2 THE BASELINE OF THE WAVEFORM MOVES WITH RESPIRATION

This reflects the transmission of intrathoracic pressures, hence the pattern of swing is reversed during IPPV.

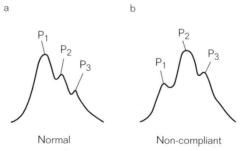

a   b

Normal   Non-compliant

Figure 14.3 The components of an intracranial pressure waveform
Although your monitoring equipment may not be sensitive enough to display them, the ICP waveform is said to have three components P_1, P_2 and P_3 that summate to produce the ICP waveform which you do see. They reflect three of the components that determine intracranial pressure at any point to different extents. P_1 varies with arterial pressure, P_2 varies inversely with compliance and P_3 with venous pressure. Thus close to the compliance threshold, the character of the waveform changes as shown.

3 THE BASELINE MOVES WITH BLOOD PRESSURE

The effects of this on cerebral blood flow as opposed to pressure are muted by autoregulation. Figure 14.4 shows cyclical changes in blood pressure reflected in an ICP trace.

4 SPONTANEOUS CYCLIC CHANGES IN THE BASELINE 'WAVES OF LUNDBERG'

- C-waves – 4 to 8 per minute.
- B-waves – frequent (1 to 2 per minute) severe elevations lasting seconds, encountered when cerebrovascular autoregulation is deranged.
- A-waves – plateau waves lasting 20 minutes or more without treatment (Figure 14.5). Ominous precursors of herniation. They are thought to occur when cerebral vasodilatation occurs in response to falls in CPP at a point close to the compliance threshold.

The consequences of raised ICP

Gradual increases in the volume of one of the intracranial compartments (e.g. by a growing brain tumour) can be compensated for by changes in CSF circulation and dynamics, for example compression of the ventricles, increase in CSF drainage and some redistribution of CSF to the subarachnoid spaces of the spinal cord. As these slow processes reach their limit, relatively small volume changes will precipitate large rises in pressure. Clinical symptoms (headache, vomiting, etc) and signs such as papilloedema may occur in this time frame. Acute or extreme changes in intracranial compartment volume cannot be compensated in the same manner. Raised ICP results, leading eventually to the ultimate neurological disaster – intracranial herniation.

14 Central Nervous System

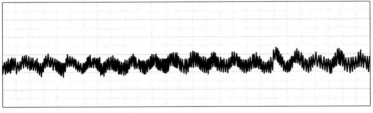

10 mmHg/div. – – 50 mm hr⁻¹

Figure 14.4 Intracranial pressure and blood pressure. Oscillations of intracranial pressure occurring with a period outside those of the Lundberg classification. In this example the frequency of 7 to 8 per hour corresponded to changes in arterial blood pressure that were probably the result of inotrope infusion by a syringe driver delivering small pulses rather than a truly continuous flow.

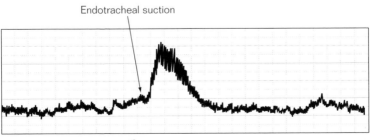

Endotracheal suction

10 mmHg/div. – – 50 mm hr⁻¹

Figure 14.5 Plateau wave in intracranial pressure. At critical intracranial elastance, plateau waves may occur spontaneously or in response to a variety of stimuli. They are ominous precursors of coning.

Two principal types of herniation are described.

1   *Tonsillar/foramen magnum herniation* in which the cerebellar tonsils and brain stem are forced into the foramen magnum. This causes loss of consciousness, a Cushing's response (hypertension and bradycardia and respiratory irregularity) leading to apnoea and death.

2   *Transtentorial (temporal lobe) herniation* where supratentorial compartment expansion causes medial displacement of the ipsilateral temporal lobe into the tentorial hiatus. This leads to compression and ischaemia of the brain stem and the ipsilateral oculomotor nerve is stretched/compressed. These events cause loss of consciousness, neurogenic hyperventilation, decerebrate posturing ipsilateral pupil dilatation and eventually will progress to tonsillar herniation.

Additionally asymmetric mass effects can cause cingulate herniation in which supratentorial herniation occurs from one side to the other underneath the falx cerebri. The treatment of RICP is discussed on pp. 229–230.

THE BLOOD–BRAIN BARRIER (BBB)

Cerebral capillary endothelial cells are separated by tight junctions with a gap that is six times narrower than other vascular beds. A unique architecture of supporting astrocytes may also act as a mechanical sieve between the cerebral circulation and the CSF. Intracranial haemorrhage and infection are both associated with a reduction in the rate of CSF bulk flow and concomitantly with an increase in CSF protein. This occurs with no structural change in the endothelial architecture.

In neonates the BBB is functionally more permeable to large polar molecules than in older children and adults although there appears to be no difference in protein diffusion coefficients between them. It is possible that this 'leaky' barrier is a corollary of reduced CSF bulk flow secondary to the structural immaturity of arachnoid villi. By 4 months of age CSF flow has reached a maximum and corresponds with the minimum CSF protein concentration.

THE CONSEQUENCES OF CELLULAR INJURY

After a neurological insult some neurones die because of physical or hypoxic trauma. Raised intracranial pressure and cerebral oedema aggravate the problem by causing secondary ischaemic and hypoxic neuronal injury. However adjacent neurones may also die from chemical reactions involving accumulation of glutamate which is an excitatory neurotransmitter. This process allows progression or expansion of the area of brain damage even if ischaemia and hypoxia are avoided. Glutamate released from damaged neurones leads to stimulation of N-methyl-D-aspartate (NMDA) receptors on the cell surface, allowing the cellular influx of calcium. This in turn starts a chain of reactions leading to cell death. Unfortunately calcium channel blockers and NMDA antagonists have not been shown to be clinically useful in preventing this process.

MEASUREMENT AND MONITORING

Intracranial pressure

Two approaches are in common use:

*   intraventricular catheter
*   intraparenchymal fibreoptic transducer.

They are contraindicated if there is significant coagulopathy (INR > 2 or platelet count <150 000). Other techniques such as epidural and subarachnoid catheters have fallen out of favour for reasons of inaccuracy, insensitivity and calibration drift.

Intraventricular catheters are considered the gold standard. They are accurate, easily calibrated and provide the therapeutic option of venting CSF to control ICP. If positioned prior to cerebral swelling and ventricular compression they retain this use subsequently. Care must be taken to ensure that the transducer is at atrial level or alternatively that the difference between the ICP transducer height (zero) and the vascular transducers has been taken into account before CPP is calculated (NB *1 mmHg = 1.36 cmH2O*).

Although it is possible to position a fibreoptic pressure transducer in other sites such as subarachnoid and extradural sites, the intraparenchymal site appears most sensitive and accurate. The transducers are easy to position, demonstrate little drift over the usual period of insertion (up to 7 days) and do not need to be recalibrated for changes in head position.

Cerebral blood flow and flow velocity

A number of techniques are available for use on the intensive care unit. None are considered standard levels of monitoring and many will continue to be used as research tools until the therapeutic manipulation of the measured parameters is proven to influence outcome.

KETY–SCHMIDT TECHNIQUE

This technique allows volumetric assessment of cerebral blood flow. It is based on the Fick principle using the arteriovenous difference in content of administered nitrous oxide (once steady state conditions have been achieved). Other indicators have also been used (such as radioactively labelled xenon).

DOPPLER ULTRASOUND

Doppler ultrasound has been used to study cerebral blood flow velocity. Although flow velocity does not quantify flow in volumetric terms, the technique can still be useful on the ICU. The pulsatility index

$$(V_{systolic} - V_{diastolic}) \div V_{mean}$$

falls as cerebrovascular resistance rises and the character of the waveform also changes as ICP rises. With decreasing CPP the diastolic flow is lost, then reversed and ultimately all forward flow is lost.

LASER-DOPPLER FLOWMETRY

This uses the frequency shift between incident and reflected laser waves from blood cells moving in the vessels within the sample area. Attempts to correlate the technique with actual CBF and to compensate for respiratory fluctuations and haemoglobin changes are not yet complete.

POSITRON EMISSION TOMOGRAPHY

This generates information about regional CBV, CBF and brain metabolism by the detection and analysis of positron emissions from radionuclides such as ^{15}O, ^{13}N or ^{11}C. The ejected positrons gradually lose kinetic energy and annihilate with electrons generating photons of a specific energy. These have great tissue penetration and are detected to generate the image.

JUGULAR VENOUS BULB OXIMETRY

Jugular venous bulb oximetry addresses the adequacy of global cerebral blood flow rather than its volume or velocity. A fibreoptic continuous oximetry probe is passed in a retrograde fashion from the internal jugular vein to the jugular venous bulb at the base of the skull. Normal jugular venous oxygen saturation (JvO_2sat) is 65 to 70 per cent. If adequate oxygen delivery is assured (anaemia and hypoxia excluded) then falls in JvO_2sat imply increased oxygen extraction. Suppression of JvO_2sat to 40 to 55 per cent suggests hypoperfusion and levels less than 40 per cent suggest global ischaemia. Samples taken from the line enable cerebral lactate production to be assayed which may increase the specificity of a low JvO_2sat. A falling JvO_2sat may be an indication to increase CPP, transfuse or otherwise increase DO_2. Rises in JvO_2sat associated with increased ICP imply cerebral hyperaemia.

NEAR INFRARED SPECTROSCOPY

Near infrared spectroscopy utilises the different absorption and reflection spectra of haemoglobin species to determine cerebral oxygenation. Near infrared wavelengths can penetrate tissue (even bone) and the spectra of oxy- and deoxyhaemoglobin can be distinguished from each other and from those of tissue cytochrome oxidase in different redox states. Cerebral blood volume is implied by total haemoglobin, and differences in supply and extraction are inferred from the ratios of oxy-, and deoxyhaemoglobin.

EEG monitoring

Children's EEGs are different from adults' and anything more than coarse interpretation requires an experienced paediatric neurophysiologist. Coarse familiarity with the paediatric EEG enables its use by the intensivist to monitor seizure activity and to titrate neurodepressant drugs (e.g. to a burst suppression sequence).

The quality of the recording may be affected by mains, ECG and electromyogram interference but in outline it reflects summated bioelectrical activity from close to the cortical surface. Normal activity is symmetrical with respect to the midline and rhythms may be distinguished by their location, frequency, amplitude, form and periodicity. The frequency (cycles per second (cps)) are counts of the number of peak-to-trough/peak-to-peak transitions. Normal EEG patterns include:

- α activity – 8 to 12 cps maximal over posterior areas, seen in awake relaxed subjects.
- β activity – 13 to 24 cps in awake subjects. More evident when α activity is suppressed and most prominent in central and frontal areas.
- δ and φ activities – slower rhythms superimposed on α and β, especially during drowsiness, which appear as bursts, primarily during drowsiness or normal sleep.

SLEEP EEG PATTERNS

Stage 1:	low voltage, fast EEG pattern
Stage 2:	sleep alpha-spindles and 'K complexes'
Stages 3 and 4:	δ activity
Stage 5	REM, similar to stage 1.

Rhythmic activity in the paediatric EEG is first evident in the precentral regions. Rhythmicity in the occipital area starts at around 4 months and is recognisably α by 2 to 3 years. The paediatric EEG is dominated by a slower rhythm than that of adults. This slower rhythm may appear in bursts, most prominent in the central and temporal/occipital regions. Their incidence and prominence decreases towards puberty. In the young, waveforms are more poorly defined and have higher amplitude.

Abnormal activity may be discrete or localised to focal injuries. Non-specific abnormal features include slowing and decrease in amplitude, increase in frequency and presence of paroxysmal activity. In general, the more severe the brain injury, the slower the EEG. Ictal activity is paroxysmal and repetitive, characteristically 'spike' or 'spike-and wave' which can be mono- or polyphasic, surface positive (i.e. pointing downwards in the EEG trace) or surface-negative (i.e. pointing upwards). Diagnostic paediatric EEGs include three per second spike-and-wave (petit mal) and hypsarrhythmia.

Cerebral function monitoring (CFM)

The CFM is a single channel mains filtered EEG trace recorded from a pair of parietal electrodes (sometimes referenced to as a midline electrode). Cumulative voltage is displayed on a paper trace. Recognisable clinical patterns include a fall in the baseline voltage which

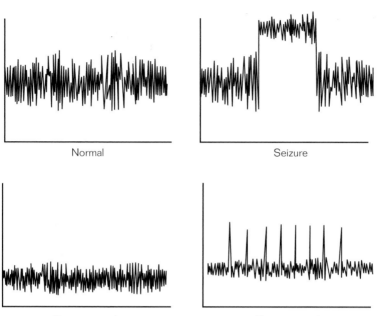

Normal

Seizure

Poor prognosis

Poor prognosis

Figure 14.6 Cerebral function monitor trace. (a) The normal trace is variable across a relatively broad bandwidth. (b) Seizures can be confidently diagnosed; they are more confined (less variable) and occur paroxysmally at a higher voltage. (c) It is possible to infer poor prognosis (although less confidently) from uniformly narrow and low voltage traces and (d) from sawtooth perturbations.

can be induced by sedation or hypothermia, but if spontaneous has a poor prognosis, as does a monotonous lack of variability. Paroxysmal changes in baseline voltage may indicate brain stem dysfunction. Seizures cause paroxysmal increases in baseline voltage with an associated narrowing of bandwidth (Figure 14.6).

Evoked potentials

With the appropriate filtering of background and spontaneous electrical activity, cortical responses to external stimuli can be detected by simultaneous EEG and are used to infer the integrity of the relevant afferent pathways, the somatosensory, auditory and visual evoked potentials for example. Somatosensory evoked potentials can demonstrate failure of peripheral, spinal (including cervical spine) and cortical conduction and are of use in trauma patients. An absent cortical response in the face of normal peripheral and spinal conduction implies a poor prognosis. False negatives may occur with bilateral subdural effusions.

SHORT NOTES ON MULTIFACTORIAL CONDITIONS
Treatment of RICP

The correct approach to raised ICP is to **resuscitate first**, then to diagnose and treat. Symptoms are unreliable in a comatose or sedated ICU patient and clinical signs are insensitive. Evidence of a Cushing's response (hypertension, bradycardia and hypoventilation) and pupil dilation with loss of the light response imply imminent herniation not just RICP. Controlled manipulation of ICP and CPP requires ICP measurement which is thus routinely undertaken to provide early detection of RICP, monitor its response to therapy, and ultimately allow prognostication. With judicious use of ICP monitoring, a therapeutic window exists particularly in traumatic brain injury where control of ICP probably improves outcome. The lack of randomised controlled trials in this field makes it difficult to be more adamant. Many aspects of care for traumatic brain injury are routinely applied to other causes of brain injury with even less justification.

A common-sense approach to treatment is to avoid anything that would make the problem worse and to treat cause rather than effect. Therefore *avoid*:

- hypoxia (and/or anaemia)
- pyrexia (keep normothermic)
- hypotension
- hypercapnia (i.e. ventilate to normocarbia, 4 to 4.5 kPa)
- high intrathoracic pressure (cough, fighting the ventilator, Valsalvas, high PEEP)
- venous obstruction (head and thorax 20° upward tilt, avoid jugular compression, e.g. neck rotation)
- excess water (relative fluid restriction, avoid hypotonic intravenous solutions. Opinions vary as to whether mild dehydration is desirable, euvolaemia certainly is however).

Remove masses as urgently as the clinical situation demands. Otherwise remove the excess blood, CSF, water or brain tissue.

- Episodic hyperaemia (raised ICP and high JvO_2) can be treated with modest hyperventilation but persistent hyperventilation will cause ischaemia.
- Ventriculostomy drains CSF.
- The brain can be depleted of water (and shrunk) by fluid restriction and/or mannitol. Mannitol is a 6-carbon sugar that does not undergo metabolism. It is not absorbed in the gastrointestinal tract and must be given intravenously. It does not cross an intact blood–brain barrier and does not enter cells. It increases plasma osmolality and expands the plasma volume by drawing intracellular water. This may relieve RICP if the blood–brain barrier is intact, and improve cerebral blood flow. Mannitol is cleared by glomerular filtration; the filtered mannitol increases the osmolality of the glomerular filtrate and prevents reabsorption of water establishing a diuresis that also removes electrolytes. Renal tubular damage (e.g. in ischaemia) can make the tubule permeable to mannitol, removing the diuretic effect.
- If all else fails and the primary insult has been addressed and/or resolved then consider surgical options. Temporal lobectomy or excision of contused brain (to create intracranial space) or craniectomy (opening the box) may prevent herniation particularly in traumatic brain injury. Treatment with moderate hypothermia may also be beneficial. The evidence base for these therapies is poor and if beneficial effects are demonstrated in children they are more likely to be at mid-range GCS scores than in the very severe or very mild injuries.

Many centres will combine these approaches to maximise efforts to reduce ICP (for example the use of ventriculostomy in traumatic brain injury when the problem is cerebral oedema not CSF accumulation). Routine hyperventilation for RICP has been avoided for many years because of evidence of aggravated cerebral ischaemia.

Cerebral oedema

Cerebral oedema occurs as the result of one of two mechanisms.

- Vasogenic cerebral oedema (e.g. surrounding a solid tumour or after traumatic head injury) characterised by cerebral blood vessel disruption and a forced leakage of fluid into surrounding tissue by hydrostatic pressure.
- Cytotoxic oedema results from cell-wall breakdown usually secondary to hypoxic-ischaemic damage, but occasionally in association with metabolic disease.

Both vasogenic and cytotoxic cerebral oedema may be further exacerbated by reperfusion injury, as blood flow is re-established. Attempts to reduce vasogenic cerebral oedema include diuretic therapies for global injury and corticosteroids for the oedema surrounding an expanding tumour.

Cell death and leakage of intracellular metabolites into the extracellular space activate inflammatory processes. There has long been hope that research into the molecular mechanisms of cell death may generate new therapeutic agents for brain injury.

Hydrocephalus

Seventy five per cent of the CSF is formed in the choroid plexi, while the remainder arises from the non-choroidal ventricular surface. Cerebrospinal fluid resides and circulates between the ventricles (lateral, third and fourth) and the subarachnoid spaces of the brain and spinal cord. The rate of production varies from 100 ml day^{-1} in the infant up to 500 ml day^{-1} in the adult. The normal total CSF volume in the adult is 100 to 150 ml. Normal CSF circulation depends on free flow through the foramina and ducts which connect the ventricles. This includes the passage of CSF from the area of the brain stem and fourth ventricle to the spinal cord through the foramen magnum. Production of CSF may be temporarily inhibited by drugs such as frusemide, steroids and acetazolamide while rises in intracranial pressure may cause an increase in reabsorption of CSF. From a therapeutic point of view, obstruction usually occurs between the third and fourth ventricles and CSF will need to be vented above this site (usually from the lateral ventricle). Communicating hydrocephalus that does not respond to conservative measures will respond to intermittent venting from any site but the pragmatic solution is a ventriculoperitoneal or ventriculoatrial shunt.

Seizures

Under normal circumstances, known epileptics having a convulsion can be expected to stop fitting spontaneously. Common patterns of paediatric seizure presentation such as febrile convulsions are, as a rule, similarly self-limiting. When these patients are fitting they warrant simple confirmation of airway patency, provision of oxygen and the attendant must also ensure the adequacy of breathing and circulation. The patients do not normally need more aggressive resuscitation but the aetiology of the fit should be determined.

Treat the cause where it can be identified. Treatable causes include:

- hypoxia
- fever
- hypoglycaemia
- meningitis or encephalitis
- poisoning
- trauma (especially that associated with haemorrhage)
- RICP
- kernicterus.

Isolated electrolyte abnormalities do not cause status epilepticus although hypocalcaemia can cause tonic clonic convulsions.

Make a diagnosis (e.g. the cause of the fever in a febrile convulsion) and initiate appropriate treatment. Although the seizure may be trivial, the cause can of course be far more serious and the differential diagnosis is far more broad reaching than the above list might imply.

Status epilepticus should be distinguished from a 'seizure' per se and is by contrast, a medical emergency. Status epilepticus is not 'any seizure witnessed by a doctor!' but is best defined as severe continuous seizure activity lasting 30 minutes or more. When dealing with status, the initial approach to resuscitation is the same as that for patients having a seizure – an ABC approach with simple airway-opening manoeuvres and administration of oxygen from the outset. Prolonged seizure activity is likely to be associated with respiratory impairment and hypoxia, which increase the risk of mortality and morbidity (e.g. cerebral oedema, cardiac arrest, etc.). Once true 'status' is recognised on the grounds of duration of seizure, then effective direct control of seizure activity becomes a priority. The target is to achieve control within 30 minutes, thus total seizure duration will have been confined to less than an hour and the risk of cerebral oedema constrained.

Drug therapy is chosen to achieve seizure control quickly and to have some lasting anti-convulsant activity while maintenance therapy is established or augmented. If intubation does not appear necessary on the grounds of airway maintenance and adequate breathing, then the usual pharmacological approach is to use benzodiazepines. They are fast acting and lipophillic, and hence distribute rapidly. Respiratory depression is however a particular problem with repeated doses and they can also cause hypotension. The choice of benzo-diazepine is influenced by the duration of anticonvulsant activity and the degree of respiratory depression. These effects increase in the order diazepam, lorazepam, clonazepam. Since anticonvulsant effects may be short lived or display tolerance, combination therapy is needed and usually achieved by loading with phenobarbitone or phenytoin, both of which can abort status as well as prevent recurrence. Diazepam exerts anticonvulsant effects for 5 to 30 minutes whereas its half-life is much longer and sedative effects can persist for over 48 hours. Lorazepam has a slightly faster speed of onset and anticonvulsant effects last for longer (48 hours). Nevertheless, tolerance can develop rapidly, leading to loss of seizure control and so dual therapy is rarely avoided. Midazolam has an even faster speed of onset of anticonvulsant activity, which lasts for up to 5 hours, but it is more sedative than diazepam or lorazepam. It has the advantage that it can be administered intramuscularly.

Alternatively phenobarbitone alone may be given to ablate the seizure. The same is probably not true of phenytoin because of the cardiotoxic risks associated with rapid loading. Furthermore rectal or intramuscular paraldehyde has a role when venous access is difficult.

In the window of opportunity usually provided by the benzodiazepine, loading doses of phenobarbital or phenytoin can be administered. Phenytoin has zero order (saturatable) kinetics, it may be difficult to achieve a therapeutic level and at any level short of this, it is rapidly eliminated. It is a negative inotrope and proarrhythmic. Fosphenytoin is a water-soluble pro-phenytoin, 1.5 mg of fosphenytoin is equivalent to 1 mg of phenytoin. It can be administered intramuscularly or by a more rapid intravenous infusion than phenytoin, and is kinder to peripheral vasculature. However after administration conversion to phenytoin (still the active drug) takes about 8 to 15 minutes negating the advantage of the faster infusion. It is not immune to cardiotoxic side effects which may occur after infusion during the conversion phase and is still not appropriate for control of status. The use of fosphenytoin is acceptable if seizures have already been controlled. Conversion to phenytoin is complete 2 hours after intravascular and 4 hours after intramuscular administration, after which conventional phenytoin assays and therapeutic ranges apply. A loading dose of phenobarbitone (20 mg kg^{-1}) does not have such severe potential toxicity and is less respiratory depressant than multiple doses of benzodiazepines. Even when the intention is to try and avoid intubation, repeated boluses of phenobarbitone (20 mg kg^{-1}) have been reportedly effective (up to 100 mg kg^{-1}) without compromising airway reflexes. However barbiturate coma induced with any agent will eventually require intubation. Coma induced by phenobarbitone is probably more haemodynamically stable than that of thiopentone, the infusion of which often requires simultaneous pressors. However it may take longer to wear off. High dose barbiturates display zero order 'saturatable' kinetics even if they have first order elimination in their normal therapeutic range.

If status persists for up to an hour then the priority for cerebral protection and treatment of potential cerebral oedema should make you abandon attempts to avoid intubation. Induce barbiturate coma with thiopentone in the form of anaesthetic induction, intubate and ventilate. The effects of thiopentone are more short lived than those of phenobarbitone and coma is maintained by infusions of 2 to 10 mg kg^{-1}hr^{-1} (best titrated to a short cycle burst suppression EEG). If there is no cerebral oedema or other indication to maintain coma however, then early weaning from ventilation is to be preferred. Most cases of recalcitrant status admitted to the intensive care unit are resolved by brief barbiturate coma and are extubated within hours. The most common cause of PICU admission in the context of seizures is when respiratory support is needed until the sedative effects of medication resolve in the post-ictal patient.

Attempts to find and potentially treat, a cause of status epilepticus can and must continue during this phase. The differential diagnosis can be narrowed by the context of the patient's age. For example pyridoxine-dependent fits, and kernicterus are not likely to present *de novo* outside the neonatal period. Similarly the likely infectious agents will be different for neonates (Group B *Streptococcus*, *Escheria coli* and *Listeria*) compared to older children (*Neisseria meningitidis*, *Haemophilus influenzae* B in non-vaccinated communities and pneumococcus).

Coma

Coma is the exact opposite of consciousness, i.e. a state of unrousable unresponsiveness without evidence of psychological awarenesss of the self or the environment. Patients in coma display no sleep–wake cycles and may:

- die
- stay in a coma (unusual)
- enter a vegetative state
- develop signs of awareness and response to the environment (and thence recover to some extent).

Progress to the fourth state is often via the third. Brain death is an important differential diagnosis of coma.

The level of consciousness is usually described using the Glasgow Coma Scale (GCS), although strictly speaking 'coma' should be reserved for patients who are GCS 3 ($E_1V_1M_1$). The GCS has been justified as a rather coarse prognosticating tool and has been adapted to paediatric practice by adaptation for preverbal stages of development and by the use of a grimace score in place of the verbal score for intubated children. With these adaptations it works well in terms of inter- and intra-assessor variability but the subsequent correlation with outcome has been less well evaluated. More rapid, yet still reproducible, assessment can be provided by the AVPU system.

States of qualitatively altered consciousness can also be distinguished. Examples include obtundation which progresses to stupor (a sleep-like state from which some degree of arousal can be stimulated) and delirium where there is often no defect in arousal but the patient is not lucid and may hallucinate.

Table 14.2 Adapted Glasgow Coma Score

	Adult and child more than 5 years old	Child less than 5 years old
Eye opening		
E4	Spontaneous	As older child
E3	To verbal stimulus	As older child
E2	To pain	As older child
E1	No response	As older child
Verbal		
V5	Orientated	Alert, babbles, coos, words or sentences to usual ability
V4	Confused	Less than usual ability or irritable cry
V3	Inappropriate words	Cries to pain
V2	Incomprehensible sounds	Moans to pain
V1	No response to pain	No response to pain

continued

Table 14.2 Adapted Glasgow Coma Score

	Adult and child more than 5 years old	Child less than 5 years old
Grimace (used in place of verbal for the intubated child)		
G5	Spontaneous normal facial / oromotor activity, for example sucks tube, coughs	
G4	Less than usual spontaneous ability, or only responds to touch	
G3	Vigorous grimace to pain	
G2	Mild grimace or some change in facial expression to pain	
G1	No response to pain	
Motor		
M6	Obeys commands	Normal spontaneous movements
M5	Localises to pain stimulus	As older child or withdraws to touch
M4	Withdraws from pain	As older child
M3	Abnormal flexion to pain	As older child
M2	Abnormal extension to pain	As older child
M1	No response to pain	As older child

Vegetative state

A vegetative state, as opposed to coma, is a state of wakeful unresponsiveness. Patients display sleep–wake cycles, eye opening and blinking. They may also chew and grind their teeth. Such activity may occasionally be interpreted or inferred as showing fragments of response (apparent brief fixing and following for example) but in reality they show no meaningful interaction. They may occasionally grunt or groan but for the most part are silent. The length of time that must elapse before a vegetative state can be described as 'persistent' has not been standardised and varies in the literature from 1 to 12 months. Non-traumatic brain injuries tend to be less responsive to treatment and so the 'persistent vegetative state' (PVS) label is sometimes attached at 6 months, whereas 12 months is most commonly used for traumatic brain injury. At any one time there are about 5 children with PVS per million people in the population. See Table 14.3.

The differential diagnosis includes akinetic mutism (conscious and attentive but with relative, not absolute, mutism and slowed or absent movements) which can result from midbrain injury, and the 'locked in' syndrome which results from damage to the ventral pons.

Table 14.3 The most common causes of PVS (listed in order of prevalence)

Children	Adults
Developmental lesion	Head injury
Hypoxic ischaemic encephalopathy	Cerebrovascular accident
Head injury	Developmental lesion
Tumour	Hypoxic ischaemic encephalopathy
	Tumour

Survival for children in PVS after traumatic brain injury is reputedly more likely than it is in adults. In truth the difference is not dramatic. It could reflect differences in the aggression of medical intervention but is more likely because of the plasticity of the developing CNS. If recovery begins before 6 months has elapsed, then a higher grade of recovery is likely. For non-traumatic brain injury, if recovery has not occurred by 3 months then it is unlikely and outcomes are similar to those for adults. There is obviously no prospect of recovery for PVS caused by degenerative diseases. Death when it occurs is usually because of aspiration or pneumonia. Table 14.4 is taken from a review presented over two articles (NEJM May & June 1994).

Critical illness polyneuropathy

The aetiology of this condition, which occurs in the aftermath of MOSF, is poorly understood. Although better described and more frequent in adults it does occur in children and

Table 14.4 Incidence of subsequent recovery of consciousness and function in adults and children, who have been in PVS for 1 month after traumatic and non-traumatic brain injury (from The Multi-Society Task Force on PVS, Medical aspects of the persistent vegetative state (1) and (2), N Engl J Med 1994 330:1499–508 and 1572–9).

Outcome	Time		
	3 months	6 months	12 months
Adult traumatic injury (n = 434)	%	%	%
Death	15	24	33
PVS	52	30	15
Recovery	33	46	52
Severe disability			28
Moderate disability			17
Good recovery			7
Adult non-traumatic injury (n = 169)			
Death	24	40	53
PVS	65	45	32
Recovery	11	15	15
Severe disability			11
Moderate disability			3
Good recovery			1
Child traumatic injury (n = 106)			
Death	4	9	9
PVS	72	40	29
Recovery	24	51	62
Severe disability			35
Moderate disability			16
Good recovery			11

Table 14.4 Incidence of subsequent recovery of consciousness and function in adults and children, who have been in PVS for 1 month after traumatic and non-traumatic brain injury (from The Multi-Society Task Force on PVS, Medical aspects of the persistent vegative state (1) and (2), *N Engl J Med* 1994 330:1499–508 and 1572–9).

Outcome	Time		
	3 months	6 months	12 months
Child non-traumatic injury (n=45)	%	%	%
Death	20	22	22
PVS	69	67	65
Recovery	11	11	13
Severe disability			7
Moderate disability			0
Good recovery			6

manifests with weakness of respiratory and limb muscles. Wasting, hyporeflexia and sensory symptoms occur frequently, but are not mandatory for the diagnosis. Investigation reveals a primary, axonal, motor and sensory neuropathy and the prognosis is good although recovery may take weeks or months.

'Junior ITU syndrome'

Movement disorders are common in children convalescing from a long period under sedation with MOSF or low cardiac output. Choreoathetoid movements, active and passive tremor and other forms of dyskinesia have been variously described. Possible aetiologies include drug withdrawal, central acetylcholine depletion or central dopamine antagonism. Nerve conduction and CNS imaging are normal, no association can be proved with any particular sedative agent and the condition fades over time (usually within 4 to 14 days). The problem can be severe enough to compromise respiratory effort and increase metabolic demand for oxygen, severely delaying attempts to wean from mechanical ventilation. Thus a number of therapies have been tried including physostigmine and clonidine without convincing evidence of efficacy.

15 Renal System

INTRODUCTION

Patients with acute or chronic 'renal' diseases, or postrenal causes of renal failure such as obstructive nephropathy, are infrequent PIC visitors. Thus the profile of renal disease on the PICU is very different from that in paediatric nephrology *per se*. Despite the relatively small numbers of renal patients, almost all PIC patients will have their renal function manipulated and closely monitored. Most of the 'renal therapeutics' used on the PICU are indicated in the context of impending or actual acute renal failure of a *prerenal* aetiology, or they form part of wider fluid, electrolyte, acid base or drug management. 'Renal replacement' therapies and allied procedures such as plasmafiltration are also used to treat problems such as drug toxicity and a mixed bag of diseases including Guillain–Barré syndrome and inborn errors of metabolism. This chapter assumes a knowledge of basic renal physiology rather than reproducing it and the coverage provided is very selective, being dictated by the need to give priority to the manipulation of renal function.

RENAL FUNCTION

In outline, renal physiology is best covered by mapping function to site in terms of the microanatomy of the nephron. This allows one to in turn consider filtration (glomerulus) and the conversion of filtrate into urine (tubule). The latter process involves the bulk reabsorption of fluid and electrolytes (proximal convoluted tubule and loop of Henle), dilution of filtrate and fine control of electrolyte exchange (distal convoluted tubule) and water conservation or excretion (distal convoluted tubule and collecting duct). Urea is added to the urine in the descending loop of Henle where it is moving along a concentration gradient. That gradient is maintained by the fact that urea permeability is restricted to this area and the papillary collecting duct which contains relatively concentrated urine. The endocrine functions of the kidney are linked to the juxtaglomerular apparatus (renin–angiotensin, vitamin D). Individual nephrons contribute to the regulation of blood flow to their own glomeruli by influencing the diameter of the afferent and efferent arterioles. This ability, combined with the sheer number of nephrons accounts for a large 'renal reserve'. Diseases that cause chronic renal failure as a result of an inexorable loss of glomeruli or nephrons do not reduce the overall glomerular filtration rate (GFR) until the limits of reserve of the remainder are exceeded. So great are these reserves that this does not occur until 80 per cent of nephrons are non-functional. The latter stages of such diseases are therefore associated with apparently plummeting GFR (Figure 15.1). Uraemia occurs when approximately 90 per cent of nephrons are non-functional and renal replacement therapy is necessary when approximately 95 per cent of function has been lost. GFR can be inferred from the plasma creatinine or creatinine clearance.

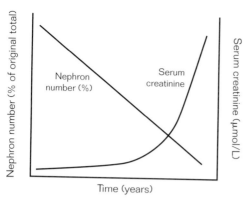

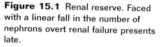

Figure 15.1 Renal reserve. Faced with a linear fall in the number of nephrons overt renal failure presents late.

Babies have immature kidneys

In early infancy the kidneys are relatively inefficient, excreting large volumes of low quality urine. This leads to higher urinary losses of sodium and potassium than adults and one should expect urine volumes of 1 to 2 ml kg^{-1} h^{-1}. Peak renal performance is reached at about 2 to 3 years, after which the inexorable age-related decline in the numbers of functional nephrons commences. 'Renal reserve' decreases at a rate of 2.5 per cent per year. Everyone develops chronic renal failure if they live long enough, but they are supposed to do it outside the paediatric age range.

A full complement of nephrons and glomeruli are present at 34 weeks but the GFR is low (≤ 0.5 ml kg^{-1} min^{-1} in preterm infants and approximately 1.5 ml kg^{-1} min^{-1} in term infants compared to 2 ml kg^{-1} min^{-1} in adults and older children). This low GFR explains the restricted ability of babies to excrete a water load. In infants born after 34 weeks gestation, the glomeruli mature at the same rate as those of a normal infant. Glomerular filtration rate increases in infancy and is normal at 5 to 6 months of age.

Maturation of the tubules lags slightly behind that of the glomeruli. At birth only the tubules of the juxtamedullary glomeruli extend into the medulla of the kidney. Tubular immaturity manifests as an obligatory urinary salt loss but the reduced ability to concentrate urine leads to water loss as well as salt. Maturation of tubules approaches the functional levels of older children and adults by 8 to 9 months of age.

At birth serum creatinine levels are markers of maternal renal function. By 5 days an appropriate balance is achieved allowing clinical use of the creatinine as a marker of the babies' GFR. Glomerular filtration rate increases in proportion with muscle mass until 1 year of age, after which it lags behind and normal creatinine levels rise slowly thereafter.

Unlike adults, the occurrence of acute renal failure during a paediatric intensive care stay usually has only a small impact on the overall ICU mortality risk. This has a lot to do with the speed with which recovery of renal function occurs. Acute renal failure in a neonate can be all over in 4 to 6 days. Part of the speed of recovery may be because of the cortical path (rather than medullary) of many of the nephrons.

TESTING RENAL FUNCTION

Although most of the time one manipulates renal function in a PIC patient to affect water balance, renal function is best described in terms of solute clearance. That is the theoretical 'volume' of plasma that is cleared of a substance per unit time.

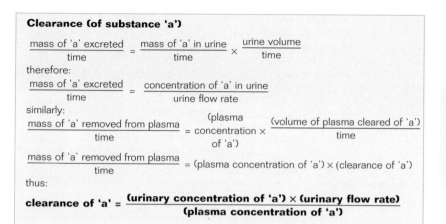

Clearance (of substance 'a')

$$\frac{\text{mass of 'a' excreted}}{\text{time}} = \frac{\text{mass of 'a' in urine}}{\text{time}} \times \frac{\text{urine volume}}{\text{time}}$$

therefore:

$$\frac{\text{mass of 'a' excreted}}{\text{time}} = \frac{\text{concentration of 'a' in urine}}{\text{urine flow rate}}$$

similarly:

$$\frac{\text{mass of 'a' removed from plasma}}{\text{time}} = \begin{array}{c}\text{(plasma}\\ \text{concentration} \times\\ \text{of 'a')}\end{array} \frac{\text{(volume of plasma cleared of 'a')}}{\text{time}}$$

$$\frac{\text{mass of 'a' removed from plasma}}{\text{time}} = \text{(plasma concentration of 'a')} \times \text{(clearance of 'a')}$$

thus:

$$\textbf{clearance of 'a'} = \frac{\textbf{(urinary concentration of 'a')} \times \textbf{(urinary flow rate)}}{\textbf{(plasma concentration of 'a')}}$$

Creatinine is assumed to be filtered but not absorbed or added to, as urine is formed from filtrate, enabling creatinine clearance to be used to estimate the GFR. Creatinine clearance overestimates GFR at low levels. It is not useful in early life and indeed in most of infancy the plasma creatinine is so low that measurement error becomes proportionately more significant leading to results that can vary widely over time without convincing evidence of a change in GFR.

Free water clearance (C_{H_2O})

This is not a true clearance in the sense of inulin or creatinine, rather it is an expression of the difference between the measured urine flow rate ($\dot{V}$) and the rate of urine flow that would be required to excrete the measured urinary osmolar load at a tonicity equal to that of plasma. Thus it is a measure of the overall concentrating/dilutional ability of the kidney.

The volume of plasma cleared of all osmotically active particles per unit time (osmolar clearance (C_{osm})) is:

(urinary osmolality (U_{osm}) × urine flow rate) ÷ plasma osmolality (P_{osm})

$= (U_{osm} \times \dot{V}) \div P_{osm}$

and free water clearance is: $C_{H_2O} = \dot{V} - C_{osm}$
so substituting we get

$C_{H_2O} = \dot{V} - ((U_{osm} \times \dot{V}) \div P_{osm})$

$\qquad = \dot{V}(1 - (U_{osm} \div P_{osm}))$ ml min^{-1}

When dilute urine is produced, C_{H_2O} is positive, implying net free water excretion. When concentrated urine is produced C_{H_2O} is negative, implying net free water conservation. At normal solute excretion rates, the capacity to excrete free water is much greater than the capacity to preserve it in dehydration. Both are limited in children. The C_{H_2O} can be used to express the severity of SIADH.

Urine protein : creatinine ratio

If one regards the glomerulus as an ultrafilter, then dysfunction will either manifest as blockage or leak (proteinuria). The molecular size of albumin means that it is normally just retained by the glomerulus. Expression of albuminuria as a clearance ratio with creatinine means that the estimation of proteinuria becomes independent of urine concentration and **239** able to be measured on a spot urine rather than 24-hour collection. Although strictly speaking, estimation of albumin and creatinine clearances requires a concomitant blood sample, in reality most variation is caused by the urinary values and so the ratio of albumin clearance to creatinine clearance is reliably predicted from the ratio of albumin and creatinine concentrations in the urine. Normal values are less than 0.1 (mg/mg). Tenfold increases represent moderate proteinuria and hundredfold increases heavy proteinuria. The most naturally proteinuric neonates are 32–34 week gestation preterm babies but even normal term infants may excrete up to 1 g albumin L^{-1} of urine in the first 48 hours of life.

One can assess total urine protein in relation to creatinine as well (normal < 20) but this test will not be as specific for glomerular dysfunction and may include tubular protein leaks.

Urine sodium

The urinary sodium concentration is a reasonably reliable predictor of extracellular fluid volume. If renal perfusion pressure falls to levels short of those that produce acute renal failure, the kidneys produce good 'quality' concentrated urine (osmolality > 300 mosm L^{-1}, urine : plasma urea ratio > 5 with a urine sodium < 20 mmol L^{-1}). The fractional sodium excretion is also low, (approximately 0.4).

$$FENa = \frac{(U_{Na} \times P_{cr})}{(P_{Na} \times U_{cr})}$$

(U_{Na}, P_{Na} = urinary and plasma sodium, U_{cr}, P_{cr} = urinary and plasma creatinine). These findings are ablated by diuretic therapy. In acute tubular necrosis the urine 'quality' is poor, urine sodium is greater than 40 mmol L^{-1} and fractional sodium excretion is equal to or greater than 7.

MANIPULATION OF URINE OUTPUT

Urine production can be doctored by manipulation of both filtration and tubular function. The usual reasons for wishing to do so are for control of the water balance irrespective of whether or not the patient is oliguric. Urine flow can protect against some renal diseases (but not many) and fluid retention is a common and unwanted corollary of many critical illnesses. Urine production is often used as a marker for the adequacy of cardiac output but can only be used as such in the absence of primary renal disease and when tubular function is preserved. The common assumption being that one is then observing the effects of haemodynamics on filtration alone.

Glomerular filtration

Filtration is a passive process regulated by glomerular blood flow. Technically the more appropriate term is 'ultrafiltration' because the fluid movement is assisted by a hydrostatic pressure gradient. The pre- and post-glomerular arterioles are the principal sites of vascular resistance across the kidney. They act to minimise the pressure drop along glomerular vessels maintaining the net hydraulic pressure in the glomerulus (the principal force behind ultrafiltration). Ultrafiltration proceeds against the oncotic pressure which rises much higher than in a normal capillary (where less fluid is filtered). Overall filtration further depends upon the surface area of the glomerular basement membrane and its hydraulic permeability. Since plasma is filtered (not blood cells), the renal plasma flow (RPF – affected by haematocrit) is a more direct determinant of GFR than the renal blood flow. The proportion of RPF that is filtered is the 'filtration fraction' (GFR : RPF). Constriction of the afferent glomerular arteriole reduces RPF and GFR. Constriction of the efferent arteriole decreases RPF but increases GFR by increasing the filtration fraction. Afferent arteriolar dilatation causes a natriuresis by increasing RPF and GFR. Provided a sufficient vascular pressure is maintained, renal autoregulation preserves the GFR in the face of wide ranges of renal blood flow.

The GFR is often estimated to be 2 ml kg^{-1} min^{-1} but can also be approximated from the serum creatinine by the formula

$$GFR = length \times (K \div P_{Cr})$$

Measured in ml min^{-1} 1.73 m^{-2}, length in cm, plasma creatinine concentration (P_{Cr}) in mg dL^{-1} (1 mg dL^{-1} = 88.5 µmol L^{-1}), and K is a constant from Table 15.1.

Table 15.1 Constants for use in calculating glomerular filtration rate.

Age	K
Infant < 1 year	0.45
Child < 13 year	0.55
Adolescent male	0.7
Adolescent female	0.55

Renal effects of low dose dopamine infusion

Low dose dopamine has predominantly (but not exclusively) β_1 effects. Like some other (non-dopaminergic) inotropes it raises RPF by increasing cardiac output. This effect is accompanied by a moderating fall in filtration fraction but a temporary natiuresis (with increased sodium excretion) predominates because of an added tubular effect which is not observed in patients with chronic renal failure. Selective renal vasodilation in response to low dose dopamine is a popular myth although it can cause a natiuresis in the face of intravascular volume depletion. This latter phenomenon is not necessarily advantageous. There is no evidence that low dose dopamine prevents renal failure in hypotensive patients. In randomised controlled studies it does not increase creatinine clearance (whereas low dose dobutamine does – without an increase in urine output). There has never been any evidence that the use of low dose dopamine affects ICU outcome and it is hard to accept that it has any advantage over appropriate volume resuscitation and other forms of inotropic support. For example in sepsis, α adrenergic stimulation from a noradrenaline (norepinephrine) infusion reverses oliguria by raising blood pressure and increasing the filtration fraction with a fall in RPF but less effect on the GFR. It does not force a natiuresis in volume-depleted patients.

Tachyphylaxis limits any potential benefits of low dose dopamine. In addition potential hazards of the infusion include: the necessity to site a central venous line for its administration, pulmonary hypertension, catabolism, impaired immune responses, suppression of growth hormone, prolactin, DHEA and thyroid function and gut ischaemia, raising the suspicion that gut bacterial translocation will be enhanced.

Tubular function

Diuretics exert their principal effects on the luminal side of the nephron hence they do not work below a minimum GFR. They may yet achieve an effect in the presence of a marginal GFR if given in higher than normal concentration. They may also exert related effects on the vascular supply to the glomerulus and nephron. Drugs that work within the site of bulk reabsorption of fluid and electrolytes, for example loop diuretics, achieve the greatest effects in terms of water loss. Thiazides work on the distal convoluted tubule and hence may have a synergistic effect when used in combination with a loop diuretic. Osmotic diuretics, such as mannitol which transiently expand plasma volume, may increase GFR during that time but their principal effect is via inhibition of water reabsorption throughout the nephron. Diuretic therapies can increase water and electrolyte loss in oliguric states. This may help fluid management and nutrition but does not avoid uraemia or rising creatinine if GFR is low. They have not been shown to decrease the incidence of acute renal failure. Furthermore drugs such as these that can induce a diuresis in hypovolaemic states must be used with extreme caution.

Summary of the approach to oliguria

- **Recognise it** ($<$ 1ml kg^{-1} hr^{-1} of urine).
- **Rule out obstruction** bladder catheterisation ($\pm$ultrasound scan). It is common practice to catheterise critically ill patients to enable close monitoring of urine output. Urine production is however unlikely to change after catheterisation of an oliguric patient. Urethral obstruction (posterior urethral valves) and anticholinergic effects on bladder emptying are rare. However, obstruction at all levels should be excluded in the oliguric patient and may necessitate an abdominal ultrasound examination.
- **Ensure adequate renal blood flow** (treat dehydration, hypotension, low cardiac output). A physiological response to prerenal restriction reverts to normal if renal blood flow is supported.
- **Distinguish prerenal and renal disease** (urine electrolytes / creatinine clearance).
- **Give a trial of diuretic therapy.** A response implies that some nephrons are functional but this will not necessarily prevent a rise in urea or creatinine. It may be possible to achieve water balance and avoid electrolyte imbalance by other medical means with diuretic drive while awaiting further renal recovery. These medical measures do not improve renal function, they circumvent renal dysfunction.
- **Consider renal replacement therapy.** Indications outlined further on pp. 242–245 include failed response to a diuretic, water overload, electrolyte abnormalities, severe uraemia. Urinary catheters are best removed during renal replacement therapy in oliguric / anuric renal failure as they represent a potential source of infection.

RENAL REPLACEMENT THERAPY

Peritoneal dialysis

In childhood the peritoneum has a greater surface area proportional to body mass making peritoneal dialysis more effective than it would be in older patients. During peritoneal dialysis, fluid movement is generated by creating an osmotic gradient through the peritoneal infusion of hypertonic fluid. A clinical choice between different dextrose strengths is used to control ultrafiltration rates. Ultrafiltration also increases with dwell time (the length of time the dialysate spends in the peritoneum) to a point. Typical volumes that are instilled with dwell times of 20 to 60 minutes, are 10 ml kg^{-1} cycle^{-1} increasing to 50 ml kg^{-1} cycle^{-1}. Solute clearance is increased by increasing dialysis fluid volume per unit time. At the upper limit of the range of cycle volumes, haemodynamically unstable patients may respond poorly to the cardiopulmonary effects of peritoneal dialysis. These include:

- decreased preload
- increased afterload
- diaphragm splinting
- reduction in lung volume.

Low-volume more-frequent cycles and continuous flow of dialysate through two peritoneal catheters represent pragmatic approaches to these problems. They may be instituted electively in haemodynamically unstable or 'at risk' patients. Both approaches increase solute clearance at the potential expense of a fall in ultrafiltration rate.

The principal risk of peritoneal dialysis is peritoneal infection. Daily samples of filtrate should be sent for microbiological surveillance and contamination and infection are treated in the first instance by adding antibiotics to the dialysate.

Extracorporeal RRT

Short-term renal replacement therapy can also be provided by extracorporeal techniques such as haemofiltration. The favoured venovenous approach minimises the haemodynamic consequences of this approach but extracorporeal RRT is never undertaken on the PICU without careful haemodynamic monitoring (at least arterial blood pressure and central venous pressure) and close monitoring of blood gases and electrolytes.

The filtration of fluid through an external filter proceeds at a rate dictated by:

- the filtration coefficient of the membrane (influenced by its surface area and permeability)
- the hydrostatic pressure gradient (which drives filtration and is affected by changes in blood flow rate)
- the colloid osmotic pressure gradient (which depends on the properties of the pores in the membrane). Colloid osmotic pressure acts to resist filtration through a haemofilter as the colloids are not filtered but persist in the blood, holding fluid back. In a plasmafilter they pass through into the filtrate and contribute to the osmotic forces that promote fluid passage into the filtrate.

The characteristics of the pores in synthetic membranes can be described by sieving coefficients for different molecules (the relative concentration in filtrate and plasma), pore size distributions or by fractal methods. The clinical choice, however, is between a 'small' pore membrane (haemofilter), a 'large' pore membrane (plasma filter) or a semi-permeable membrane for dialysis (although in reality these allow some ultrafiltration as well). In the context of extracorporeal RRT the term **ultrafiltration** is sometimes reserved for occasions when filtration is occurring without the administration of a replacement fluid. **Slow continuous ultrafiltration** (SCUF) at filtration rates of 1 to 2 ml kg^{-1} hr^{-1} is thus principally a process for removing water. Modern 'kidneys' (dialysis membranes) are cheaper than haemofilters and allow ultrafiltration rates in this range. They have therefore been used routinely in this role for some time. Naturally solute clearance is negligible at such filtrate flows without a dialysate.

HAEMOFILTRATION

Haemofiltration is a generic term for processes involving the use of a haemofilter. Haemofilters have a much greater ultrafiltration rate than dialysis membranes and can clear significant amounts of water. The exchange of a large volume of ultrafiltrate with replacement fluid permits bulk clearance of solutes as well. Even at lower ultrafiltration rates there is an opportunity to use the water loss to generate 'space' within an overall fluid restriction for TPN, drug infusions, flushes, blood products, etc. Such an approach is particularly useful in oliguric states. Net fluid removal is assured by adjusting the rate of ultrafiltration in relation to the infusions (including the replacement fluid).

HAEMODIAFILTRATION

Haemodiafiltration refers to the addition of a countercurrent flow of dialysate across the haemofilter. By increasing the diffusion gradient, solute clearance is expected to increase at a rate proportional to the dialysate flow. The technique is superfluous if one uses high ultrafiltration rates such as those that are made possible by adding replacement fluid pre-filter – 'pre-dilution'.

CLEARANCE

The clearance of a substance during filtration depends on the proportion of its total volume of distribution that is in the plasma. It also depends on the sieving coefficient of the membrane for that solute and the rate of ultrafiltration. The solutes move by convection driven by the bulk flow of fluid. The membranes in haemofilters allow the passage of molecules with a molecular weight of less than 30 000 Da. Thus ions and small chemicals such as sodium, potassium, calcium, magnesium, bicarbonate, phosphate, glucose and ammonia are filtered freely. Also included are endogenous substances such as myoglobin, insulin and interleukins, and some exogenous substances such as vancomycin, heparin and many toxins (including endotoxin). However molecules that are bound to plasma proteins are not filtered effectively.

PLASMAFILTER

The membrane in a plasmafilter contains larger pores which allow albumin, globulins and protein bound substances to be filtered while retaining cellular components. Plasmafilters will remove particles of molecular weight up to 3 000 000 Da including endotoxins and exotoxins and all the substances listed in Table 15.2.

Table 15.2 Examples of molecules that pass unimpeded across a plasmafilter.

Albumin	66 000 Da
α_1 acid glycoprotein	40 000 Da
α_1 antitrypsin	50 000–55 000 Da
α_2 macroglobulin	820 000 Da
Complement initiators (C_{1qrs}, C_2, C_4, properdin)	86 000– 400 000 Da
Complement effectors (C_{3-9})	24 000–184 000 Da
Complement inhibitors	90 000–300 000 Da
Elastase	26 000
TNFα	17 000
IgG	150 000 Da
IgA	160 000 or 400 000 Da
IgM	900 000 Da
IgD	180 000 Da
IgE	190 000 Da
Myoglobin	17 000 Da
Haemoglobin	69 000 Da

Plasmafiltration has little effect on high affinity tissue bound antibodies, activated T cells or deposited immune complexes.

PLASMAPHERESIS

Plasmapheresis is a different technique with similar results to plasmafiltration. It uses centrifugation and therefore density-dependent cell separation to separate cellular components from plasma.

DIALYSIS

Dialysis uses a semi-permeable membrane. In addition to a low rate of ultrafiltration, solutes and water move across the membrane by diffusion and osmosis. Large countercurrent flows of dialysate up to 800 ml min^{-1} are used to maximise diffusion gradients and therefore solute clearance.

Table 15.3 Choice of filter (products are quoted as examples only)

Weight	Access (Dual lumen catheter)		Haemofilter (examples)			Plasmafilter (examples)		Blood pump speed
	Gauge	Length	Code	Area	Priming	Code	Priming	
< 2 kg	6.5F	10 cm	Mini filter	0.021m²	6 mL	PN1000	23 mL	10 ml min⁻¹
3–6 kg	6.5F	10 cm	FH 22	0.2 m²	13 mL	PN1000	23 mL	25 ml min⁻¹
5–15 kg	8F	12.5 cm	FH 22	0.2 m²	13 mL	PN1000	23 mL	25 ml min⁻¹
10–20 kg	8F	15 cm	FH 22	0.2 m²	13 mL	P1S	33 mL	40 ml min⁻¹
10–20 kg	10.8F	12.5 cm	FH 22	0.2 m²	13 mL	P1S	33 mL	40 ml min⁻¹
20–40 kg	11F	12.5 cm	FH 66	0.6 m²	55 mL	P1S	33 mL	75 ml min⁻¹
20–40 kg	11F	15 cm	FH 66	0.6 m²	55 mL	P1S	33 mL	75 ml min⁻¹
> 40 kg	11F	15 cm	FH 66	0.6 m²	55 mL	P1S	33 mL	150 ml min⁻¹

The choice between the various approaches is fairly straightforward.

Common clinical scenarios

Oliguric patient, fluid overloaded with minor electrolyte disturbance
but not responding to less invasive measures:
- ultrafiltration (CVVH) at a rate determined by the desired water loss rate but tempered by the haemodynamic state and not to exceed 5 ml kg⁻¹ hr⁻¹.

Electrolyte disturbance predominates:
- CVVH (ultrafiltration with pre-filter replacement fluid). Ultrafiltration at 20 ml kg⁻¹ hr⁻¹ with up to 100 per cent replacement. Ultrafiltration rate can be increased up to 50 ml kg⁻¹ hr⁻¹ for severe electrolyte derangement or other circumstances where high solute clearance is desired (e.g. poisoning).

Fulminating sepsis with or without immunological disease:
- plasma filtration (exchange 3.5 plasma volumes within the first 4 hours)

Haemodynamically stable patient with established renal failure:
- intermittent haemodialysis or peritoneal dialysis.

CIRCUIT

The standard circuit for paediatric RRT uses double lumen venovenous access, which is strongly preferred over arteriovenous circuits because of greater haemodynamic stability. Separate catheters can be used but need to be at least 5 Fr (in neonates) and as short as possible to permit the necessary blood flow. Unlike arteriovenous circuits, venovenous circuits require pumps to generate sufficient blood flow. These increase the extracorporeal fluid volume but provide the ability to closely regulate blood (and therefore filtrate) flow, prolonging the lifespan of the filter and making the whole process easier to regulate. Within these constraints, extracorporeal volume is kept to a minimum. The circuits include safety features such as bubble detectors, downstream clamps to prevent air embolism and pressure sensors to prevent suction or high driving pressures, both of which would cause haemolysis. Heat loss can be significant and is of greater concern with smaller children and infants. The problem can be addressed by including a heat exchange column in the circuit, insulating or warming the circuit, or using warmed replacement fluid.

ANTICOAGULATION

During filtration, filter lifespan is often sufficient without anticoagulants, particularly if there is adequate blood flow and there are no areas of stasis in the circuit. Routine anticoagulation with heparin to (ACT) activated clotting time levels of 150 to 180 seconds is however customary if the patient has a normal clotting profile. Patients with coagulopathy tend not to receive heparin, although the threshold for a prostacyclin infusion is lower in such cases. Prostacyclin reduces platelet activation and prolongs platelet survival. Anti-platelet doses of less than 5 ng kg^{-1} min $^{-1}$ administered pre-filter are not normally associated with significant vasodilatation. Platelet supplementation may still be necessary even when prostacyclin is being given. Heparin is usually administered pre-filter in doses around 20 units kg^{-1} hr^{-1} after a loading dose of 30 units kg^{-1}. Thus a significant proportion of the dose passes out in the filtrate. In clinical situations where filter survival has been problematic but systemic anticoagulation is contraindicated, heparin can be administered pre-filter in larger doses and protamine infused post-filter, both doses titrated against ACTs from the circuit and patient. The starting dose for protamine is 1 mg for every 100 units of heparin.

HAEMOFILTRATION REGIME

Blood flow rates of 25 ml min^{-1} are used for neonates, 50 ml min^{-1} for infants and older children, and up to 100 ml min^{-1} for adolescents; this requirement determines the size of the vascular access cannula. Fluid is usually removed at rates of 10 to 50 ml kg^{-1} h^{-1} (maximum 1.2–2 L hr^{-1}). The net loss to the patient is compensated with replacement fluid so that it rarely exceeds 5 ml kg^{-1} hr^{-1}. Rates of fluid loss as high as 12 ml kg^{-1} hr^{-1} are used during intermittent haemodialysis, but patients must be haemodynamically stable and may not manage to shift fluid fast enough into the vascular space to accommodate any further increase. If the filtration rate exceeds the plasma flow rate (which is calculated as extracorporeal blood flow × (1 − haematocrit)) then red cell sludge will block the filter. This can be avoided by the addition of replacement fluid pre-filter. A preference for high rates of ultrafiltration (using the process for solute clearance) makes this the norm. Conversely if one chooses to administer replacement fluid pre-filter then it is advisable to increase the ultrafiltration rate to counteract the effect of dilution on the clearance of agents that one is trying to remove. Such considerations are superfluous if the aim is merely to remove water.

Filters are changed when they clog (manifested by a decrease in the ultrafiltration rate or an increased resistance to blood flow) or electively after 72 hours.

HAEMOFILTRATION REPLACEMENT FLUID

The composition of the replacement fluid is adjusted to meet changing requirements. The most important choices in the type of fluid are related to its buffering and potassium content. Physiological levels of calcium and phosphate can be added to the replacement solution by using acetate in place of conventional lactate buffer but they will otherwise precipitate. For acidotic patients requiring the addition of bicarbonate to the dialysate, the calcium concentration of the solution is further limited making appropriate supplementation necessary elsewhere. Otherwise a good rule of thumb is to prescribe as near to a physiological concentration of electrolytes as possible and to increase parenteral nutrition to allow for the increased losses of amino acids, trace elements and minerals.

PLASMAFILTRATION REGIME

The clearance profile of native plasma during plasma exchange (including the 'evil humor' contained within it) follows an exponential decay. Exchange of one plasma-volume clears approximately 50 per cent of the native plasma but larger volume exchanges achieve diminishing returns. It is not feasible to aim for 100 per cent exchange. The active components that plasma exchange is targeting are often not restricted to the vascular space and have varying distribution profiles outside the plasma, varying rates of synthesis and varying natural rates of clearance or metabolism. These profiles are also drastically altered by disease states such as MOSF. After plasma exchange, redistribution of extravascular or tissue-bound substances leads to plasma profiles that change in the manner displayed in

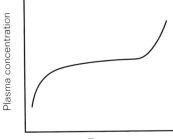

Figure 15.2 Plasma profile after plasma exchange. After plasma exchange, tissue-bound proteins and other moieties dissociate and move into the ECF and then the vascular compartment at a rate determined by many factors including the dissociation constant (varies with pH etc.) and molecular size, the latter particularly influencing the rate of entry into the vascular compartment. The blood concentration rises but reaches a plateau. Continued generation accounts for the second rise which continues until the next exchange.

Figure 15.2, at rates dependent on their tissue affinity. Ideally one therefore repeats the plasma exchange at intervals, rather than changing the exchange volume protocol or the ultrafiltration rate used during exchange. For maximum benefit repeat exchange should occur shortly after the phase of rapid concentration increase, but this may not be clearly defined for a given disease. Diseases mediated by agents that are mainly intravascular with a short half-life can receive continuous exchange but diseases mediated by agents with longer half-lives and larger volumes of distribution require repeated intermittent exchanges.

PLASMAFILTRATION REPLACEMENT FLUID

When performing plasmafiltration the patient is at risk of significant fluctuations in plasma albumin and globulin concentrations depending on the chosen fluid replacement regime. For intermittent plasmafiltration replace the filtrate volume with a 50:50 or 75:25 mix of 4.5 per cent human albumin solution and fresh frozen plasma. Longer-term plasmafiltration is better performed with a specifically prescribed replacement fluid, for example acetate buffered haemofiltration replacement fluid with 40 gL^{-1} of albumin added. These patients still require supplemental clotting factors. Longer-term plasmafiltration may also necessitate immunoglobulin supplementation. Fibrinogen deficiency may still occur even when FFP is included in the replacement regime. It manifests as a high activated clotting time that does not reduce with decreasing dosage of heparin (or even protamine) and is treated with additional cryoprecipitate.

PLASMAFILTRATION IN GUILLAIN–BARRÉ

This therapy is usually reserved for patients with poor prognostic factors, including rapid onset and the need for mechanical ventilation. It is difficult to distinguish the 10 per cent of cases where the problem is axonal and therefore not inflammatory. For the remainder, steroids still do not work and plasmafiltration, plasmaphoresis and intravenous gamma globulin all improve the percentage of patients that recover (to about 60%). The advantage of plasmafiltration and plasmaphoresis is that they demonstrate much quicker recovery in responders, reducing the time on ventilation and therefore the length of PICU stay. The time until they walk again and the percentage recovery by 6 months are also improved.

HAEMO-/PLASMAFILTRATION IN SEPTIC SHOCK

This subject is discussed in Chapter 17, Host Defence (see page 277). As yet consistent improvements in survival have not been proven. The justification for this approach is therefore empirical. Its proponents reserve it for the sicker cases and appear to get better results if the technique is applied soon after the onset of symptoms.

Both haemofiltration and plasmafiltration provide significant clearance of complement components. They can also remove large amounts of cytokines but without reliable changes in the plasma profile of these chemicals. Variable clearance despite sieving coefficients close to one implies that the rate of release of cytokines into the circulation exceeds that of their elimination. The effects of filtration or exchange on the cytokine profile are certainly short lived, hence the argument in favour of continuous filtration. The author's current approach is to exchange 3 to 4 plasma volumes over 4 to 6 hours and to repeat if necessary at daily intervals for 2 to 3 days. In the presence of oliguria or severe illness, patients are reverted to haemofiltration between and after plasma exchanges. Continuous plasmafiltration is a more pragmatic approach.

The systemic inflammatory response, caused by contact of blood with the artificial surfaces in the circuit, is usually small scale during RRT; this may (or may not) be because of the process of filtration itself.

Even without changes in the chosen ultrafiltration regime, large differences have been demonstrated in the clearances of different vasoactive mediators between different patients using the same type of haemofilter. It is already possible to tailor both filter and filtrate volume to the type and amount of mediators to be cleared. However the further adaptation of these techniques will inevitably be delayed until more knowledge has been gained about the specific relationships between illness severity and the inflammatory cascades. Also proof of their fundamental efficacy is still lacking. In the meanwhile plasmafiltration is preferred over haemofiltration for sepsis because the presumed mechanism of benefit is by clearance of inflammatory mediators and the clearance profile of a plasmafilter is more comprehensive.

PATTERNS OF RENAL DYSFUNCTION

Acute renal failure

Acute renal failure usually presents with oliguria and is most commonly the result of a prerenal insult. Despite luxurious perfusion, renal oxygen consumption is directly related to renal blood flow. This is because low renal blood flow is usually associated with a low GFR and hence less requirement for active reabsorption from the glomerular filtrate. Renal perfusion pressure drops with hypotension which ultimately causes acute renal failure. The process may be accelerated by high venous pressures which further compromise renal perfusion. In the face of hypotension the kidney responds as if intravascular volume depletion were the cause. Afferent glomerular arteriolar constriction occurs, reducing RPF and GFR eventually causing medullary ischaemia (acute tubular necrosis) and even cortical damage. Cellular debris enters the filtrate and urine and blocks the tubules. Back leakage of filtrate from the tubules contributes to cortical oedema. The appropriate response to this scenario is to treat the cause, which usually (as above) means the restoration of normal blood pressure and renal blood flow. Then provide adequate nutrition since energy requirement may be 50 per cent above baseline. Protein restriction causes catabolism and should be avoided. After these two manoeuvres one waits for spontaneous renal recovery and uses renal replacement therapy.

The other less common causes of acute renal failure seen by the intensivist are nephrotoxic drugs (perceptively less common since the widespread adoption of 24 hour dosing regimes for aminoglycosides) haemolysis and tumour lysis syndrome. Urine output is preserved in some forms of acute renal failure such as those induced by osmotic diuresis, diabetes insipidus or post-obstruction uropathy. The need for RRT is judged by the criteria above, rather than the aetiology per se. However it is often useful to institute RRT early, to allow adequate nutrition and pre-empt severe electrolyte imbalance or water overload. Recovery is usually rapid in neonates, for whom acute renal failure rarely lasts more than a week but is more prolonged in older children or in cases of renal toxicity.

Chronic renal failure

Patients with chronic renal failure commonly experience growth failure so do not assume that a 25 kg patient is an 8 year old! These patients are prone to a constellation of different complications that affect the way inter-current illnesses are managed, including the following.

- *Cardiovascular problems* – patients may present in a variety of intravascular volume states depending upon their recent fluid intake and haemodialysis regime. Nevertheless their well-known haemodynamic fragility is aggravated by impaired autonomic reflexes. There is a tendency to hypertension (sodium and water overload, high intravascular volume, Goldblatt and other renin–angiotensin mechanisms, resistance to atrial naturetic factor, atheroma, high intracellular calcium levels, catecholamine release). Patients may also suffer from cardiomyopathy and a mixed bag of other problems including accelerated atherosclerosis and pericarditis.
- *Fluid, electrolyte and acid–base disturbances* – most typically hyperkalemia and metabolic acidosis but also fluid shifts (dysequilibrium) and abnormalities of calcium and phosphorous metabolism (see below). Chronic thirst is difficult for children to resist and the most common problem in oligo- and anuric patients is water overload.
- *The inability to activate vitamin D* – this leads to phosphate retention and hypocalcaemia. Secondary hyperparathyroidism contributes to renal osteodystrophy and osteomalacia.
- *Anaemia* – low erythropoietin levels, increased red cell fragility and a haemorrhagic tendency aggravated by poor platelet function all contribute. Beware of covert gastrointestinal bleeding.
- *Immunosuppression.*
- *Pancreatitis.*
- *Glucose intolerance.*
- *Neurological disturbance* – for example dysequilibrium and hypertensive encephalopathy, but also peripheral neuropathy including impaired autonomic reflexes.

Haemolytic uraemic syndrome

Nephritic presentations usually include hypertension, haematuria and renal insufficiency. Most glomerulonephritides are relatively chronic diseases and manage to avoid PICU admission. Haemolytic uraemic syndrome is a common exception, usually because it is missed and complications such as fluid overload have already occurred by the time the diagnosis is made. The condition is a microangiopathy causing glomerulonephritis, enteritis and microangiopathic anaemia with characteristic fragmentation of red cells on the blood film. Coagulation tests are usually normal but a bleeding tendency can result from thrombocytopaenia. More severe presentations include myocarditis and cerebral vasculitis and atypical cases may develop hepatitis. Epidemic haemolytic uraemic syndrome is usually caused by enteric infection from verocytotoxin-producing *Escherichia coli*. The genetic information required to produce the toxin is shared through plasmid transfer which may lead to proliferation of the ability to cause haemolytic uraemic syndrome in the future. Non-infective causes are also recognised and genetic factors probably account for the apparent variation in patient susceptibility. Most patients, up to 70 per cent, recover completely, detectable renal abnormalities persist in less than 25 per cent of patients, and fewer than 5 per cent remain in renal failure and require transplant. Poor prognostic indicators include recognition of cerebral involvement, exposure of the Thomsen antigen on red cells as occurs in haemolytic uraemic syndrome secondary to neuraminidase positive infections, and allied to this, the absence of a diarrhoeal prodrome. There is no specific therapy directed at the microangiopathy (prostacyclin, antiplatelet drugs and immunoglobulins have all been tried without convincing benefit). Treatment requires early recognition, appropriate fluid restriction and support with renal replacement therapy where necessary.

Nephrotic syndrome

This term refers to a condition of hypoalbuminaemic oedema where the protein loss occurs as the result of nephropathy. Most cases in paediatrics are caused by minimal change nephritis and most of these are steroid responsive. When symptomatic (oedematous) oedema is aggravated by secondary hyperaldosteronism and sodium retention, it may respond to sodium restriction and thiazide diuretics. These patients are at increased risk of pneumococcal infections, peritonitis, urinary tract infection, pneumonia, cellulitis, hyperlipidaemia, and thrombotic complications. Those that are not steroid responsive or who lose steroid responsiveness may respond to cytotoxic therapy. Other aetiologies such as focal segmental glomerular sclerosis carry a much worse prognosis but become easier to handle in terms of intravascular volume as the GFR deteriorates. Hypovolaemic crises usually reflect accelerated protein loss and ultimately will recur unless this root cause is treatable and treated. Acute responses to volume replacement are improved if the albumin is raised but the benefits may be short lived. Because the total body water is high and the non-glomerular capillaries are healthy, many will take the opportunity to administer a loop diuretic and establish a diuresis when volume and albumin support are necessary.

SECONDARY RENAL FAILURE

Haemolysis

Severe widespread haemolysis can be seen in blood dyscrasias (such as the porphyrias, spherocytosis and sickle cell), tranfusion accidents or errors, inborn metabolic errors (such as glucose–6-phosphate dehydrogenase deficiency), infections (hepatitis), in association with extracorporeal circulation (ECMO, cardiopulmonary bypass and haemofiltration) and cardiac abnormalities (intravascular devices, artificial valves, VSD/regurgitant jets imping-ing on valve apparatus). It can also be a feature of vasculitides and microangiopathy (e.g. haemolytic uraemic syndrome) and can occur in some forms of poisoning.

During severe acute haemolysis the oxygen-carrying capacity can be supplemented by red cell transfusion. Tubular renal function may be preserved by high urine flow rates but the glomerular damage from sludged red cell stroma cannot be treated directly and may lead to acute renal failure.

Tumour lysis syndrome

Tumour lysis occurs spontaneously in rapidly proliferating tumours such as T cell leukaemias, or otherwise when large tumour bulks rapidly respond to chemotherapy. The main toxic solutes are potassium, phosphate and uric acid. Preventative therapy is the mainstay of treatment. Allopurinol inhibits xanthine oxidase, an enzyme that catalyses the conversion of hypoxanthine and xanthine to uric acid. Urate oxidase (uricozyme), a natu-rally occurring proteolytic enzyme in many mammals, degrades uric acid to allantoins, which are ten times more soluble than uric acid and easily eliminated by the kidneys. The dosage of allopurinol is limited in renal failure. Pre-hydration (200–400% fluids) with alka-line fluids encourages a diuresis that limits deposition of calcium phosphate and uric acid precipitation in the kidney. This treatment may preserve renal function but it aggravates pulmonary oedema and requires invasive haemodynamic monitoring in marginal cases. Renal replacement therapy should be started early, especially in the presence of hyper-kalaemia since more conservative measures are unlikely to be effective. If necessary, acute tubular necrosis because of tumour lysis can be distinguished from other causes by a urine uric acid : creatinine ratio greater than one.

16 Gastro-Intestinal System

- **Background**
- **Short notes on specific conditions**

BACKGROUND

Macroscopically, gastro-intestinal structures are all present by 6 weeks of gestation, however even in term infants the microscopic structure and function are immature continuing their development during childhood. For example, small intestinal mucosal villi are leaf like rather than finger shaped in children and present a lower luminal surface area. Normally blood flow to the intestine is increased by the increased metabolic demands of digestion. However when this process fails, the countercurrent arteriovenous plexus within the villus can still render the tip vulnerable to ischaemia as in older patients.

Although the gut of the newborn infant is capable of absorbing sufficient nutrients to sustain life, functional maturity develops during childhood. Gastric acid production increases greatly over the first 10 days of life and then decreases to normal values. There is a reduced capacity for fat absorption, and intestinal glucose transport is about 25 per cent of adult values. Significant quantities of intact proteins (such as maternal immunoglobulin) can cross neonatal gut mucosa. The transport of solutes is adequate but there is little functional reserve. Relatively minor gut disease processes (e.g. viral infection) can result in severe functional disturbances (diarrhoea and dehydration) and diarrhoea and vomiting are almost universal symptoms of a diversity of illnesses in children from salt losing congenital adrenal hyperplasia to meningitis.

Pancreas

In infants pancreatic secretion of amylase and lipase is low, contributing to *relative* starch and fat intolerance. However fat malabsorption only results after a further reduction in lipase secretion.

Liver

At birth the liver comprises 5 per cent of body weight, compared to 2 per cent in adults. Features of its relative immaturity include low levels of bile acid secretion, low activity of microsomal enzymes (responsible for drug metabolism and conjugation reactions) and reduced synthetic function. These factors contribute to a reduced ability in neonates to absorb fats, breakdown drugs, conjugate bilirubin and synthesise albumin. The fetal liver's glycogen stores are 2 to 3 times adult values at term, but are used up in the immediate postnatal period rendering the infant intolerant of subsequent prolonged fasting. Hepatic gluconeogenesis develops rapidly during the first few days of life.

The liver's role in drug metabolism and the impact of maturational issues has been discussed in Chapter 9, Pharmacology. Although the presence of liver dysfunction and co-administered drugs should be carefully considered when prescribing drugs for children, the liver has considerable functional reserve and impaired drug elimination is, in general terms, not an early feature of liver dysfunction. However the assessment of the degree of liver dysfunction can be problematic. Classic liver 'function' tests (measuring blood levels of transaminases and alkaline phosphatase) are very poor indicators of hepatic synthetic, metabolic, immune, nutritional and other functions. Rises in circulating enzyme levels can be delayed by several hours in acute liver injury and the extent of the rise is dependent on the number of active hepatocytes present at the outset. The prothrombin time is the best routinely performed test of hepatic synthetic ability and the serum bilirubin is an important marker of metabolic function, provided it is interpreted in context. The bilirubin level has further connotations in terms of albumin drug binding capacity. Hypoalbuminaemia is a frequent corollary of hepatic dysfunction.

Minor degrees of liver dysfunction are common in critically ill children. The liver blood supply is subject to some degree of autoregulation where changes in portal venous flow, the major component of liver blood flow, lead to reciprocal changes in hepatic arterial flow keeping the total liver blood flow constant (the 'hepatic arterial buffer' response). However liver blood flow is reduced during shock and right heart failure and may also be reduced by mechanical ventilation depending on the cardiovascular circumstances. Recovery of hepatic function with resolution of the underlying critical illness is usual.

SHORT NOTES ON SPECIFIC CONDITIONS

Gastro-oesophageal reflux

Gastro-oesophageal reflux (GOR) is common in neonates and need not lead to symptomatic disorders such as poor feeding or bleeding from oesophagitis or indeed aspiration. The extent of GOR declines sharply by 1 year of age partly because of the effect of gravity as an upright posture is adopted. GOR can persist or recur in the context of acute or chronic underlying disease because of effects on posture, oesophageal motility, position and coordination of the components of the lower oesophageal sphincter, gastric luminal pressure and the organisation of gastric peristalsis and emptying. Reflux episodes are more common in the horizontal supine position and can produce apnoea, vagal responses such as bradycardia, laryngospasm and bronchospasm, recurrent stridor and potentially, sudden infant death syndrome. Symptomatic GOR is more common after repair of oesophageal atresia and congenital diaphragmatic hernia and in patients with severe neurological impairment. The best available method for objective quantification of reflux is oesophageal pH monitoring but the correlation of the results with symptomatology is imperfect. Barium swallow can also be used to make the diagnosis. Medical therapy includes the use of thickened feeds and alginate gels, drugs which increase gastric pH (ranitidine, omeprazole) and prokinetic agents. Surgical management (fundoplication and/or gastrostomy) is necessary in some patients.

PIC patients are at increased risk of GOR for a variety of reasons including supine positioning, nasogastric tube placement, coma and drug effects on the lower oesophageal sphincter. During mechanical ventilation, coughing and tracheal suctioning may precipitate GOR as well as vomiting. GOR occurs less frequently in patients receiving muscle relaxants. Pulmonary aspiration can occur around uncuffed endotracheal tubes (that is not to imply that cuffed tubes entirely prevent it).

Cisapride can be associated with prolonged QTc interval on the ECG and associated ventricular arrhythmias. Drugs that inhibit cytochrome P450, such as erythromycin or fluconazole, increase the risk of such effects. The pharmacokinetics of cisapride in premature neonates are unpredictable. Caution should be exercised in its use and it has recently been withdrawn in the UK.

Gastro-intestinal haemorrhage

Severe gastro-intestinal (GI) haemorrhage is a well-recognised complication of critical illness in childhood but it has a lower incidence than in older patients. In patients with head trauma, the classic Cushing's ulcer presents about 1 week after the injury. In burns patients Curling's ulcer classically develops 2 or more weeks after the injury. More commonly stress gastritis occurs within 4 days of injury. Periods of shock and acidosis lead to mucosal damage and ulceration, which can lead to bleeding. Upper GI bleeding is often confirmed by the finding of fresh or altered blood (coffee grounds) on nasogastric tube aspiration. Malaena stool is associated with larger upper GI bleeds. Rectal fresh blood is usually caused by lower GI haemorrhage, but may occur with rapid major bleeds from higher sites. Potential sites of upper GI bleeding include oesophageal varices in patients with portal hypertension and gastric ulcers and erosions. Bleeding can occur from islands of gastric mucosa associated with a Meckel's diverticulum and intussusception produces a bloody 'red currant jelly' stool.

MANAGEMENT

RESUSCITATE

Treat shock by restoring the circulation with appropriate fluids and control haemorrhage where you can. The commonest cause of bleeding in a patient with known varices is variceal although there may be a peptic ulcer. This is the reverse of the adult situation where the ulcer is the more likely source. Paediatric sizes of Sengstaken-Blakemore tubes are readily available. In all cases coagulopathy and thrombocytopaenia should be corrected rapidly with fresh frozen plasma, and/or cryoprecipitate, and platelet transfusions as necessary. Establish cardiovascular monitoring and site a large bore nasogastric tube if a Sengstaken-Blakemore is not indicated.

DIAGNOSE

Endoscopy can be performed at the bedside in PICU and may identify the site of upper or lower GI bleeding. Angiography, isotope scans and barium studies may also aid in diagnosis.

TREAT

In many cases bleeding will stop spontaneously especially if any concurrent coagulopathy and thrombocytopaenia are corrected. It is important to keep up with blood losses but in variceal bleeds avoid driving filling pressure too high. Local control of bleeding may be accomplished endoscopically, for example sclerosing or banding of varices or injection of a bleeding vessel. Bleeding vessels identified angiographically may be amenable to embolisation. Vasopressin and octreotide infusions reduce splanchnic blood supply and can help control bleeding. Surgical intervention is indicated when medical management has failed to stop bleeding in a surgically accessible site.

PROPHYLAXIS

The mortality from *massive* GI haemorrhage is high and most clinicians feel this necessitates attempts at prophylaxis for 'at-risk' groups (i.e. not all admissions). These include patients with significant burns, major trauma, shock, coagulopathy and renal failure. Prompt restoration of splanchnic perfusion and enteral feeding may have some protective effects, particularly for patients receiving glucocorticoids or non-steroidal anti-inflammatory drugs. Ranitidine and sucralfate are the most frequently prescribed drugs for prophylaxis although omeprazole raises gastric pH very effectively. Sucralfate's efficacy in preventing GI haemorrhage has not been rigorously tested and aluminium toxicity is common where renal function is compromised.

Short gut syndrome

This term describes a pattern of malabsorption and malnutrition occurring as a consequence of small bowel resection, usually after surgery for neonatal necrotising enterocolitis, or gastroschisis. Decreased luminal surface area, enzyme depletion and short transit times all contribute to the clinical manifestations of failure to thrive, diarrhoea and abdominal distension with undigested food or reducing substances in the stool. After surgery it is difficult to predict the nutritional future even with detailed knowledge of the quantity and quality of remaining bowel. However malabsorption is probable if more than 50 per cent of the small bowel has been removed and preservation of the ileocaecal valve significantly prolongs the transit time. Ileal resection has more profound effects than higher resection and involves the loss of active transport sites for nutrients (particularly fat), vitamin B_{12} and conjugated bile salts. Patients may require antacids, cholestyramine and motility decreasing agents like loperamide. Fat malabsorption is associated with fat-soluble vitamin deficiency. Bacterial overgrowth can aggravate diarrhoea and translocation can lead to septicaemia. Ileostomies are associated with chronic sodium and bicarbonate losses. Loss of the large bowel is a potent cause of water loss. Long-term vascular access for PN increases the risk of sepsis and prolonged TPN administration is associated with cholestasis that can lead to cirrhosis. Enteral formulae which rely on medium-chain triglycerides as a fat source, and which contain carbohydrate as glucose polymers, are preferred. Dietary supplements of vitamins (including the fat soluble A, D, E and K), trace elements, calcium, iron, B_{12} and folate are advisable.

The gut and SIRS

In addition to its absorptive functions, the gut has a pivotal role in the body's host defence systems. Gastrointestinal contents include vast numbers of micro-organisms in a rich nutrient broth of partly digested food and naturally-shed epithelial cells. In addition the gut lumen contains many potentially antigenic proteins. The primary mucosal barrier to these organisms is backed up by abundant lymphoid tissue (Peyer's patches).

There are a number of theories linking the gut to the development of the systemic inflammatory response syndrome (SIRS). Normally the splanchnic circulation contains about 30 per cent of circulating blood volume. However during shock, perfusion is greatly reduced or sacrificed to preserve flow to the brain, heart and lungs. These effects are mediated by endogenous catecholamines, vasopressin and angiotensin II and can be compounded by inadequate fluid resuscitation and the therapeutic use of α agonists. It is speculated that damage to the gut mucosal barrier leads to translocation of bacteria and endotoxin into the blood stream causing a persistent inflammatory stimulus, neutrophil activation and subsequent SIRS. Where such damage results from a reperfusion injury, for example from free radical generation, it is possible to conceptualise an escalating cycle of inflammatory damage. Such theories have led to the postulate that the gut is the 'engine' of SIRS. Data from studies using gastric tonometry (pHi) in general support an association between poor perfusion and/or a failure of perfusion to improve with resuscitation, with a poor prognosis, though in these cases the poor prognosis has not necessarily been as a result of persistent SIRS.

Pancreatitis

Acute pancreatitis is rare in paediatric medicine. A grumbling neonatal pancreatitis occurs in patients with cystic fibrosis generating high immune reactive trypsin levels. A variety of congenital malformations affecting the exocrine ducts can occur. Inborn errors of metabolism, trauma, viral infections, drugs and toxins and gall stones (e.g. in patients with sickle cell anaemia or hyperlipidaemia) account for the remainder. The diagnosis is made on the basis of history, clinical features, imaging (abdominal X-ray – Sentinel loop or ultrasound) and laboratory results (elevated amylase and lipase levels). Treatment consists of ceasing enteral feeds, nutritional support with parenteral nutrition and prompt recognition and treatment of complicating factors such as pseudocyst or abcess formation, hypocalcaemia, hyperglycaemia, metastatic fat necrosis, metabolic acidosis, coagulopathy, shock and ARDS.

Fulminant hepatic failure

Acute severe liver cell dysfunction can occur abruptly during the presentation of disease or as a complication of chronic liver failure. There is a clinical as well as a philosophical distinction however from end-stage chronic liver failure. The diagnosis usually follows a typical history of clinical features such as nausea and malaise, followed by jaundice and coagulopathy (unresponsive to vitamin K). Encephalopathy occurs later in the spectrum of severity than in adults and is therefore more ominous. The most rapidly progressive cases develop hypoglycaemia, metabolic acidosis and hyperammonaemia in association with coma before jaundice is detected.

The context and severity of the presentation affect the prognosis. Poor prognostic factors include:

- aetiology (e.g. worse when caused by paracetamol overdose or non-A non-B viral hepatitis); paracetamol overdose does not normally cause fulminant hepatic failure in paediatrics thus fulminant hepatic failure when it does occur usually represents exceptionally high dose poisoning
- speed of progression
- age of the patient (worse when the patient is less than 10 years old)
- concurrent renal failure
- prothrombin time greater than 90 seconds
- severe encephalopathy.

To put this in context; the mortality without transplantation is 50 to 80 per cent but rises to more than 90 per cent with severe encephalopathy or coagulopathy.

Table 16.1 Hepatic encephalopathy.

Grade	Clinical features
I	Minor functional disturbance
II	Drowsy but rousable, responds to commands
III	Aggressive, agitated or incoherent.
IVa	Unrousable but may exhibit a pain response
IVb	Unrousable and unresponsive

Typical supportive laboratory findings include high serum transaminases although falling levels (such as shrinking liver size) can represent deterioration rather than improvement. In most cases histologically there is massive hepatocellular necrosis, although severe liver cell dysfunction may occur without cell death in some conditions. The presence of marked coagulopathy however makes liver biopsy hazardous.

The differential diagnosis includes infective, metabolic, vascular, toxic (and idiosyncratic) causes. Worldwide viral hepatitis is the commonest cause. In teenagers and adults, paracetamol poisoning, generally with suicidal intent, is prominent. Young children may be accidentally or deliberately overdosed with paracetamol by a carer or assailant. Although children are at less risk of fulminant hepatic failure after high dose paracetamol exposure, their prognosis is still poor if it does develop. In many patients the cause is not identified and if hepatic failure is severe enough then the diagnosis is largely academic unless it is likely to recur in a transplanted liver or contraindicate treatment by transplantation. Patients are listed for transplantation if:

- their liver failure is sufficiently severe. This is where most variation occurs between units but it is often judged purely on coagulopathy (e.g. INR > 4, prothrombin time > 60 seconds)
- they are not actively septicaemic, too sick, or beyond help (e.g. severe cerebral oedema with raised intracranial pressure or extensive involvement or failure of other organ systems)
- they have suitable vascular anatomy.

The limited supply of donor organs is a complicating factor.

Complications
COMA

Comatose patients (grade III/IV encephalopathy) will require intubation for airway protection and ventilation. Nasotracheal tubes are avoided in the presence of coagulopathy. Treatable causes of coma such as hypoglycaemia or subclinical status epilepticus should be identified and treated. CT scanning can be useful to exclude cerebral haemorrhage as the cause of acute neurological deterioration. Flumazenil and plasmapheresis have been used to temporarily improve encephalopathy, but do not alter outcome. Attempts to alter gut pH and flora to reduce the number of urea splitting organisms present, are common.

CEREBRAL OEDEMA

Cerebral oedema is present in 75 per cent of patients with grade IV encephalopathy (i.e. not all patients!) and is frequently the cause of death. It is much rarer in acute-on-chronic liver failure. The interpretation of CT scans is an insensitive approach to recognising mild cerebral oedema, which is the manifestation of a diffuse ongoing brain injury (cytotoxic cerebral oedema). In most cases it is reasonable to assume that cerebrovascular autoregulation is correspondingly impaired (see below).

RAISED INTRACRANIAL PRESSURE

Neither CT nor MRI can reliably detect raised intracranial pressure until mass effect occurs. Neurological recovery from cerebral oedema is generally good if liver function is restored and the ischaemic consequences of raised intracranial pressure can be avoided. Therefore, where possible, measure intracranial pressure (this may necessitate aggressive correction of coagulopathy first and subsequently). The treatment priorities are as follows.

- Preserve cerebral oxygen delivery.
  Maintain cardiac output and haemoglobin concentration. Ventilate with high FiO_2 with a minute volume sufficient to run low normal $PaCO_2$ and assume that cerebral blood flow will bear a linear relationship with cerebral perfusion pressure. Maintain CPP above 50 mmHg principally by cardiovascular support. Avoid rises in ICP by a policy of minimal handling, nursing with head midline and a 20° head up position, and paralysis to avoid coughing and straining. Aggressive treatment of raised intracranial pressure using procedures such as craniectomy has not yet been shown to improve outcome in cerebral oedema caused by 'metabolic coma' such as this.
- Minimise cerebral swelling.
  Impose a therapeutic fluid restriction even to the point of hypernatraemia as high as 150 mmol L^{-1}. The role of mannitol in an ongoing cerebral insult such as this is equivocal and it should not be given in the presence of oliguric renal failure (see below).
- Minimise cerebral oxygen demand
  Principally by recognising and controlling seizures and avoiding hyperthermia. Barbiturate coma is preferred and is induced by thiopentone infusion in doses sufficient to cause a burst-suppression EEG.

RENAL FAILURE

Renal failure presents with oliguria, it can lead to fluid overload and complicates both the management of cerebral oedema and the correction of coagulopathy. Treatable causes of prerenal failure such as hypovolaemia or hypotension caused by haemodynamic instability should be corrected, but a low threshold exists for haemofiltration. Even in the face of marginal renal dysfunction the fluid exchange required to allow correction of coagulopathy without aggravating cerebral oedema (e.g. when a donor becomes available) may be beyond the ability of drug-induced diuresis.

HAEMODYNAMIC INSTABILITY

This is common, particularly a low systemic vascular resistance and variable (but usually raised) cardiac output. Invasive cardiovascular monitoring (CVP, arterial line ± Swan–Ganz catheter) is essential and inotropic support commonly includes α agonists. Vigilance is required to detect hypovolaemia caused by occult or acute haemorrhage.

COAGULOPATHY

Coagulopathy is typical of fulminant hepatic failure. Levels of factors II, V, VII, IX and X and antithrombin III are all reduced. Thrombocytopaenia also occurs and should be corrected if the platelet counts fall below 50×10^9 per litre in the presence of concurrent coagulopathy. The prothrombin time is the best prognostic liver function test and coagulopathy should only be corrected with fresh frozen plasma (and/or cryoprecipitate) if there is a therapeutic indication such as bleeding, the need to establish intracranial pressure monitoring or imminent surgery.

METABOLIC ACIDOSIS

This results principally from increased lactate production because of impaired oxygen delivery or extraction and impaired metabolism. It can impair the response to inotropes and recurs inexorably if the cause cannot be treated. Ideally, problematic acidosis should be treated with moderate volume haemofiltration using a bicarbonate buffered replacement fluid.

HYPOGLYCAEMIA

Hypoglycaemia is common as a result of impaired liver gluconeogenesis and reduced uptake of insulin by the failing liver. It should be anticipated, appropriately supplemented with intravenous dextrose (without compromising the fluid restriction) and closely monitored.

ELECTROLYTE DISTURBANCES

Electrolyte disturbances such as hyponatraemia are more common if there has been a history of chronic hepatic dysfunction and secondary hyperaldosteronism.

SEPSIS

Sepsis is a considerable risk in these patients. The risk is aggravated by the use of invasive treatments and impaired cellular and humoral immunity. A high index of suspicion for infection results, requiring limited septic 'screens' in response to fluctuations in the patient's clinical condition. This approach should be extended to starting blind therapy with broad spectrum antimicrobial and antifungal agents when dramatic changes in clinical condition occur.

THERAPY

There is no definitive treatment available for fulminant hepatic failure and management depends on supportive care, with liver transplantation in selected cases. Early transfer to a specialist centre with a transplant programme is advisable. The results of a transplant series for fulminant hepatic failure can be improved with more stringent case selection but there will have been no real improvement for the treatment of fulminant hepatic failure if the non-transplanted patients still die. It is important to identify early those causes of liver failure (e.g. paracetamol poisoning) for which specific therapies exist, although N-acetyl cysteine is currently being used more generically in liver failure.

The best signs of clinical improvement are spontaneous improvement in the coagulation profile, a fall in serum bilirubin or evidence of resolution of cerebral oedema.

There is currently considerable interest in the development of artificial liver devices to enable support of patients either as a bridge to transplantation or hepatocellular recovery.

Liver transplantation

Paediatric liver transplantation *per se* is now claimed to be associated with 1 year survival as high as 90 per cent, although survival is much lower for high risk groups such as neonates and patients in preoperative fulminant hepatic failure. Morbidity increases with delay in transplantation. In particular, neurological outcome is significantly worse if cerebral oedema occurs prior to transplant, even without raised intracranial pressure. Technical sophistication in hepatic transplant surgery has been improving rapidly over the last 10 years but activity is still constrained by the availability of donor organs. Cut down techniques, split liver grafts and even living related donor techniques have evolved as a consequence. 'Elective' orthotopic liver transplant patients routinely visit the intensive care unit postoperatively but in the absence of surgical complications their stay is brief. Priorities in management are:

- the maintenance of haemodynamic stability
- immune suppression
- assessment of graft function and the quality of vascular anastomoses.

Early graft failure is usually the result of a preservation injury (primary non function) or ischaemia (e.g. portal vein or hepatic artery occlusion). Hyperacute rejection still takes days to present. Recipients who were in fulminant hepatic failure prior to transplantation (particularly neonates) naturally run a more complicated course.

17 Host Defence

- **Detection and recognition of infection**
- **Protection from infection**
- **Treatment of infection**
- **Problems with host defence**

When using an organ system structured approach to a PIC patient (as opposed to a diagnostic or problem orientated one) the 'host defence' issues are often grouped together as a distinct category for discussion. These issues include injury, inflammation and healing as well as immunity, but they commonly concentrate on 'infection risk' as well as the investigation, treatment and prophylaxis of specific infections and infectious diseases. This chapter cannot provide a comprehensive overview of these diverse subjects and therefore presents a mixture of core knowledge, common issues and clinical protocols with a few specific examples.

DETECTION AND RECOGNITION OF INFECTION

Most topologically external surfaces in the body (skin, upper respiratory and gastrointestinal tracts) are liberally colonised with micro-organisms within 24 hours of birth. But this does not mean that the patient is infected. A definition of 'infection' at one of these sites requires:

- overgrowth of a known or potential pathogen and
- clinical symptoms or signs.

Microbiologists make distinctions between 'colonisation' and 'overgrowth' by the magnitude of the growth expressed by counting the numbers of 'colony forming units' per millilitre or gram of body sample from these sites. They rarely report further any growth of organisms regarded as normal flora. However when organisms grow from sites that are normally sterile (lower respiratory tract, blood, urine, cerebrospinal fluid) then there is either infection or there has been contamination of the sample. Furthermore the decision about what represents a potential pathogen rather than normal flora must be context sensitive in terms of the age and immunological susceptibility of the patient.

Most intensive care units conduct some degree of microbiological surveillance to identify carriers of multi-resistant pathogens. Some go a lot further. The most common situation however is to seek a microbiological explanation for a deterioration in condition, laboratory results or fever. This process involves some form of 'septic screen' where culture samples are obtained from the relevant, normally sterile, sites. This usually involves blood and urine but may involve pleural or peritoneal fluid and cerebrospinal fluid (CSF) depending on the context.

The main role of lumbar puncture (LP) is primarily to *exclude* meningitis, i.e. to establish a population that does not need antibiotic therapy, hospital admission, etc. Sick children (including the haemodynamically unstable or those with respiratory compromise) and anyone with a possibility of raised intracranial pressure should not be subjected to LP for fear of acute deterioration. If necessary these patients should be treated as if they have got meningitis until they are well enough to tolerate lumbar puncture. Currently for most age groups in most parts of the world this does not involve a change in antibiotic regimen anyway.

If you experience technical difficulty while performing an LP then you may be faced with recognising and interpreting a traumatic tap (the degree of blood staining usually reduces **259** in successive bottles). Calculate a WBC:RBC ratio from the peripheral blood count and compare it to the ratio in the least contaminated CSF. Alternatively one can allow one white blood cell for each 700 red blood cells. Blood contamination to the degree of a CSF red blood cell count of 1000 red blood cells can raise the CSF protein by as much as 1 mg dL^{-1}.

There are a number of indirect ways of detecting infection or improving the sensitivity of diagnostic investigations such as polymerase chain reaction and the detection of bacterial antigens in body fluids. Infection may also be implied with varying predictive power by changes in acute phase indices such as C-reactive protein (CRP) or immature:total neutrophil ratio. The white cell count alone is a remarkably non-specific marker.

Temperature and illness

The normal diurnal variation in body temperature (peaks at midday and midnight) ranges across 1°C. This is not present in babies but it is established by 2 years of age. The rhythm is influenced by sleep, bathing and eating (and ovulation in post-pubertal females) and is probably determined by two thermoregulatory centres in the hypothalamus. Definitions of 'normal' temperature increase over the first 7 months of life and fall again by the age of 3 years giving wide 95% confidence intervals (36.6°C to 38.4°C) during this time. Exaggerated peaks of diurnal rhythm are an early non-specific sign of inflammation even if they do not reach a magnitude that one would accept as fever.

Skin temperature can be measured at various sites (forehead, axilla, etc.) and depending on the site used should be regarded as 'peripheral' (extensively influenced by environment and perfusion) or 'core'. Core temperature is also approximated by measurement at various sites which deliver different results depending on circumstances (open chest, mid-laparotomy, recent administration of suppository, etc.). Differences in measurement technique can also make substantial differences to the recorded result especially with rectal temperature. Since measurement error will almost always lead to underestimation, core temperature is best defined pragmatically as the highest measurable temperature from any central site. The clinical preference is for appropriately measured rectal values. In adults, body temperature is usually highest in the rectum, bladder, brain and liver, and is progressively lower in the right ventricle, pulmonary artery, oesophagus, tympanic membrane, mouth, axilla and forehead. In children axillary temperature is commonly regarded as 1°C below rectal. In newborns the rectal temperature is approximately equal to the axillary temperature plus 0.2°C for each week of age up to 5 weeks.

The toe–core temperature difference is a commonly used clinical marker of perfusion (but not necessarily sepsis). It widens in cold environments, some forms of shock and after administration of α adrenergic agents. It falls in warm environments, and after administration of vasodilators. As a consequence it can be remarkably insensitive in the PICU patient and should always be interpreted alongside other clinical and physiological parameters.

Fever is a part of an inflammatory response. It does not necessarily indicate infection and is widely assumed to be beneficial in the host defence against disease. In fact this presumed evolutionary advantage has been difficult to prove (with specific exceptions including indirect evidence that antipyretics worsen the outcome in severe sepsis). Fever is one of the criteria which contribute to a diagnosis of the 'systemic inflammatory response syndrome'. Various factors (e.g. environmental temperature, age and prematurity of the patient) must be taken into account when interpreting body temperature. Of particular importance are direct sunlight and the use of servo-controlled temperature devices. Non-infective causes of fever also include:

- transfusion reactions to blood, plasma, platelets or other blood products
- drug reactions including malignant hyperpyrexia
- neoplasms such as lymphoma
- systemic inflammatory response syndrome (SIRS)
- CNS diseases including haemorrhage

- non-infective phenomena such as intracranial air, thrombosis, tissue damage (e.g. after a crush injury)
- non-infective inflammation (e.g. pancreatitis) or inflammatory diseases such as Kawasaki's disease
- endocrine causes (e.g. phaeochromocytoma, thyrotoxicosis and carcinoid)
- inherited metabolic disorders (e.g. porphyria).

After cardiac, neurological and abdominal surgery, fever is to be expected and does not necessarily indicate bacteraemia or other infection. However once 48 postoperative hours have elapsed, the occurrence of fever *de novo* cannot be confidently ascribed to the surgery. Taken the other way, infection cannot be confidently excluded perioperatively because of the presence of fever from other causes. This is part of the reasoning in favour of antibiotic prophylaxis for some surgical procedures.

Clinical thermometry is an art that is rarely referenced in modern PIC. The required reaction time for investigation and treatment of the feverish patient is often too short to allow recognition of fever patterns other than the Jarisch–Herxheimer reaction (a sharp rise in temperature associated with cardiovascular lability occurring some hours after the start of antibiotic therapy ascribed to a pulse of endotoxin release from dying micro-organisms). Other recognised patterns of fever include:

- continuous sustained fever with slight remissions occurring in lobar pneumonia, Gram-negative infections, ricketsial diseases, typhoid, falciparum malaria and CNS disorders (not necessarily infective)
- intermittent 'picket fence' fever with evening peaks occurring in localised pyogenic infections, bacteraemia and endocarditis
- quotidian, tertian and quartan malarias (these are well described).
- double quotidian fever (two daily spikes) occurring in salmonellosis, miliary TB, gonococcal and meningococcal disease
- saddle back 'biphasic' fever (several days of fever, then a 24-hour gap followed by several more days of fever) occurring in dengue, yellow fever, Colorado tick fever, Rift Valley fever, influenza and other viral diseases such as polio
- Charcot's fever (sporadic episodes) typical of cholangitis
- Pel–Ebstein fever (weekly cycles of fever and relapse) occurring in Hodgkin's disease and brucellosis
- reversal of diurnal rhythm of fever occurs occasionally in miliary TB, salmonellosis, liver abscess and endocarditis.

Treatment of fever

The routine treatment of even moderate fever cannot be justified unless metabolic rate oxygen demand and delivery are critical, or until extreme temperatures are reached (>40°C) introducing the danger of encephalopathy, acidosis, rhabdomyolysis and non-specific increased mortality risk. Antipyretic doses of paracetamol are larger than analgesic doses and topical cooling is only effective if accompanied by elective paralysis. If topical approaches do not work, central cooling can be achieved using cold peritoneal lavage.

PROTECTION FROM INFECTION

Non-specific host defences

NON-SPECIFIC PROTECTION

Non-specific protection from infection is afforded by the skin and mucous membranes which act as mechanical barriers to the entry of organisms. The physical features that contribute to these barriers are their pH, dryness, oiliness and the presence of secretions with specific antimicrobial or antiseptic properties, these secretions are lavaged or toileted by ciliary action. Microbiological contamination occurs when these surfaces are bypassed by intravenous cannulae, urinary catheters, endotracheal tubes, etc. The character of this con- tamination depends on the environment and flora and changes reflect both external and internal (e.g. hormonal) environmental circumstances. Normal commensal flora compete with potential pathogens for resources and survival and as such form part of the passive (for the host) protection from infection. Patients who regularly inhabit hospital areas are likely to be colonised with organisms of a type (and resistance pattern) that reflect this fact. An individual's nutritional state and the presence of chronic disease may also change the pattern of colonisation or infection.

COMPLEMENT

Complement is a system of soluble proteins found in normal serum and interstitial fluid and on mucosal surfaces. When activated via the alternative pathway it mounts a non-specific, i.e. poorly targeted, toxic response culminating in lysis of cells and organisms, neutrophil activation and increased endothelial permeability. Complement fragments bound to microbes facilitate the adherence of phagocytic cells. Other fragments trigger anaphylactic degranulation of mast cells releasing acute inflammatory mediators such as histamine, neu- trophil chemotactic factor, platelet aggregating factor, interleukins, leukotrienes, prostaglandins and proteases.

ACUTE INFLAMMATION

This is a generic term for the process of capillary dilatation, exudation of plasma proteins, margination and migration of neutrophils, lysis and bleeding that produces pain, redness, swelling and heat. Acute inflammation can be activated by complement, tissue macrophages and mast cells but is crucially effected by neutrophils. The generalised acti- vation of such processes in a SIRS produces multi-organ system failure (MOSF). Even when inflammation is localised there are systemic responses of diagnostic and host defence significance. Endotoxin, tumour necrosis factor α (TNFα) and interleukins all stim- ulate the liver to produce opsonins such as CRP and other 'acute phase' proteins.

PHAGOCYTIC CELLS

Phagocytic cells (macrophages, eosinophils and neutrophils) act alone or in concert, triggered by the chemotactic factors that they produce when activated or that are released from lym- phocytes. Macrophages are additionally involved in antigen presentation to T lymphocytes. Other mediator cells may enhance the activity of phagocytic cells, responding either directly to antigen or to complexed immunoglobulins such as IgE.

The specific immune response

The specificity of the immune response is a consequence of specific antigen recognition, ultimately by lymphocytes. B lymphocytes produce five classes of immunoglobulin (IgA, IgD, IgE, IgG and IgM), and T lymphocytes provide a cell-mediated response. Defence against extracellular organisms is largely via antibody, complement and polymorphs. Intracellular infections are combated by T cells, soluble cytokines and natural killer (NK) cells which can locate antibody bound to cell surfaces and then kill those cells by a variety of techniques. B and T lymphocytes cannot be distinguished morphologically but by surface markers identified by specific monoclonal antibodies. These clusters of differentiation (CD) markers are used to define both B and T lymphocytes and NK cells. They also contribute to antigen recognition in a cell-type-specific way. T_{helper} cells are CD4 antigen positive, $T_{cytotoxic}$ cells are CD8 antigen positive and B lymphocytes are CD19, 20 and 21 positive.

The recognition of the characteristic 'self' attribute of cells relies on their surface expression and recognition of major histocompatability antigens (MHC). The MHC in humans are often referred to as human leucocyte associated (HLA) antigens. HLA class I and II molecules form grooves that function as antigen binding sites and are the molecular location of the specificity of the cellular immune response. Class I are found on all nucle- ated cells and class II on antigen-presenting cells. Superantigens (such as the toxic shock syndrome toxin, TSST–1, responsible for staphylococcal-induced toxic shock syndrome) generate polyclonal activation by binding outside these sites.

In generic terms the 'specificity' of the immune response starts with exposure to recognition structures, which are immensely variable, thereby providing a breadth of cover. There is then selection and proliferation or production of the immune species (cellular or humoral) involved in a matched receptor–antigen pair. These 'recognition' structures are:

- the variable region of free and bound immunoglobulins
- the variable regions of the major histocompatability complex (discussed above)
- the variable regions of the T cell receptor chains (which detect processed antigen on antigen-presenting cells).

B LYMPHOCYTES

B lymphocytes each make a specific antibody and express it on their surface. Antigen binding to this site triggers clonal proliferation and differentiation into plasma cells which secrete specific antibodies. Intitial responses largely produce IgM, a high valency antibody and subsequent responses produce IgG. Clonal proliferation includes the production of memory cells, which respond rapidly to subsequent antigen exposure by producing IgG (the logic behind vaccination). IgA is the major immunoglobulin in the serous secretions at mucosal surfaces. IgD is mainly restricted to lymphocyte surfaces (acting as an antigen receptor) and IgE binds to mast cells where its role is in combating parasitic infections and producing atopic reactions. Antigen antibody complexes activate complement via the classical pathway.

T CELLS

When exposed to matching antigen, T cells undergo clonal proliferation and produce memory cells like B cells. T_{helper} cells activate both macrophages and B lymphocytes expressing altered class II MHC. They also 'help' the interaction between $T_{cytotoxic}$ cells and their targets. $T_{cytotoxic}$ (CD8 antigen positive) cells attack cells expressing the appropriate altered class I MHC. Their targets are destroyed by exocytosis of granules containing enzymes and TNF that perforate cell membranes and induce apoptosis.

CYTOKINES

After the initial exposure of T cells to antigen (via antigen presenting cells) subsequent responses are orchestrated by T_{helper} cells via cytokines. T_{helper} cells' 'help' for $T_{cytotoxic}$ /target interactions, and clonal proliferation is also mediated by cytokines. Cytokines are low molecular weight proteins that typically have a short half-life suiting them to their role as mediators. They are pleiotropic (have multiple effects) interacting with each other and with inflammatory cells in cascade reactions. Examples include the interleukins IL–1 to IL–13, colony stimulating factors such as granulocyte macrophage colony stimulating factor, tumour necrosis factors, interferons and others.

Paediatric immunology

The pattern, presentation and aetiology of infectious disease in paediatrics is radically different to that in older patients and the principal reason for the difference is the immaturity and 'ignorance' of the immune system.

Neonatal susceptibility to (and inability to localise) infection is well known and accentuated in the preterm infant. Non-specific mechanisms apply, such as the fact that physical barriers to micro-organisms are less effective, and immediately post partum colonising pathogens experience no competition from existing flora. Complement levels are lower than in adults and older children and there is absolute IgA and IgM deficiency. Maternal IgG may also be deficient in preterm infants. $T_{cytotoxic}$ cell function is reduced compared to that in adults. The T cells also proliferate slowly after some types of stimuli and generate cytokines less efficiently. B cell responses are augmented if the relevant maternal antibody is present but a relative hypogammaglobulinaemia occurs at 3 to 4 weeks even in the immune-competent term infant. Neonatal neutrophils are less responsive to chemotactic stimuli and less adherent when activated. Poor opsonisation of non-self antigens also results in marked reduction in their phagocytic activity.

Marrow suppression occurs earlier and infections can more easily fulminate in neonates and children. Falling white cell counts can therefore be more worrying than rising ones especially if accompanied by thrombocytopaenia. Patients with recurrent infections, infectious diseases that run an atypically severe course or that are caused by otherwise opportunistic organisms should be formally investigated for congenital and acquired immune deficiency. Some so-called 'opportunistic' infections in adults are not so in children.

TREATMENT OF INFECTION

Localised infections benefit from localised treatments such as removal of an infected vascular access catheter, drainage of pus, irrigation and debridement, but all will require concurrent systemic antibiotic therapy.

Antibiotic prescribing

No 'new' antibiotics (i.e. no new class of drug) have become available for many years but new preparations and refined versions of existing species continue to proliferate. In the face of this proliferation it is wise to restrict prescribing patterns to a manageable number of agents. New broad spectrum agents are almost invariably expensive and despite having few differences in spectrum from their predecessors are actively promoted by the pharmaceutical industry. Appropriately targeted narrow spectrum agents are often cheaper and just as effective. The widespread use of broad spectrum antibiotics in the medical and agricultural spheres has lead to the rapid evolution of resistant strains of bacteria. These are conveniently adapted to survive in an ICU where their competitors are, in theory, being methodically eradicated. Misuse of antibiotics in hospital, particularly the over-prescribing of broad spectrum antibiotics is directly related to the emergence of multi-resistant nosocomial pathogens. Despite the recognition that, historically, antibiotic usage has been too liberal and often for trivial indications, neutropaenic patients, those undergoing transplants and those with other types and causes of immune deficiency are still treated regularly with blind courses of powerful broad-spectrum agents. These patients act as incubators for the development of drug resistance and are frequently the source of ICU contamination. Such organisms are notoriously difficult to eradicate from an ICU and profoundly affect the operation and reputation of the unit, since ICU contamination is potentially self-perpetuating. Nosocomial infection can only be averted by cleanliness, attempted decontamination and meticulous hand washing.

It is therefore useful to negotiate an antibiotic prescribing policy with local microbiology and pharmacy departments to try and minimise these effects, achieve a cost-effective approach and to take account of local flora and patterns of resistance. By their very nature such policies will not transfer well between institutions but examples follow in Tables 17.1 and 17.2.

Antibiotic prophylaxis

This should not be provided routinely to cover ICU admission or 'sterile' or 'clean' procedures such as intubation, siting of peripheral or central vascular lines, urinary catheterisation or the insertion of surgical drains. Antibiotic prophylaxis is reasonable for abdominal surgery and is customary for cardiac surgery although popular regimes are poorly supported by randomised controlled trials. Standardised unit protocols for the cleansing of vascular access sites (soap and water is best) and the maximum permissible dwell time for cannulae are also useful. New adjuncts such as antibiotic-impregnated cannulae are currently being evaluated.

Table 17.1 A suggested antibiotic prescribing policy by site of infection for use while awaiting culture and sensitivity results.

Infection	Likely organisms	Suggested treatment
Respiratory system		
Pneumonia (community acquired)	*Streptococcus pneumoniae, Haemophilus influenzae, Moraxella catarrhalis* and 'atypical' organisms.	cefuroxime ± erythromycin
Pneumonia (hospital acquired and no recent exposure to broad spectrum antibiotics)	Above + coliforms, *Pseudomonas, Acinetobacter.*	cefuroxime + gentamicin
Pneumonia (hospital acquired with recent exposure to broad spectrum antibiotics)	Above + coliforms, *Pseudomonas, Acinetobacter.*	amoxicillin + ciprofloxacin
Pneumonia (neonatal)	Group B streptococcus, *Staphylococcus aureus,* coagulase negative *Staphylococcus, Escherichia coli,* enterococci.	amoxicillin + cefotaxime
Pneumonia (aspiration)	Oral flora including anaerobes.	cefuroxime + metronidazole
Epiglottitis Bacterial tracheitis	*H. influenzae* type B, *Staphylococcus aureus, Streptococcus pneumoniae,* group A streptococcus.	cefuroxime
Cardiovascular system		
Intravascular device related infection	Coagulase negative *Staph., Staph. aureus,* coliforms, *Pseudomonas.*	cefuroxime (+ vancomycin for resistant *Staph.*)
Endocarditis	Viridans Streptococci *Staph. aureus.*	amoxicillin + gentamicin
Endocarditis (postoperative)	*Staph. aureus,* coagulase negative *Staph.*	flucloxacillin + gentamicin or vancomycin + gentamicin
Gastrointestinal tract and urinary tract		
Intra-abdominal infection	Coliforms, enterococci, anaerobes.	amoxicillin + gentamicin + metronidazole or cefuroxime + metronidazole
Urinary tract infection	Coliforms	cefuroxime
Skin and soft tissue, bone and joint infection		
Surgical wound infection (post laparotomy)	*Staph. aureus,* faecal flora.	cefuroxime + metronidazole
Surgical wound infection (other sites)	*Staph. aureus*	flucloxacillin (if no response and no positive culture result progress to cefuroxime ± metronidazole then if still no positive culture with sensitivities and no clinical improvement after 5–7 days change to amoxicillin, ciprofloxacin and metronidazole

Table 17.1 A suggested antibiotic prescribing policy by site of infection for use while awaiting culture and sensitivity results.

Infection	Likely organisms	Suggested treatment
		to cover *Staph.*, *Strep.* spp., enterococci, coliforms and anaerobes)
Wound infection, human or animal bite	Oral flora.	co-amoxiclav orally or cefuroxime + metronidazole
Cellulitis	Group A streptococcus, *Staph. aureus.*	benzylpenicillin and flucloxacillin
Cellulitis (immuno-compromised patient)	Group A streptococcus, *Staph. aureus*, coliforms, *Pseudomonas*, anaerobes.	benzylpenicillin + cefuroxime (or ceftriaxone) + gentamicin + metronidazole
Necrotising fasciitis	Group A streptococcus, anaerobes, coliforms.	benzylpenicillin + cefuroxime + metronidazole
Osteomyelitis (neonatal)	Group B streptococcus, coliforms *Staph. aureus*, *Listeria*	amoxicillin + cefuroxime
Osteomyelitis (age <5 years)	*H. influenzae*, *Staph. aureus*, *Strep. pneumoniae*, Group A streptococcus.	cefuroxime
Osteomyelitis (age >5 years)	*Staph. aureus*, . *Strep. pneumoniae*, Group A streptococcus	flucloxacillin + fusidic acid
Septic arthritis (all ages)	As for osteomyelitis.	as for osteomyelitis
Intracranial sepsis		
Meningitis	*Neisseria meningitidis*, *Strep. pneumoniae*, *H. influenzae.*	cefotaxime
Meningitis (neonatal)	Group B streptococcus. *E. coli*, *Listeria*	amoxicillin + cefotaxime
Meningitis (immunocompromised)	*N. meningitidis*, *Strep. pneumoniae*, *H. influenzae*, *Listeria*	amoxicillin + cefotaxime + acyclovir (in case of herpes)
Meningitis (VP shunt)	Coagulase negative *Staph.*, *Staph. aureus*, coliforms.	cefotaxime ± intrathecal vancomycin (if organisms on Gram stain look like *Staph.*)
Brain abscess	*Strep. milleri*, anaerobes, coliforms.	amoxicillin + cefotaxime + metronidazole
Septicaemia		
Suspected septicaemia with no focus of infection	*N. meningitidis*, . *Strep. pneumoniae*, *H. influenzae*, group A streptococcus, coliforms	cefotaxime + gentamicin

continued

Table 17.1 A suggested antibiotic prescribing policy by site of infection for use while awaiting culture and sensitivity results.

Infection	Likely organisms	Suggested treatment
Suspected septicaemia with no focus of infection (neonates)	Group B streptococcus, *Staph. aureus*, coliforms, *Listeria*, enterococci.	amoxicillin + cefotaxime
Suspected septicaemia with no focus of infection (neutropaenic)	*Staph. aureus*, coliforms, *Pseudomonas*	ceftriaxone + gentamicin (progressing to vancomycin and ceftazidime)

Table 17.2 A suggested antibiotic-prescribing policy for the initial treatment of positive culture results (clinically judged to represent significant infection) pending specific sensitivity results (from Shann 1998 *Drug Doses Collective Pty Ltd*).

Organism	Therapy
Acinetobacter	ticarcillin or imipenem ± tobramycin
Actinomyces	benzylpenicillin
Aeromonas	co-trimoxazole
Bartonella kenselae (cat scratch)	ciprofloxacin or co-trimoxazole
Bacillus anthracis (anthrax)	benzylpenicillin
Bacteroides	oral: benzylpenicillin. GI: metronidazole
Bordetella pertussis	erythromycin
Borrelia burgdorferi (Lyme disease)	doxycycline or amoxycillin
Brucella	tetracycline + gentamicin or co-trimoxazole
Calymmatobacterium granulomatis (granuloma inguinale)	tetracycline
Campylobacter fetus	imipenem ± gentamicin
Campylobacter jejuni	ciprofloxacin or erythromycin
Chlamydia pneumonia	tetracycline or erythromycin
Chlamydia psitacci (psittacosis, ornithosis)	tetracycline or chloramphenicol
Chlamydia trachomatis	erythromycin. Trachoma: azithromycin lymphogranuloma venereum: tetracycline
Clostridia	benzylpenicillin *Cl. difficile*: metronidazole or vancomycin botulism: oral vancomycin
Corynebacteria	erythromycin JK group: vancomycin
Elkenella corrodens	amoxycillin ± clavulanic acid
Enterobacter	cefotaxime or imipenem + amikacin
Escherichia coli	cefotaxime ± gentamicin
Francisella tularensis (tularaemia)	gentamicin

continued

Table 17.2 A suggested antibiotic-prescribing policy for the initial treatment of positive culture results (clinically judged to represent significant infection) pending specific sensitivity results (from Shann 1998 *Drug Doses Collective Pty Ltd*).

Organism	Therapy
Fusobacterium	benzylpenicillin
Gardnerella vaginalis	metronidazole
Haemophilus ducreyi (chancroid)	erythromycin
Haemophilus influenzae	co-trimoxazole severe infection: cefotaxime or ceftriaxone
Helicobacter pylori	colloidal bismuth subcitrate + metronidazole + clarithromycin (< 8 years) or tetracycline (> 7 years)
Klebsiella pneumoniae	cefotaxime ± gentamicin
Legionella	erythromycin ± rifampicin
Leptospira	benzylpenicillin
Leptotrichia buccalis	benzylpenicillin
Listeria monocytogenes	amoxycillin ± gentamicin
Moraxella catarrahalis	co-trimoxazole or cefotaxime
Morganella morganii	cefotaxime ± gentamicin
Mycobacterium avium	clarithromycin ± rifampicin ± ethambutol ± clofazimine
Mycobacterium fortuitum	amikacin + doxycycline
Mycobacterium kansasii	isoniazid + rifampicin ± either ethambutol or streptomycin
Mycobacterium leprae (leprosy)	dapsone + rifampicin ± clofazimine
Mycobacterium marinum (balnei)	minocycline
Mycobacterium tuberculosis	isoniazid + rifampicin + pyrazinamide ± ethambutol
Mycoplasma pneumoniae	erythromycin or tetracycline
Neisseria gonorrhoeae	ceftriaxone
Neisseria meningitidis	benzylpenicillin
Nocardia	co-trimoxazole
Pasturella multocida	benzylpenicillin
Proteus	cefotaxime ± gentamicin. Indole negative: amoxycillin
Providencia	cefotaxime ± gentamicin
Pseudomonas aeruginosa	ticarcillin + tobramycin. Urine: ciprofloxacin or ticarcillin and/or tobramycin
Pseudomonas cepacia	co-trimoxazole
Pseudomonas mallei	streptomycin + either tetracycline or chloramphenicol
Pseudomonas pseudomallei	ceftazidime

Table 17.2 A suggested antibiotic-prescribing policy for the initial treatment of positive culture results (clinically judged to represent significant infection) pending specific sensitivity results (from Shann 1998 *Drug Doses Collective Pty Ltd*).

Organism	Therapy
Rikettsia	tetracycline or chloramphenicol
Rochalimaea henselae (bacillary angiomatosis)	erythromycin
Salmonella	cefotaxime *S. typhi*: ceftriaxone or ciprofloxacin
Serratia	cefotaxime ± gentamicin
Shigella	ciprofloxacin or co-trimoxazole or amoxycillin or ceftriaxone
Spirillium minus (rat bite fever)	benzylpenicillin
Staphylococcus	flucloxacillin ± gentamicin. Resistant strains: vancomycin ± gentamicin and/or rifampicin
Stenotrophomonas maltophilia	co-trimoxazole
Streptobacillus moniliformis (rat bite fever)	benzylpenicillin
Streptococcus	benzylpenicillin. Enterococcus: benzylpenicillin + gentamicin or amikacin *S. viridans*: benzylpenicillin ± gentamicin
Treponema pallidum (syphilis)	benzylpenicillin
Treponema pertenue (yaws)	benzylpenicillin
Ureaplasma urealyticum	erythromycin
Vibrio cholerae	tetracycline or cefotaxime
Vibrio vulnificus	tetracycline or cefotaxime
Yersinnia enterocolitica	co-trimoxazole
Yersinnia pestis (plague)	streptomycin

PROBLEMS WITH HOST DEFENCE

Multi-resistant organisms

There are many different serotypes of methicillin-resistant *Staphylococcus aureus* (MRSA) only some of which spread in epidemic fashion. Treatment agents are effectively limited to vancomycin, though some strains are sensitive to imipenem. Vigilance consists of routine surveillance, cultures of contacts with MRSA-positive patients, isolation of colonised patients wherever possible and treatment of colonised staff. Unprotected exposure to MRSA usually results in colonisation and in many institutions the battle with this organism has been lost, making such measures impractical. It is only good fortune that makes MRSA infections (as opposed to colonisation) rare.

The increased use of vancomycin for treating MRSA has probably contributed to the increase in infections amongst hospitalised patients due to vancomycin-resistant enterococcus (VRE). The incidence has increased rapidly since first reports in the late 1980s. Colonisation with VRE in the community is common, the human reservoir being increased by the presence and consumption of livestock treated with avoparcin, an antibiotic used as a feed additive for growth promotion. Nosocomial transmission is common and colonisation precedes most infections. Strict isolation of infected patients and meticulous hand washing and cleaning of contact surfaces is necessary. VRE can transfer vancomycin resistance to other bacteria and a vancomycin-resistant MRSA would be untreatable. No effective antimicrobial therapy is available. Pristinomycin (ointment) and streptogramins like quinupristin and dalfopristin (currently unlicensed) have been proposed.

The problem does not stop with these organisms. Medicine is also threatened by penicillin-resistant pneumococci, multi-resistant *Acinetobacter* spp. and even multiple-drug-resistant forms of tuberculosis.

Multi-organ system failure

SIRS AND MOSF

Multi-organ system failure (MOSF) is a potential outcome of a systemic inflammatory response. By consensus, the terminology for what was previously known as 'sepsis syndrome' has been changed along these lines because of the recognition that sepsis is only one of many possible causes of this well-known clinical scenario. The systemic inflammatory response syndrome (SIRS) is a pathophysiological process that represents a broad common pathway for many adults and children with critical illness. It can be initiated by a 'single' insult such as cardiopulmonary bypass, major trauma, sepsis or burns, or alternatively it can occur as a consequence of the recognisable clinical progression of other illnesses such as autoimmune disorders. The outlook depends on reducing exposure to the inflammatory stimulus as much as anything else.

SIRS is further defined (by consensus) by the detection of acute, otherwise unexplained alterations in two or more clinical observations of respiratory rate, heart rate, temperature or white cell count (WCC) (preferably immature : total neutrophil ratio). Fischer and Fanconi have proposed a paediatric adaptation to the adult values for these parameters which is summarised in Table 17.3.

Table 17.3 Diagnosis of SIRS requires the presence of two or more of the following conditions (from Fischer and Fanconi 1996 *Intensive care in childhood: a challenge to the future.* Update in intensive care and emergency medicine 25 D, Springer Verlag).

	Respiratory rate (breaths per min)	Heart rate (bpm)	Temperature (°C)	WCC[a] ($\times 10^9$ L^{-1}) or immature neutrophil count[b]
Adults[a] (>15 years)	> 20	> 90	< 36 or > 38	< 4 or > 12 or > 0.1 bands
12–15 years	> 25	> 100	< 36 or > 38.5	< 4 or > 12 or > 0.1 bands
5–12 years	> 30	> 120	< 36 or > 38.7	< 4 or > 12 or > 0.15 bands
2–5 years	> 35	> 130	< 36 or > 39	< 4 or > 15 or > 0.15 bands
1–2 years	> 40	> 140	< 36 or > 39	< 4 or > 15 or > 0.15 bands
1–12 months[c]	> 45	> 160	< 36 or > 38.5	< 4 or > 15 or > 0.2 bands
< 1 month[c]	> 60	> 190	< 35.5 or > 38	< 4 or > 20 or > 0.25 bands
< 5 days[c]	> 60	> 190	< 35.5 or > 38	< 4 or > 35 or > 0.3 bands

[a] Consensus definition
[b] Adjust to local laboratory reference ranges
[c] For respiratory rate, heart rate and temperature use gestational age
   WCC – use postnatal age

MOSF represents a spectrum of disease, the description of which varies depending upon the organ systems affected. At least two organ systems should be affected for a minimum of 24 to 48 hours in order to make the diagnosis. A common practice in adult ICU is to define the respective organ failures in numerical terms that are lifted from the APACHE II mortality prediction model. This has the conceptual appeal that the parameters and values used have some relation to changes in mortality risk. However the use of APACHE thresholds in this manner is still a somewhat arbitrary approach. A parallel system has not evolved for paediatrics though there are mortality prediction models that use the necessary parameters. Even with rigid numerical definitions for organ failure, the terms 'multi-organ system dysfunction syndrome' (MODS) and MOSF are interchangeable.

The 'common path' of SIRS and MOSF is best described in terms of the immunological and inflammatory processes involved and the elucidation of these has been one of the most rapid growth areas of modern intensive care research. However a working knowledge of the microcirculation is required to put the widespread capillary leak and cellular oxygen deficit involved in MOSF into context and to understand its consequences.

ANATOMY AND FUNCTION OF THE MICROCIRCULATION

The structure of the capillary endothelium varies according to site but there are common features in the basic structure that persist throughout. There is a layer of thin endothelial cells, one cell thick, lining the luminal surface of a basement membrane. The luminal surfaces of these cells bear a negative charge imparted by a layer of glycosaminoglycans (these species restrict the permeability of the membrane with regard to negatively charged molecules such as albumin). The cellular lining may be fenestrated (depending on the site) and there are numerous clefts between cells and tubular channels that traverse the endothelial cells themselves. Endothelial cells may change shape with changes in pressure and have physiological responses to blood flow and shear stress, including the release of vasoactive mediators and anticoagulants.

There is no smooth muscle component to the capillary wall. The precapillary region does retain smooth muscle and because of its regulatory effects on the capillary bed is often termed the 'precapillary sphincter'. In some capillary beds (but not skeletal muscle) there are channels, accessed via precapillary sphincter controlled vessels, through which blood can bypass the whole capillary bed. Postcapillary venules have no smooth muscle either but nevertheless contribute to venous capacitance. The interplay of the various factors that affect precapillary sphincter activity is being closely scrutinised. The identification of the nitric oxide radical as the significant 'endothelium derived relaxation factor' is one aspect of this research that has potential therapeutic consequences.

Transcapillary exchange

The major process driving solute movements across the intact capillary membrane is diffusion (not filtration). Small, lipid-soluble molecules move freely through endothelial cells and capillary pores. Water and water-soluble materials pass mainly through intercellular pores in the endothelium or through a facilitative transport mechanism mediated by special proteins – aquaporins. For the diffusion of small water-soluble molecules (e.g. sodium chloride, glucose) pore size is not rate limiting and movement is dictated by blood supply, i.e. 'flow limited'. These movements are dictated by the Fick equation (diffusion rate = blood flow ÷ arteriovenous concentration difference). Movement of water across the membrane is also influenced by the Gibbs Donnan effect. This explains small electrolyte differences that occur across membranes when a non-diffusible ion (e.g. a plasma protein with anionic charge) is present on one side of the membrane. The drive to maintain electrical neutrality then causes movement of diffusible ions (Na^+ in our example) against their own concentration gradient. The number of diffusible ions that move increases disproportionately as the concentration gradient of protein rises. The movement of protein itself across capillary membranes is resisted by a negative charge on the luminal surface of the vascular endothelium largely generated by glycosaminoglycan molecules. The osmotic effect exerted by colloids (colloid osmotic pressure or oncotic pressure) is quantitatively small but nevertheless it may be crucial in the fine balance of fluid movement across capillary beds. Larger lipid-insoluble molecules (e.g. sucrose) are limited by pore size and they move at rates inversely proportional to their molecular size, i.e. they are 'diffusion limited'.

Diffusion between intravascular and interstitial fluid is affected by concentration gradient, capillary permeability, capillary surface area, intercapillary distance and blood flow. The first three of these are linked by Fick's law of diffusion which relates the diffusion rate of a material:

- directly to its diffusion coefficient (related to molecular size and therefore weight)
- directly to the area of the capillary membrane
- directly to the concentration gradient
- inversely to the thickness (and hence permeability) of the membrane.

Capillary diffusion gradients can be conceptualised as longitudinal and radial. The longitudinal diffusion gradient along the capillary changes from arterial to venous ends. It is affected by capillary length, the rate of consumption or production of solute in the interstitial fluid and the blood flow. The gradient at any particular point along the capillary (radial gradient) depends on the radius of the capillary, the radial size of the tissue cylinder surrounding the capillary (Kogh), the diffusion coefficient of the solute concerned and its concentration at a given distance from the capillary. Thus as intercapillary distances increase, even marked capillary recruitment cannot prevent islands of tissue where, for example, the supply of oxygen becomes inadequate.

In addition to solute diffusion, bulk movement of fluid across membranes (filtration) also carries solutes across the membrane or through its pores. This occurs irrespective of whether it is initiated by hydrostatic or osmotic influences. The anatomical variation in the size and number of clefts between endothelial cells is thus related to their filtration properties. By far the most important homeostatic mechanism controlling this process is the vasomotor control of precapillary vessels. Glomeruli are specialised exceptions where control is exerted over pre- and postcapillary vessels. The filtration of fluid is a passive process proceeding at a rate dictated by:

- the filtration coefficient of the membrane (influenced by its surface area and permeability)
- the hydrostatic pressure gradient (greater within the arterial end of the capillary but consistent across a glomerulus)
- the colloid osmotic pressure gradient

in a relationship described by Starling's law of ultrafiltration. The net filtration is out of the capillary at the arterial end and into the capillary at the venous end.

PATHOPHYSIOLOGY OF MOSF

In the evolution of MOSF a sequence of events leads to reduced tissue perfusion. Increased vascular permeability allows colloid and water to leak into the interstitial space (manifested in the kidney by an increased albumin excretion rate). Fluctuations in vasomotor tone alter the haemodynamic state by affecting pulmonary and systemic vascular resistance. Thrombi form in the microcirculation and blood pools in postcapillary capacitance venules. The reduced blood volume reduces venous return and diminishes cardiac output. Any associated cardiomyopathy limits the cardiovascular response and compensatory vasoconstriction can further limit peripheral perfusion. This is the so-called 'ebb' phase of the response to injury. The noxious stimuli initiating this response often do so by processes that involve free radical production. They include direct tissue injury, exotoxin production by bacteria, the shedding or release of cell wall and intracellular components of bacteria (endotoxin) or neutrophil activation by other causes such as exposure of blood to artificial surfaces, hypothermia and reperfusion injury.

In the subsequent 'flow' phase cardiac output returns to normal or supranormal levels, oxygen consumption is increased, end organ perfusion is increased but catabolism continues. However, high cardiac output with low systemic vascular resistance can occur without improvement in the microcirculation. Pulmonary hypertension may seriously affect cardiopulmonary status. In the systemic circulation the diversion of blood through peripheral arteriovenous shunts tends to make mixed venous oxygen content high while tissue hypoxia persists. In this circumstance the mixed venous oxygen content does not reflect the $VO_2 : DO_2$ relation (see Chapter 11, Respiratory System page 140) and the cellular position with regard to oxygen supply is akin to that within a limb which has had a tourniquet applied. Such a position is, not surprisingly, hard to interpret as recovery. Even in patients whose 'flow' phase is part of recovery (and oxygen delivery is improving allowing an increase in oxygen consumption), other abnormalities such as insulin resistance persist. Weight loss during this phase occurs both as a result of catabolism and as a result of a diuresis, which accompanies the loss of oedema fluid as the capillary endothelial integrity is restored. Catabolism is an adaptation to starvation and may therefore be amenable to adequate nutrition in which case lactic acidosis, hyperkalaemia, uraemia and hyperphosphataemia can all be minimised.

MOSF as a disease of the microcirculation

The **vascular endothelium** normally provides an inert interface to the immune system. The high concentrations of anionic glycosaminoglycans on the luminal surface serve to localise important molecules such as antithrombin III. Endothelial cells also secrete prostacyclin, Von Willebrand factor and the plasminogen activators tPA and uPA. Both endothelial cell destruction and damage to the basement membrane occur in MOSF. The high negative charge imparted by the glycosaminoglycans is reduced partly as the result of the release of cationic proteins from activated platelets, macrophages, neutrophils and eosinophils. The loss of charge increases the permeability of the endothelium to albumin. An interstitial oedema of relatively protein-rich fluid results.

Endothelial damage can be initiated and/or aggravated by activated **neutrophils**, which stick to the endothelium and migrate through it. They undergo a respiratory burst and degranulate releasing proteolytic enzymes such as elastase, and reactive oxygen species in addition to the cationic proteins referred to above. These cause further endothelial cell destruction and local damage reducing the luminal charge and stripping glycosaminoglycans from the luminal surface. Plasma normally contains serine protease inhibitors such as α_1 antitrypsin and α_2 macroglobulin that inactivate neutrophil proteolytic enzymes, however in severe MOSF or septic shock this reserve can be overcome and enzymes such as elastase 'leak' from the microcirculation into the circulating blood. These enzymes lead to widespread complement activation, platelet dysfunction and disseminated intravascular coagulation.

Within the tissues **macrophages** release soluble inflammatory mediators such as tumour necrosis factor, interleukins, interferons and platelet activating factor. They also degranulate like neutrophils releasing proteolytic enzymes, reactive oxygen species, cationic proteins and prostaglandins. These actions can occur independently of their role in the recognition of 'self' and presentation of 'non-self' antigens to the rest of the immune system.

Many of the acute phase reactants can activate platelets causing them to become 'sticky', aggregate and degranulate. They release vasoactive mediators such as prostaglandins and thromboxane, growth factors and proteolytic enzymes. Their surface glycoprotein receptors, which are essential in anchoring them at sites of injury, are disrupted by elastase. Activated platelets that remain in the circulation are mopped up by the reticuloendothelial system.

Initiators and mediators of MOSF

The most popular of the proposed mechanisms by which SIRS progresses to MOSF involves inappropriate host regulation of endogenous inflammatory mediators, the peptide members of which are called cytokines. In models of Gram-negative sepsis this is initiated by endotoxin and in Gram-positive sepsis by exotoxins.

Endotoxin is a lipopolysaccharide which has antigenic and glycolipid components. The latter is a key component of its toxicity since it enables penetration of cell membranes. Endotoxin is produced in small amounts by most Gram-negative organisms. Pulses of release occur when significant numbers of bacteria are lysed by the immune system or by antibiotics. Endotoxin triggers release of TNFα most of which comes from macrophages. The release of other inflammatory mediators such as platelet activating factor is also triggered. Complement deficiency aggravates endotoxic shock.

Exotoxins may be secreted by a variety of Gram-positive organisms. An example is the α haemolytic toxin of *Staphylococcus aureus*, which directly activates complement.

TNFα can produce all of the manifestations of septic shock (hypotension, acidosis, haemorrhagic infarction) and endotoxin is a potent stimulus for its release. It is not clear how many of its effects are direct and how many are the result of other mediators. Coincidentally it raises serum triglycerides which can bind endotoxin.

Interleukins IL–1, 6 and 8 are proinflammatory. IL–1 is a pyrogen which stimulates acute phase protein synthesis, neutrophil production in the marrow and local degranulation. IL–1 and 6 stimulate production of other cytokines by T cells and IL–8 is a neutrophil chemoattractant. IL–4, 10 and 13 are inhibitory.

Arachidonic acid derivatives such as prostaglandins are vasoactive compounds with a variety of cellular effects and effects on platelet adhesion. They may modulate the effects of TNFα.

Nitric oxide is a gaseous free radical, which is synthesised from the essential amino acid L-arginine by the cleavage of a terminal nitrogen group which then combines with oxygen. The reaction is catalysed by a family of enzymes – nitric oxide synthetases (NOS) and requires several co-factors. Constitutive NOS are found in neural and endothelial tissue and inducible NOS is expressed by many cells after exposure to cytokines, TNFα and endotoxin. Nitric oxide moves between cells and binds to the haem group of guanylate cyclase stimulating the conversion of cGTP to cGMP which in turn reduces the intracellular calcium level. In vascular smooth muscle this causes relaxation. Nitric oxide release is the final common pathway of many physiological and pharmacological influences on tissue and organ blood flow. Its release is influenced by shear stress and pulsatile flow in the vessels and can be blocked using competitive NOS inhibitors such as I-NMMA. Free nitric oxide in the blood reacts with oxyhaemoglobin to form methaemoglobin and inorganic nitrate.

Free radicals generically are extremely short-lived, highly chemically reactive species characterised by the presence of an unpaired electron. Their production is increased in reperfusion injury and has been implicated in all manner of molecular damage and membrane disruption. There are many mechanisms of production and although evidence of free radical damage is readily acquired, the potential generic benefits of antioxidant chemicals and enzymes are unproven.

CLINICAL PERSPECTIVE

The mortality risk associated with MOSF is related to the number of organ systems involved. The significance of failure in each organ system on cumulative mortality risk, increases with age. The difference in mortality risk from MOSF is therefore most dramatic between adults and patients under 2 years (the majority of PICU patients). MOSF is also less common in PICU than it is in adult practice. The onset of additional organ dysfunction in a critically ill child should be investigated and explained. Aetiologically it may represent disease progression, a consequence of treatment, new disease or a manifestation of SIRS.

The clinical management priorities in the treatment of SIRS and MOSF are:

- resuscitation from shock
- supporting cellular oxygen delivery
- control of disseminated intravascular coagulation
- control of sepsis
- other organ-specific support (generally covered elsewhere in this text)
- nutritional support (see Chapter 8, Nutrition).

Resuscitation from shock

Shock must be recognised early while it is still compensated (i.e. before blood pressure falls). Resuscitation from shock involves restoration of the plasma volume and appropriate inotropic support. The most common error during resuscitation is to underestimate the required volume of intravenous fluids or the rapidity with which the patient's condition is deteriorating. Repeated boluses of 20 ml kg^{-1} are recommended in resuscitation protocols based on indications of haemodynamic response (tachycardia, blood pressure, liver size, etc.). On the PICU the selection of appropriate inotropes and judgement of circulatory filling is enhanced if one is able to employ invasive cardiovascular monitoring. Swan–Ganz catheterisation is practicable in children over 18 months of age and the routine use of pulmonary artery and left atrial lines after cardiac surgery is inordinately useful. Problems with myocardial contractility are probably best supported with adrenaline (epinephrine) but in high output low systemic vascular resistance states, noradrenaline (norepinephrine) is more appropriate. Neonatal myocardium is more dependent on circulating ionised calcium than myocardium in older patients and the inotropic benefits of calcium infusion continue even as supranormal levels of calcium are reached. There are also beneficial effects supplying calcium as a co-enzyme in the coagulation cascade. Case reports are occurring where children with septic shock and recalcitrant low systemic vascular resistance show dramatic responses to angiotensin II infusions (0.05–0.3 μg kg^{-1} min^{-1}). Angiotensin II is a potent pressor, not liable to tachyphylaxis that also stimulates secretion of adrenocorticotropic hormone, aldosterone and antidiuretic hormone. There are sound physiological reasons to suppose that children will prove to be more responsive to this agent than adults.

Supporting cellular oxygen delivery

Supplemental oxygen and early intubation are also part of the ABC of elementary resuscitation and should be instituted long before shock or respiratory failure supervene. Once ventilated on the PICU, cellular oxygen delivery is further enhanced by red cell transfusion to haemoglobin concentrations of 14 or 15 g dL^{-1} combined with appropriate support of the cardiac output. Transfusion is frequently necessary after resuscitation with clear fluids or colloids and red cells do not leak as much from the circulation. The author does not subscribe to 'alternative' schools of thought such as favouring lower haematocrits (to reduce viscosity and encourage flow in the microcirculation) or attempting to boost cardiac output (and therefore oxygen delivery) to supranormal levels with excess inotropic drive.

In the microcirculation all efforts to minimise oedema will reap rewards in terms of cellular oxygen delivery. Pulmonary involvement in MOSF is characterised by non-cardiogenic pulmonary oedema (Adult Respiratory Distress Syndrome). Ventilatory strategies that address this include high end-expiratory pressures to reduce alveolar water and frequent postural changes to redistribute lung water. These have the most success when combined with attempts to minimise barotrauma and volutrauma such as permissive hypercarbia and pressure limited ventilation (which may necessitate the use of inverse I : E ratios).

Disseminated intravascular coagulation

Cytokines, arachidonic acid derivatives, enzymes such as elastase, and liberated or consumed tPA and antithrombin III have many complex interactions with platelet function and the coagulation cascades. The relative importance of each in pathogenesis is difficult to determine and not all are stimulant, but the net result is widespread activation of both coagulation and fibrinolysis, consumption of clotting and fibrinolytic factors and inhibition of platelet function. This leads to microvascular thrombosis and haemorrhage. The clinical approach must be to remove the cause where possible and in the interim to replace or supplement the clotting factors with fresh frozen plasma and cryoprecipitate. No clear role has been established for:

- serine protease inhibitors
- anticoagulants such as heparin
- antifibrinolytics
- additional supplements of specific factors such as proteins C and S.

Control of sepsis

Sepsis as a cause or complication of MOSF is best controlled by the administration of appropriate antibiotics. The most popular example of MOSF to cite in paediatrics is that precipitated by meningococcal septicaemia. Although it accounts for only about 2 per cent of PICU admissions (whereas SIRS occurs in as many as 80 per cent of admissions), the fulminant nature of the presentation and rapidity of deterioration make prompt recognition and administration of antibiotics (penicillin, cefotaxime or ceftriaxone) mandatory to all suspected cases. Otherwise the choice of antibiotic for cases of MOSF where a septic origin is suspected, is made easier if the organism or likely organisms are known (see Table 17.1 & 17.2).

Patients with MOSF are exposed to further infective risks from compromised host defences and invasive therapies. However fever and raised levels of acute-phase reactants are features of SIRS in the absence of sepsis and may not demand antibiotic therapy, especially since blind, broad spectrum antibiotic therapy encourages microbial resistance. The most common clinical problem is in fact to distinguish a group of patients in whom blind antibiotic therapy can be avoided. Protocol demands a low threshold for repeated cultures of blood, urine, endotracheal secretions, vascular access sites, etc. in what has become known as the 'sepsis screen'. Such cat-like observation has to accompany any policy of masterly inactivity in antibiotic prescribing.

Patients with MOSF may also be at risk from 'translocation' of organisms from the gut to the blood stream and this has been one of the arguments used to support a policy of selective decontamination of the digestive tract (SDDT). Most proponents of SDDT work in adult ICU's where nosocomial pneumonia is commoner and has far greater significance than in PIC's.

There are two components to a policy of SDDT. The first is to institute a policy of enhanced microbiological surveillance. In contrast to the 'septic screen' where diagnostic samples are taken from normally sterile areas when one suspects an infective cause for deterioration, this level of surveillance involves routine sampling from sites that are not normally sterile. Colonisation and overgrowth can therefore be scrutinised and a carrier state defined by the detection and confirmation of the asymptomatic presence of a potential pathogen. Proponents of this approach assert that 50 per cent of ICU infections can be categorised as 'primary endogenous', where the causative organism is a germ that was present before admission to ICU and that primary endogenous infections are more likely to occur early in the ICU stay. The word 'early' in this context does not have a precise definition and the time span where a primary endogenous infection is most likely, will vary with the degree of immune suppression. The flora of previously 'well' patients, as determined by surveillance, is likely to differ from that of patients with known premorbid disease or predisposing conditions. In the first instance they are likely to be *Streptococcus pneumoniae*,

Haemophilus influenzae, Moraxella catarrhalis, Escherichia coli, Staphylococcus aureus or a yeast, whereas for patients with premorbid disease or hospital residents it would be *Klebsiella, Proteus, Morganella, Enterobacter, Citrobacter, Serratia, Acinetobacter* or *Pseudomonas*. If the causative organism colonised a patient during the ICU stay, then the term 'secondary endogenous' is used to describe subsequent infection. The remaining infections are classified 'exogenous', where the first isolate is the one that diagnoses the infection. SDDT proponents treat patients, in whom surveillance detects a potential pathogen, with intravenous antibiotics to prevent primary endogenous infection and they use an oral paste of polymixin E, tobramycin and amphotericin in the hope of preventing secondary endogenous infections. There is no convincing evidence to support the application of this approach to the PICU. On the PICU nosocomial pneumonia is less common than in AICU and has a lower mortality. Even the policy of routine microbiological surveillance has not been rigorously justified.

Another approach to the recognition of infection utilises acute phase reactants and differential neutrophil counts (band counts or immature : total neutrophil ratios). Antibiotics are reserved for patients who demonstrate an abrupt rise in the chosen index. In all cases, routine surveillance of these parameters is required because the baseline level is high in MOSF anyway. It is likely to be the change (increase) in value in each case, rather than its absolute level, that is of most significance in terms of the positive predictive power for culture-proven sepsis.

In the future it is widely hoped that methods of modulating the inflammatory response and the microcirculation will be of proven benefit in MOSF. Many attempts have been made to find a useful agent to administer in this regard. Some of these agents include:

- nitric oxide synthase inhibitors (such as l-NMMA),
- nitric oxide antagonists such as methylene blue (a soluble guanylate cyclase inhibitor)
- procoagulant proteases such as Protein C
- protease inhibitors such as aprotonin and antithrombin III
- platelet-preserving vasodilator agents such as prostacyclin
- antiendotoxin antibodies
- monoclonal anti-TNFα antibodies
- steroids
- free radical scavengers and iron chelating agents.

Most of these have been hailed as 'magic bullets' at one stage or another. Many of these therapies are effective in experimental models when the therapeutic agent is administered prior to the insult that generates MOSF. This is particularly frustrating since this pattern often cannot be reproduced in the clinical setting and later administration often appears to be of reduced, little or no benefit (but watch this space!).

Many freely circulating inflammatory mediators (endotoxin for example) can be removed by haemofiltration. Additionally protein bound acute phase reactants, can be cleared by plasmafiltration. These approaches have the advantage of allowing tight control of fluid balance, helping the management of oedema, and can be easily accompanied by accelerated solute clearance and aggressive supplementation of clotting factors. Filtration may be impracticable in the very small infant for whom exchange transfusion represents a similar approach. Plasmafiltration has been attempted as a therapy for MOSF since the late 1970s and has been associated with dramatic haemodynamic responses in some cases of early fulminant Gram-negative sepsis. In animal studies, the ultrafiltrate from pigs with septic shock produces shock when infused into healthy pigs. High levels of endotoxin and inflammatory mediators correlate with the severity of illness and all these species are amenable to removal by filtration. Animal studies also show lower mortality than predicted in treated groups and reduced or no effect if plasma exchange is delayed. Randomised controlled trials of plasmafiltration are indicated in children but like the supplemental approaches, face difficulties in controlling for the time interval between the onset of symptoms and the start of treatment.

18 Physics for the Intensivist

- **States of matter**
- **Pressure**
- **Measurement of pressure**
- **Flow**
- **Measurement of flow and volume**
- **Temperature**
- **Oximetry**
- **Exponential functions**
- **Appendix: basic and derived SI units**

In the eternal debate, 'medicine an art or a science' most intensivists would put their speciality at the scientific end of the clinical spectrum. Practising intensivists have to have a working scientific knowledge. This chapter is a series of short notes that have applications across the organ systems that are covered in the rest of the book. While the emphasis is on the physical principles, clinical and physiological examples will hopefully serve to put them into context and demonstrate their utility.

STATES OF MATTER

Matter exists as phases, solid, liquid or gas, depending upon the mobility of the molecules within that phase. For a solid the molecules are unable to alter their positions, relative to each other, and oscillate about a fixed point. Within liquids the molecules are free to move but do not get very far before colliding with another molecule. For gases, the molecules can travel much further and collide less often. Both gases and liquids are called 'fluids' as they do not have a fixed shape.

If a gas is compressed, the molecules are pressed closer together causing the gas to condense into a liquid, provided that the gas molecules are not so energetic as to prevent this from happening. The energy of molecules increases with temperature. At and above a particular temperature (the 'critical temperature') a gas cannot be compressed into a liquid no matter how much pressure is applied. Gases below their critical temperatures are called vapours. The physical behaviour of a vapour is the same as that of a gas until it is compressed sufficiently to condense. Once in the presence of its liquid phase a gas behaves very differently. Under these circumstances, irrespective of changes in the volume of the closed container, the pressure will remain the same. This pressure is the saturated vapour pressure (SVP) (saturated because it is in contact with its liquid). At a fixed temperature SVP is constant and does not change with volume. As the temperature increases, a greater proportion of the molecules have the energy to leave the liquid phase and the SVP increases. When the SVP reaches atmospheric pressure the liquid boils. The 'boiling point' of a liquid is that at which vapour forms throughout the liquid and not just at its surface. At this point the SVP equals atmospheric pressure. The temperature at which this happens is pressure dependent, such that at normal atmospheric pressure water boils at 100°C but at the top of Everest it boils at a lower temperature. If a liquid under pressure is heated above the critical temperature it becomes a gas. If it does this within the confines of a restricted volume (e.g. a gas cylinder) then an enormous increase in pressure occurs.

As the temperature rises, the SVP rises, because more molecules have the energy to escape the liquid phase and become vapour (evaporate). As these higher energy molecules evaporate, the energy (temperature) of the liquid falls. Hence evaporation causes cooling. When liquid molecules enter the vapour phase, extra energy is required if the temperature of the remaining liquid is to stay constant. The amount of energy required to vaporise a kilogram of water while keeping it at the same temperature is called the latent heat of vaporisation. The latent heat of water at 20°C and 100°C is 2.43 and 2.26 MJ kg^{-1} respectively. As the temperature rises less additional energy is required to vaporise it. At the critical temperature, no more energy is necessary as it is physically impossible to exist as a liquid above this temperature (the latent heat of vaporisation is zero). Importantly, when vapours below their critical temperature condense back into liquid, this heat is released.

Relevant consequences include the following.

- The critical temperature of water is over 400°C and it behaves as a vapour in the alveolar gas equation (see p. 281).
- The critical temperature of nitrous oxide is 36.5°C and full cylinders of nitrous oxide contain liquid.
  - Nitrous oxide cylinders are never completely filled. In temperate climates the filling ratio (mass of nitrous oxide divided by the mass of water that would completely fill the cylinder) is 0.67. This equates to about 90 per cent full of liquid nitrous oxide. In hot climates the filling ratio is less than this.
  - The pressure gauges on nitrous oxide cylinders read a constant pressure until they are only a quarter full at which point they are empty of liquid.
  - Entonox cylinders contain gaseous nitrous oxide and gaseous oxygen even at room temperature. The nitrous oxide 'dissolves' in the oxygen and its critical temperature falls to −7°C, a 'pseudo-critical' temperature. If the temperature falls below −7°C, the nitrous oxide liquifies. In this state, the cylinder will initially discharge more oxygen than nitrous oxide. As the oxygen is discharged, increasing concentrations of nitrous oxide will be discharged which may result in a hypoxic mixture being delivered to the patient. It is therefore recommended that if an Entonox cylinder gets cold, it should be stored on its side at above 5°C for at least 24 hours before use so the nitrous oxide can redissolve into the oxygen.
- Wet babies get cold quickly.
- Thermal injuries from steam are much worse than those from hotter, dry gases. The heat required to raise the temperature of 1 g of air by 100°C is 100 J but the release of heat from 1 g of water vapour as it condenses is 2260 J. Steam inhalational injuries often cause very severe laryngeal and tracheal burns.

PRESSURE

Pressure develops when a force is applied over an area, i.e. the greater the force or smaller the surface area, the greater the pressure.

$$\text{pressure (Pa)} = \frac{\text{force (N)}}{\text{area (m}^2)}$$

The internationally approved unit of Pressure is the Pascal (Pa) or Newtons m^{-2}. Other units that relate to the Pascal are:

$$1 \text{ mmHg} = 133 \text{ Pa} = 1.36 \text{ cmH}_2\text{O}$$

thus if one is measuring pressure via a water column, for example cerebrospinal fluid pressure at lumbar puncture or ventriculostomy, the conversion must be applied to generate compatible units for calculations such as the cerebral perfusion pressure where it has to be subtracted from the blood pressure (mmHg). The other factor that should be standardised in such circumstances is the 'reference point' – the height of the transducer. All circulatory pressures are referenced to transducers at atrial level and for cerebral perfusion pressure, the cerebrospinal fluid pressure should be too.

Another practical example is the pressure generated in a syringe as you apply your thumb. As syringes have different cross-sectional areas, the pressure delivered varies enormously. Take 2 ml, 20 ml and 50 ml syringes and a standard thumb pressure (25 N). The cross-sectional areas of the plungers are 5×10^{-5} m^2 (2 ml), 2.5×10^{-4}m^2 (20 ml) and 5×10^{-4} m^2 (50 ml). Therefore the pressures generated are 500 kPa (2 ml), 100 kPa (20 ml) and 50 kPa (50 ml). In practice this means:

- the pressure generated by a 2 ml syringe exceeds systolic arterial blood pressure; manually flushing an arterial line produces retrograde flow as far back as the aorta and can cause thrombo/gas bubble embolism, therefore *flush arterial lines gently*
- a small syringe generates high pressure and may unblock rigid cannulae but should not be used with silastic catheters which can rupture and embolise; the risk is reduced if a larger volume syringe (10 ml) is used with minimal force
- for rapid volume infusion there is a balance between ease of injection and the volume infused. In children, with relatively small bore cannulae (20–22G) *in situ*, better overall infusion rates can often be achieved with more 10 or 20 ml boluses than with fewer 50 ml boluses
- if rapid infusion is performed manually with a syringe it is advisable to use a Luer lock to prevent disruption of the connection at high pressure.

Boyle's law

At a constant temperature the volume of a fixed quantity of gas is inversely proportional to the pressure.

$$P \propto \frac{1}{V}$$

Gas cylinders have a fixed volume; the pressure on the gauge is therefore directly proportional to the amount of gas left in the cylinder. A size E oxygen cylinder, full at a pressure of 137 bar (13 700 kPa) contains the equivalent of 680 litres of oxygen (at atmospheric pressure). When the gauge reads 68.5 bar, the cylinder is half full.

Dalton's law of partial pressures

In a mixture of gases the pressure exerted by each gas is that which the gas would exert if it was alone in the container. The total pressure is the sum of these components. The alveolar gas equation uses this law.

$$P_AO_2 = P_iO_2 - \left(\frac{PaCO_2}{R} \right) + F$$

- The P_iO_2 equates to the FiO_2 at sea level because atmospheric pressure is approximately 100 kPa and the FiO_2 is a percentage. Such a substitution would not be appropriate at altitude where barometric pressure (P_B) is lower, or during IPPV.
- If we are going to use substitutes for P_iO_2 then we have to take account of the pressure attributed to water vapour. As alveolar air is fully saturated with water vapour, the pressure exerted will be its SVP at 37°C, which is 6.3 kPa.
- F (the correction factor for volume changes between inhaled and expired gas) can be dropped for the normally respired gases.
- R is the respiratory quotient which we can approximate to 0.8.

Thus we have

$$P_AO_2 = [F_iO_2 \times (P_B - P_{H2O})] - (PaCO_2 \div 0.8)$$

At sea level and breathing air

$$P_AO_2 = [0.21 \times (101.3 - 6.3)] - \left(\frac{5.3}{0.8} \right) = 13.3 \text{ kPa}$$

Allowing for physiological shunt, the patient's arterial PaO_2 would be around 12.5 kPa.

At an altitude of 5000 metres, $P_B = 58$ but P_{H2O} will still be 6.3. Breathing air at 21% gives

$$P_iO_2 = [0.21 \times (58 - 6.3)] = 10.9 \text{ kPa}$$

and

$$P_AO_2 = 10.9 - \left(\frac{5.3}{0.8}\right) = 4.3 \text{ kPa}$$

Laplace's law

Where there is a pressure gradient between the inside and outside of a chamber (e.g. gas cylinder, artery, ventricle), tension is produced in the wall. Laplace's law relates the two:

$$P = \frac{2Th}{R}$$

where T is wall tension, R is the radius of the vessel and h is the thickness of the vessel wall. This can be rearranged to:

$$T = \frac{PR}{2h}$$

Practical examples where Laplace's law applies include:

- the collapse of alveoli as they shrink below a critical volume where the tension in their walls exceeds the distending pressure
- tension in the wall of the heart changes as the ventricle dilates; if the radius doubles twice the work is required to generate the same pressure. Wall tension during systole is the true expression of afterload
- during positive pressure ventilation the positive pleural pressure can be considered to be squeezing the ventricle from the outside thereby reducing afterload. The magnitude of this effect is given by

$$T = \frac{[P_{vent} - P_{pl}] \times R}{2h}$$

Positive pleural pressure also establishes a pressure gradient between the thoracic and abdominal aorta that reduces aortic input impedance.

MEASUREMENT OF PRESSURE

Mercury manometers measure pressure by raising a column of mercury. Theoretically, providing the column tubing is tall and strong enough, any pressure could be measured but their range is usually limited up to atmospheric pressure. They are very accurate as the mercury is not compressible and the pressure relates directly to the height of the column.

Aneroid gauges (from the greek 'a-neros' meaning 'without liquid') rely on an expansion chamber connected to the dial. They need regular calibration but are very accurate. They are compact and can measure pressures up to many hundreds of atmospheres. Examples include the pressure gauges on gas cylinders (Bourdon gauges).

Transducers convert one form of energy to another. Pressure transducers generate an electrical signal in proportion to the applied pressure, they are the most common approach to pressure monitoring used in the ICU. However all transducers are prone to inaccuracies because of resonance and damping. Furthermore, depending on how they are used, their measurements may be compounded by physical effects such as the kinetic component of pressure measurement.

Resonance and damping

An arterial pressure transducer can be considered as a weight suspended from a spring. When stretched and released, the weight will oscillate at a certain frequency, the 'natural' frequency f_0. When the system is cyclically driven, as the frequency of stimulation approaches f_0 the amplitude increases. Theoretically amplitude increases to infinity, at a frequency just below f_0, the so-called 'resonant frequency'. In reality it is restrained from these dizzy heights by friction, i.e. damping, in the system. A biological pressure waveform such as an arterial pulse comprises the sum of a fundamental frequency (lowest frequency) and multiple higher frequency harmonics. If the resonant frequency of the transducer approaches that of the harmonics (normally about 20 Hz), then resonant effects predominate on the trace and the waveform is less accurate. This effect is usually recognised by a spiky trace and causes over-reading of systolic and under-reading of diastolic pressures. The mean pressure should still be accurate. The resonant frequency of the system can be calculated from the formula:

$$f_0 = \frac{r}{2} \sqrt{\frac{E}{\pi \rho l}}$$

where r is the radius of tube, l is its length, ρ is the fluid density and E is the elastance (the reciprocal of compliance) of the system.

To maximise the f_0, the catheter should be short and wide and the diaphragm and tubing should be as stiff as possible; f_0 is decreased by air bubbles which reduce E, and by clots, fibrin or kinks in the system which reduce r. A standard arterial transducer has a resonant frequency of 100 Hz, but with the narrow arterial catheter and long, compliant tubing, this frequently falls to below 20 Hz. Damping of the system (β) can improve the usefulness of the waveform. So-called optimal damping ($\beta = 0.64$) produces the most accurate waveform by achieving the flattest frequency response over the range of physiological frequencies.

An optimal waveform can be determined with a step test. The transducer is open to the flush system for a second and then released. This sets up resonant oscillations in the waveform which rapidly fade away. For optimal damping, the amplitude of successive oscillations should be 5 per cent of the preceding oscillation. More than this and the system is said to be under-damped. Less than this and the system is over-damped and will under-read systolic pressure and over-read diastolic pressure.

Kinetic effects

When fluids flow they exert pressure in the direction of flow. In the absence of flow, pressure is still exerted but the pressure is the same in all directions (Pascal's law). The pressure exerted in the direction of flow is known as the kinetic component of pressure and is given by the formula

$$P = \frac{1}{2} (\rho v^2)$$

where ρ stands for the density of the fluid and v for its velocity.

In circulatory monitoring, the systolic, end systolic, mean and diastolic blood pressures are all 'static' pressures. Even though our concept of physiology is that vascular pressures change over time, at each instantaneous measurement point they are static – residual pressures exerted in all directions. However the fluid (blood) is in motion. Similarly the inspiratory and expiratory pressures in the gas circuit of a ventilator may be regarded as static pressures but in each phase the gas may be in motion.

Hence when trying to measure pressure changes in the circulation or in the gas circuit described, the kinetic energy component of pressure (a consequence of velocity) is an important potential source of variation. The effects can be demonstrated in the circulation as they manifest upon the arterial line transducers. Pressure effects of kinetic energy are maximal when flow is directed at (perpendicular and towards) a transducer and minimal when directed away from it. When systolic pressure measurements need to be made accurately, side hole catheters are used to minimise the effects of kinetic pressure. With an end hole catheter, as flow increases there is a greater increase in peak pressure than mean pressure because of the increase in the kinetic component. Since flow varies at dif-

Table 18.1 Pressure relations to flow at different arterial sites.

Site (pressure point)	Pressure at baseline flow	Pressure at 3 × baseline flow (% of original pressure)
Aorta (systolic)	120	180 (150%)
Aorta (mean)	100	140 (140%)
Distal artery (systolic)	110	120 (109%)
Distal artery (mean)	95	100 (105%)

ferent sites in the circulation so the confounding effects vary depending upon the site of measurement. Table 18.1 demonstrates these confounding effects by comparing pressures in the aorta and distal arteries at two different flow states (one 3 times the other). These effects are separate and distinctly different from the exaggeration of pulse pressure in distal vessels caused by the superimposition of reflected harmonics.

FLOW

Flow is the quantity of a substance, liquid or gas, passing a given point per unit time. It is a rate. Flow will only occur if there is a gradient between two points. Depending on the circumstances this gradient may be voltage or pressure. Pressure gradients provide the energy for fluid flow. Both liquids and gases are fluids.

In the consideration of pressure measurement we had to take account of effects related to the velocity of flow but velocity is not the only interesting feature of flow. Its character can also vary and at its extremes flow is either turbulent or laminar.

Laminar flow

Under conditions of laminar flow, the viscosity of fluids (including gases) is their only physical property that affects flow. The remaining parameters of interest are features of the tube, vessel or conduit rather than the fluid. The absence of turbulence means that such flow is characteristically inaudible. It does not produce heart murmurs or contribute to breath sounds. Laminar flow is much more efficient than turbulent flow, i.e. there is greater flow per unit pressure. With laminar flow

pressure difference (ΔP) = flow rate × resistance

and the resistance to laminar flow of a Newtonian fluid obeys Poiseuille's law

$$resistance = \frac{8\eta l}{\pi r^4}$$

Laminar flow is:

- proportional to the pressure difference (ΔP)
- proportional to the fourth power of the internal radius of the tube (r)
- inversely proportional to the length of the tube (l)
- inversely proportional to the viscosity of the fluid (η).

Hence

$$flow = \frac{\pi \Delta P r^4}{8\eta l}$$

The most important determinant of laminar flow is tube diameter. A doubling of tube radius increases flow by 16 times for the same pressure gradient. Halving its length only increases flow 2 times.

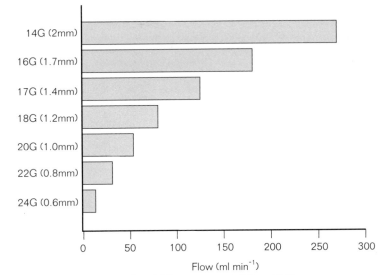

Figure 18.1 Flow through cannulae of different gauges at 100 cms/H_2O pressure.

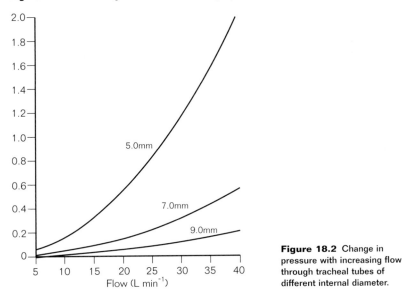

Figure 18.2 Change in pressure with increasing flow through tracheal tubes of different internal diameter.

In Figure 18.1, note how maximal flow increases exponentially with increasing catheter size, but the increase is less than expected as the larger cannulae are also longer.

Similar flow changes with radius can be seen with endotracheal tubes (Figure 18.2).

During respiration, peak inspiratory flow rates approximate to 3 times the minute volume per minute. An adolescent will have a normal peak inspiratory flow of 15 to 30 L min^{-1}. Too small a tube greatly increases the work of breathing, an effect that is further exaggerated if the patient is already tachypnoeic from respiratory disease.

Laminar flow streams in stable layers which, when they flow through a tube, can be visualised as concentric cylinders sliding over each other. The fastest flows are at the centre making the advancing front streamlined. This means, for example, that with laminar gas flow, tidal flow through a tube can occur at volumes significantly lower than the dead space. This phenomenon is particularly relevant during high frequency ventilation.

It is often considered expedient to overlook the fact that blood is a non-Newtonian fluid and to use Poiseuille's law to describe intravascular blood flow. Poiseuille's law reveals how the physiological manipulation of blood flow, by pressure gradients, is most effectively achieved by changes in vessel radius. Such a gross simplification (blood as a Newtonian fluid and the vascular bed likened to a rigid tube) particularly breaks down when one tries to consider complex flow patterns or regional flows. Changes in blood viscosity (e.g. as a consequence of increasing haematocrit in response to sustained hypoxia) affect flow but are best thought of as effect rather than cause. They certainly do not represent a rapid physiological response to influence regional blood flow.

Turbulent flow

Turbulent flow is fundamentally different. It commonly occurs where sudden changes in velocity occur, such as through a narrowing or orifice, or around a sharp bend (turbulent flow is much more likely with right angle bends rather than smooth curves). The advancing wave front of a turbulent flow is flat which makes it more reliable when, for example, trying to purge a ventilator circuit of anaesthetic vapour. However compared to a laminar stream it takes greater pressure to generate the same flow, making turbulent flow much less efficient. Resistance to turbulent flow is in fact inversely proportional to the fifth power of the radius and

$$\Delta P = \text{flow rate}^2 \times \text{resistance}$$

The greater pressure required for flow means more work. Furthermore, to double the flow rate, the pressure must increase fourfold, i.e. it is non-linear. In turbulent flow, viscosity is irrelevant and the resistance is proportional to the density of the fluid. Hence in airway obstruction, helium–oxygen mixtures can be used to achieve better flow. A mixture of 80% helium and 20% oxygen has the same viscosity as 100% oxygen but less than a third of its density.

$$\text{Flow} \propto \sqrt{\frac{P}{l\rho}}$$

where P is the pressure gradient, l is the length of tube and ρ is the density of the fluid.

Mixed flow

Flow need not be totally laminar or completely turbulent. Mixed flow can be considered as being impeded by a resistance that has two components

$$\Delta P = b_1(\text{flow}) + b_2(\text{flow})^2$$

Alternatively resistance can be modelled as $b(\text{flow})^n$ where $1 \leq n \leq 2$. When the value of n approximates to 1 the flow is more laminar and when it approximates to 2 the flow is more turbulent. Mixed flows can also be described by the Reynolds number. For flow in a straight unbranching tube

Reynolds number = (linear velocity of fluid × tube diameter × fluid density)

$\div$ fluid viscosity = $\dfrac{\upsilon\rho d}{\eta}$

Where υ = linear velocity of fluid, ρ = density, η = viscosity and d = diameter of the tube.

A value of less than 1000 means the flow is laminar, 1000 to 1500 is mixed and more than 1500 it is turbulent.

Mixed flows are common in respiratory gases under clinical and physiological conditions. For gas mixtures with different ratios of density : viscosity, flows may tend to be more or less turbulent. The use of helium makes turbulent flow less likely to occur as well as reducing the associated resistance. This is another reason for its use in inspired gases when treating upper airway obstruction or as the shuttle gas in intra-aortic balloon pumps. The velocity at which flow changes from laminar to turbulent is called the critical velocity.

Bernoulli equation

A number of the effects that have been described above are usefully coordinated in the Bernoulli equation. For a steady flow of fluid of a constant density in a streamline, without friction and with negligible viscosity, the appropriately 'contracted' Bernoulli equation summarises the total mechanical energy of the fluid as

$$P_s + 1/2 \, (\rho v^2) + \rho gh = \text{constant}$$

where:

- P_s is static (or residual) pressure found in a fluid filled vessel, static pressure is independent of flow and is exerted in all directions (Pascal's law)
- $1/2 \, (\rho v^2)$ is the kinetic pressure component. The ρ stands for the density of the fluid and v for its velocity
- ρgh is the component of pressure difference that results from a difference in height between the measurement site and any arbitrary reference point (such as the height difference between a transducer and a catheter tip).

In fact the Bernoulli equation represents the application of the law of conservation of energy to a non-compressible fluid. Since energy is neither created nor destroyed; when flow increases, energy is stored as an increase in pressure or as a change in velocity but the total energy remains constant.

Conceptually this is not hard to understand or to model. When a fluid flows through a narrowing, the smaller cross-sectional area means that for the same volume to flow, the fluid must increase its velocity, i.e. its kinetic energy. In order to conserve energy there must be concomitant fall in potential energy, i.e. a fall in pressure within the narrowing.

An example of the utility of the Bernoulli equation is in the assessment of obstructions or stenoses where it relates the velocity increases to the pressure drop across the obstruction. If you know the velocity (as you might from a Doppler signal), the Bernoulli equation tells you the change in pressure (ΔP), a standard medical way of grading stenoses or obstructions. The contraction of the Bernoulli equation in clinical use is:

$$\Delta P \approx 4 \, V_2^2$$

where V_2 is the highest measured velocity. The derivation is not intuitively obvious and so is shown below.

Contracted Bernoulli equation

With the caveats mentioned above (a steady flow of fluid of a constant density in a streamline, without friction and with negligible viscosity) the terms in the Bernoulli equation for flow acceleration and viscous friction are discounted. The term for convective acceleration is adapted to represent the change from the flow velocity (V_1) to the accelerated distal flow velocity (V_2). Thus

$$\Delta P = P_1 - P_2 = 1/2 \text{ density } (V_2^2 - V_1^2)$$

For ease of calculation V_1 is assumed to be very low compared to V_2 and so $(V_2^2 - V_1^2)$ equates to V_2^2.

ΔP thus far is in mmHg, convert to Nm^{-2} by multiplying by 133.3. The density of blood is 1060×10^2 kg m^{-3}. So the equation further simplifies as follows

$$\Delta P = 0.5 \times \text{density} \times V_2^2$$
$$\Delta P \times 133.3 = 0.5 \times 1060 \times V_2^2$$
$$\Delta P = ((0.5 \times 1060) \div 133.3) \times V_2^2$$
$$\Delta P = 3.97 \times V_2^2$$
$$\Delta P \approx 4 \, V_2^2$$

The pressure gradient associated with the change in velocity produces suction that draws in the walls of an elastic vessel exaggerating the stenosis. Suction produced in this way is a Venturi effect (used in nebulisers, oxygen delivery systems and portable suction equipment). After the obstruction the pressure is again higher than within it (although lower than it is proximal to the obstruction) and the flow is turbulent. These factors combine to produce a radial force leading to post-stenotic dilatation in blood vessels. The dilatation leads to lower velocity (higher pressure) and is hence progressive.

MEASUREMENT OF FLOW AND VOLUME

Remember that flow and volume are inextricably linked. Volume per unit time is flow, while flow measured over a period of time will give volume. Therefore devices that measure volume can measure flow and vice versa.

Gas flows – continuous

The main continuous gas source on the intensive care unit is from wall outlets, oxygen cylinders and anaesthetic machines. These flows are measured using a variable orifice flow meter (rotameter) which consists of a bobbin in a conical tube. With increasing flows, the bobbin is pushed further up the tube. The increasing annular orifice around the bobbin counteracts the increasing flow and the pressure on the bobbin remains constant. The flow around the bobbin has both laminar and turbulent elements and therefore depends on both the density and viscosity of the gas concerned. A flowmeter calibrated for a particular gas will therefore give inaccurate flows if used for different gas.

Gas flows – intermittent

A pneumotachograph consists of a mesh or bundle of small-bore tubes that form a resistance to flow. As the flow increases, the measured pressure difference across it increases. Within the flow range of the device, the flow is designed to remain laminar and therefore linearly related to the pressure gradient. Higher flows become more turbulent and non-linear. The device has a very rapid response time and is ideal for variable flows, such as those in ventilator circuits. The area under the pressure–time curve is calculated by integration to give total flow throughout the respiratory cycle.

A hot-wire anemometer works on the principle that a gas of known heat capacity, flowing through a tube of known dimensions, will cause cooling of two heated resistance wires (part of a Wheatstone bridge) in proportion to the rate of gas flow. The change in temperature of the wires alters their resistance and unbalances the Wheatstone bridge. The degree of imbalance is proportional to flow and is displayed electronically.

Gas volumes

Spirometry is the simplest method of measuring respiratory volume and is the commonest respiratory function test used. Vital capacity (VC) is often reduced in intensive care patients, because of pneumonia, atelectasis, pain, sedation, residual neuromuscular paralysis, muscular weakness and neuromuscular diseases. Measurement of VC requires the child's cooperation but can be useful in assessing respiratory muscle strength when weaning or assessing the need for mechanical ventilation (e.g. in progressive neuromuscular diseases, such as Guillain–Barré or myasthenia gravis).

Turbine flowmeters measure volume during intermittent or cyclical flow. They are not accurate for the measurement of continuous flow. The Wright's respirometer is a mechanical turbine flowmeter and is widely used for measuring tidal volume during mechanical ventilation. It can also be attached to a facemask to measure vital capacity in the absence of a spirometer. Unlike electronic turbine flowmeters, the Wright's respirometer only measures flow in one direction. The patient should not be allowed to both inspire and expire through the device.

Liquid flows

Measurement of liquid flow takes many forms in the intensive care unit including intravenous infusions and blood flow, particularly cardiac output. This section will concentrate on the measurement of cardiac output, particularly using the 'Fick principle'.

The Fick principle states that for a constant stream (of liquid or gas), when a substance is added to or removed from that stream, the flow is proportional to the concentration difference produced. It is the basis for many methods of cardiac output and organ blood flow measurement, including the direct Fick method (oxygen consumption) and the indicator-dilution methods of thermodilution, dye dilution and radionuclide dilution.

The direct Fick method assumes that during the study period (usually several minutes) oxygen consumption remains constant. Arterial and mixed venous ($C_{\bar{v}} O_2$) blood samples are necessary, the latter taken from the pulmonary artery to assure adequate mixing. Oxygen consumption is measured, either using a Benedict Roth spirometer, and rebreathing through soda lime, or with a metabolic monitor. The method is very accurate but requires cumbersome equipment and pulmonary artery catheterisation. In addition, any gas leaks in the system reduce its accuracy. This can be a particular problem with uncuffed endotracheal tubes used in children

$$\text{Cardiac output} = \dot{V}O_2 \div (CaO_2 - C_{\bar{v}} O_2)$$

The indicator-dilution method involves the sudden injection of a bolus of indicator (indocyanine green, cold intravenous fluid or radionuclide) and the measurement of the resulting gradient from baseline as the indicator passes a sensor (light absorbance meter, thermistor or Geiger counter respectively). The thermodilution method (cold intravenous fluid) is the commonest method of measuring cardiac output and many consider it to be the benchmark. Multiple estimations may be made easily as there is no recirculation of indicator. It usually requires a pulmonary artery catheter. A bolus of known volume and temperature is rapidly injected into the right atrium and completely mixes with the blood passing through the heart. The resulting temperature gradient is measured by a thermistor on the tip of the catheter, in the pulmonary artery. A curve of temperature gradient against time is plotted. The area under the curve represents the product of mean temperature gradient and time.

TEMPERATURE

Heat is kinetic energy in a form that will transfer from a hotter body to a cooler body. Temperature is the relative thermal state of a body that determines whether it will receive heat from, or donate it to, other bodies. There is an inverse relationship between temperature and volume. For a given amount of energy, if volume expands temperature falls (this is the way the universe cooled after the big bang). Conversely if volume contracts then temperature rises. This effect is quite different from the expansion that occurs when a body receives additional energy in the form of heat.

The heat energy in a patient is a balance between energy production and the interaction with the environment. Heat is generated by cellular respiration (increased in exercise) and lost by radiation (40%), convection (32%), and conduction (28%). The majority of conductive heat loss occurs heating surface water to a vapour (latent heat of vaporisation), 30% of this surface water being in the respiratory tract.

When heat energy is given to a body, the temperature of the body rises until either both bodies achieve the same temperature (and net heat transfer ceases) or a new steady state is achieved between this energy input and the other energy exchanges that are occurring. Excessive warming of small babies may exceed their homeostatic capabilities and lead to an equilibrium greater than 37°C, i.e. hyperthermia.

'Heat capacity' is the amount of energy required to raise temperature by 1°C. Specific heat capacity is heat capacity per kilogram. A small child has a small heat capacity by virtue of his low mass and will cool down or heat up much more quickly than an adult for a given amount of heat. Small animals and young babies have a high surface area : volume ratio and therefore interact with their environmental temperature to a greater degree. Heat distribution is largely about blood flow and so it is no surprise to find the heart and metabolic rates of young animals and babies to be faster than those of their larger or older counterparts to compensate for the increased losses.

Measurement of temperature

Temperature measurement has many uses in PICU. In addition to measuring temperatures that change relatively slowly, such as body temperature, it is often necessary to measure rapidly changing temperatures, such as thermodilution cardiac output measurement or respiratory monitoring.

Types of thermometer include mercury thermometers, resistance thermometers, thermocouples, thermistors and dial thermometers such as bimetallic strips.

The mercury-filled clinical thermometer is very accurate within the physiological temperature range. Its use is limited by taking several minutes to equilibrate and by its fragility.

Resistance thermometers make use of the small increase in resistance seen when a metal is heated; usually a platinum wire is used. When accurately calibrated at one temperature, usually 0°C, and used within a Wheatstone bridge, it may be accurate to within several thousandths of a degree centigrade.

Thermocouples make use of the Seebeck effect. When two different metals are put in contact, a potential difference is generated. If the two metal wires form a loop and one junction is kept at a constant temperature, the potential difference is proportional to the temperature at the other junction.

Thermistors are semiconductors. These show an exponential fall in resistance as temperature rises. They can be made very small and have a very rapid response rate. This means that they are particularly useful for measuring rapidly changing temperatures or as intravascular temperature probes. Thermistors are used for thermodilution cardiac output determination. They are damaged by high temperatures and generally cannot be autoclaved.

OXIMETRY

Oximeters rely upon the Lambert law; when light passes through a homogenous semitransparent medium, the amount of light transmitted decreases exponentially in relation to the distance travelled

$$I_t = I_0 \, e^{\,-Ecd}$$

where I_t is the intensity of transmitted light, I_0 that of incident light, c is the concentration of the substance, d is the distance travelled through the substance and E is the extinction coefficient. The absorbance is the reciprocal of I_t and, like I_t, it is specific for different wavelengths of light in different media.

Under normal circumstances only two species of haemoglobin are found, oxyhaemoglobin and reduced haemoglobin. By comparing the absorption of two different wavelengths of incident light (660 and 940 nm), it is possible to separate out the relative contributions of oxyhaemoglobin and reduced haemoglobin by their different absorption spectra (Figure 18.3).

The absorption spectra of methaemoglobin and carboxyhaemoglobin cause major inaccuracies with devices using just two wavelengths. Carboxyhaemoglobin's absorption spectrum is similar to that of oxyhaemoglobin at 660 nm. The pulse oximeter reads carboxyhaemoglobin as oxyhaemoglobin. Therefore, despite high levels of carboxyhaemoglobin the pulse oximeter will give a normal pulse oximeter saturation. Methaemoglobin's absorption spectrum is nearly identical to reduced haemoglobin at 660 nm but closer to that of oxyhaemoglobin at 940 nm. This causes the pulse oximeter to tend towards 85% saturation irrespective of the concentration of methaemoglobin, again leading to the risk of severe unrecognised tissue hypoxia. Accurate determination of the concentrations of haemoglobin species requires a co-oximeter. These instruments use four wavelengths of light and can separate out the different species.

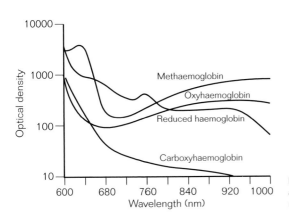

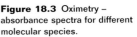

Figure 18.3 Oximetry – absorbance spectra for different molecular species.

EXPONENTIAL FUNCTIONS

Many natural processes have an exponential time course. An exponential function is one where the rate of change depends on its present state rather than its initial condition. An exponential that proceeds in discrete steps is a geometric progression. For example, a bag of intravenous fluid will drain into a patient through an unmetered giving set. The rate of flow into the patient is related to the volume of fluid remaining in the bag, i.e. the head of pressure. As the volume falls so does the head of pressure and therefore the rate of flow.

It is often worth taking a little time to derive such exponential functions (some clinical examples follow). Taking the example of the bag of intravenous fluid. If the volume of fluid left in the bag is y we can graph it against time t. This is called a die-away curve and has the formula (the minus sign in this case is because the bag is emptying):

$$y = be^{-kt}$$

where b and k are constants. If we differentiate this formula: the rate of change of y at any given point is given by the gradient of the curve (dy/dt) at that point. If we take logarithms on both sides to make the maths easier, we get

$$\ln y = \ln b - kt \quad (1)$$

Differentiating (1) we get

$$\frac{1}{y} \frac{dy}{dt} = -k$$

which can be rearranged to

$$\frac{dy}{dt} = -ky$$

where k is a constant that defines the speed of this particular function. Notice that the rate of the process is dependent on the amount of y left at any particular time. So what happens at time zero? If we take equation (1), at time zero y = b, i.e. b is the value of y at time zero, which we can call y_0 so we can rewrite the formula as:

$$y = y_0 e^{-kt}$$

Tao (τ), the time-constant, is the reciprocal of the rate constant k and the equation may be rewritten as

$$y = y_0 e^{-t/\tau}$$

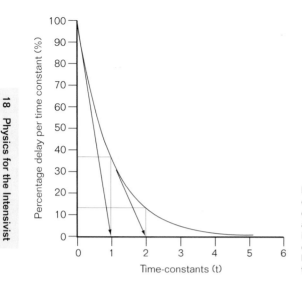

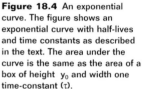

Figure 18.4 An exponential curve. The figure shows an exponential curve with half-lives and time constants as described in the text. The area under the curve is the same as the area of a box of height y_0 and width one time-constant (τ).

τ is a theoretical value for the time the process would have taken to complete had it continued at its present rate (i.e. the time from that point to the intercept at y_0. It represents the time the process takes to fall to 37 per cent (e^{-1}) of its present level. Two time-constants represent the time to fall to 37 per cent of 37 per cent, i.e. 13.5% and so on (Figure 18.4).

Half-life refers to the time a process takes to fall to 50 per cent of its current value. Two half-lives to 25 per cent and so on. 'Half-life' is easier to understand but 'time-constant' is more useful when the area under the curve is required.

The interest in exponentials stems from several factors.

- Many biological processes are exponential in nature including many metabolic processes, renal elimination of certain drugs, air flow during spontaneous respiration, first order pharmacokinetics, tumour growth and bacterial multiplication.
- An exponential function will give a straight line when plotted on semilogarithmic paper. The slope of the line is k or $1/\tau$. If the line is extrapolated back to the y axis, the inter section is y_0. Note this refers to $\log_e$. For $\log_{10}$, the slope is $\dfrac{k}{2.3}$ or $\dfrac{1}{2.3 \times \tau}$ y_0 remains the same. It is therefore simple to predict the value of an exponential function at any particular time or steps, as in a geometrical progression.
- The area remaining under an exponential curve equals the product of τ and y. Therefore if you know y_0 and τ, you know the total area under the curve to infinity. This is especially useful for washout curves for cardiac output or organ blood flow measurement.
- Many biological processes can be described in terms of the relationship between two physiological variables, such that if the value for τ (for the particular process) can be ascertained and you already know one of the variables, you can work out the second.

Exponential functions can be used to help with all sorts of problems. Take for example a patient with sickle cell disease who needs protection from a crisis during a hypoxic illness. If we consider the safe end-point of an exchange transfusion to be the point where the patient has 80 per cent of their total red cells of donor origin, how much blood are we going to have to exchange?

The answer depends on the relationship between the volume of the syringe that you use and the circulating blood volume:

- if C_0 = the original quantity of a substance in the blood

- and C_D = the desired quantity of the same substance in the blood
- and V_S = the volume of blood in the syringe to be used
- and V_{CBV} = the circulating volume of blood

then the number of syringes (n) to be exchanged is given by

$$n = \log (C_D \div C_O) \div \log [1 - (V_S \div V_{CBV})]$$

So if the patient is 10 kg (V_{CBV} = 800 ml) and we use a 20 ml syringe (V_S = 20) then:

$$n = \log (0.2) \div \log (78 \div 80)$$
$$= 64 \text{ syringes.}$$

The same formula can be used to predict haemoglobin concentration after dilutional exchange transfusion. The formula assumes that the substance is confined to the vascular space so it tends to overestimate the potential effectiveness of exchanges for removal of substances such as bilirubin where the whole point is that the volume of distribution extends outside the vascular space.

Alternatively, if you did not have the above formula, you could have started the exchange transfusion and then plotted your progress on semilogarithmic paper, with percentage of original haemoglobin on the y axis and number of cycles on the x axis. You would find the same answer by extrapolating the line to your desired percentage original haemoglobin and reading off the number of cycles. A more common example is to calculate when to give the next dose of gentamicin. In order to minimise both toxicity and unnecessary treatment delays waiting for random trough levels, measure two random levels, say 6 to 12 hours apart. Plot them on semilogarithmic paper and you can read off the time when the level falls to your chosen trough where a further dose is due.

Appendix: Basic SI Units

There are seven basic SI (Système International) units, from which all other units of measurement can be derived. It is important to note the case (upper or lower) of the abbreviated units. The seven basic units are:

Length	metre	m
Mass	kilogram	kg
Time	second	s
Current	ampere	A
Temperature	kelvin	K
Luminous intensity	candela	cd
Amount of substance	mole	mol

Derived SI units are:

Force	newton	N	$1\ N = 1\ kg\ m\ s^{-2}$
Pressure	pascal	Pa	$1\ Pa = 1\ N\ m^{-2}$
	mmHg		$7.5\ mmHg = 1$ kilopascal (kPa)
	cmH_2O		$1\ cmH_2O = 98\ Pa = 0.7\ mmHg$
	bar		$1\ bar = 100\ kPa = 750\ mmHg$

Standard atmospheric pressure   101.325 kPa

Energy	joule	J	$1\ J = 1\ N\ m$
calorie	cal		$1\ cal = 4.18\ J$
			$1000\ cal = 1\ kcal = 1\ Cal$ (NB uppercase)
Power	watt	W	$1\ W = 1\ J\ s^{-1}$
Temperature	Celsius	°C	$°C = K - 273.15$
			$0°C = 273.15\ K$
Volume	litre	L	$1\ L = 0.001\ m^3$
	millilitre	ml	$1000\ ml = 1\ L$

Prefixes for SI units

deci	d	10^{-1}	deca	da	10^{1}
centi	c	10^{-2}	hecto	h	10^{2}
milli	m	10^{-3}	kilo	k	10^{3}
micro	μ	10^{-6}	mega	M	10^{6}
nano	n	10^{-9}	giga	G	10^{9}
pico	p	10^{-12}	tera	T	10^{12}

19 Ingestion and Poisoning

- **General management**
- **Notes on specific agents**

Childhood poisoning accounts for about 18 000 UK hospital admissions per year. Over 90 per cent of deaths from poisoning are caused by inhalation of carbon monoxide or other gases or fumes. The main substances ingested (as opposed to inhaled) are iron, tricyclic antidepressants, benzodiazepines, paracetamol and oral contraceptives. Tricyclics, opiates, barbiturates, salicylates and lead however account for the majority of deaths. The 'Notes on Specific Agents' in this chapter are listed in alphabetical order.

GENERAL MANAGEMENT

Resuscitate

AIRWAY

Many drugs impair airway patency and reflexes, reduce ventilation and thence depress the cardiovascular system. Watching for signs of these problems (and intervening where necessary) is fundamental to the management of all cases of poisoning.

BREATHING

Hypoxia is rapidly fatal. In addition, it exacerbates the toxicity of many drugs and must be avoided at all times. Hypoventilation leads to hypoxia and hypercarbia. The resulting acidosis increases the toxicity of many drugs (e.g. aspirin and tricyclic antidepressants). Remember: if a patient is receiving supplemental oxygen then the pulse oximeter is not a monitor of ventilation. Significant hypoventilation will occur before the oxygen saturation falls. Record the respiratory rate and apparent tidal volume, and look for paradoxical breathing or Kussmaul's respiration.

CIRCULATION

Check the rate, rhythm and volume of the pulse. Look for evidence of vasoconstriction or vasodilatation and confirm hyper- or hypotension by measuring the blood pressure.

DISABILITY

CONTROL SEIZURES

Seizures may be a toxic effect or caused by hypoxia or hypoglycaemia. They must be aggressively investigated and treated. In general terms treat the cause then the seizure (benzodiazepines are usually the best first line). Poisoned patients who are convulsing need intubation and ventilation.

TREAT HYPOTHERMIA

Measure the patient's temperature and treat hypothermia.

CHECK NEUROLOGICAL SIGNS

Make an assessment of conscious level, look for irritability/hyperreflexia, decerebrate/decorticate movements. Look at the pupils for mydriasis, miosis, strabismus or nystagmus. Remember:

- loss of brainstem reflexes mimicking the signs of brain death can occur in severe poisoning with tricyclic antidepressants, carbamazepine and phenytoin, where full recovery is common

- lateralising neurological signs are rarely due to poisoning alone and another cause should be sought (e.g. intracranial haematoma from a head injury).

EXPOSURE

Further examination should include inspection of the skin looking for blisters, burns or bruising and look inside the mouth for lesions or ulceration. Look for evidence of abdominal discomfort.

Diagnose

GET A HISTORY

Bear in mind that this may be unreliable. Find out what was ingested, how much and how long ago. As a general rule assume that what was ingested is the difference between what is left in the bottle or blister pack and the total amount that was prescribed. Ostensibly single drug ingestion in teenagers may actually involve multiple drugs, particularly alcohol. Toxicology tests should routinely include paracetamol and salicylates (especially if a metabolic acidosis is present).

GET SPECIALIST ADVICE

National poisons advice centres are available 24 hours a day and should be used for up-to-date advice. UK telephone numbers are listed below. If you are dialling from outside the UK then dial the international code, which is 44 and drop the first 0.

National Number	0870 600 6266
Belfast	02890 240503
Birmingham	0121 507 5588 or 507 5589
Cardiff	02920 709901
Edinburgh	0131 536 2300
London	0207 635 9191
Newcastle	0191 282 0300

PSYCHOSOCIAL REVIEW

It is necessary to ascertain whether the ingestion was accidental, deliberate self harm or perpetrated by an assailant, and appropriate action must be taken to protect the child.

Treat

PREVENT FURTHER ABSORPTION

INDUCED EMESIS

This has no role in the hospital management of poisoning. It should be limited to treatment of a very recent ingestion by a patient in a remote area where there may be a significant delay in transfer to hospital. Even then contraindications include a child with an actual or potential depressed level of consciousness or a risk of seizure or ingestion of a volatile hydrocarbon.

GASTRIC LAVAGE

Gastric lavage recovers 20 to 30 per cent of the drug at best. It is reserved for recent overdoses of large amounts where even a small reduction in absorption might be lifesaving, or for drugs which are not adsorbed to charcoal such as iron. There is a theoretical risk of increasing drug absorption by flushing drug through the pylorus. This may be reduced by giving activated charcoal before and after the lavage. It is essential that the patient's airway be protected during the procedure.

ACTIVATED CHARCOAL.

The majority of drugs are adsorbed by charcoal. Exceptions include iron, alcohols (ethanol, methanol, ethylene glycol), caustics and acids and lithium. A single dose of 1 g kg^{-1} effectively reduces drug absorption. Repeat doses, every 4 hours, may be useful for some agents (carbamazepine, theophylline, phenobarbital, aspirin and tricyclic antidepressants), both by increasing intraluminal drug adsorption and by intestinal dialysis of drug from the blood back into the gut. Bowel sounds must be present before repeat doses are given, otherwise the volume of repeat doses can lead to gastric distension with risk of regurgitation and aspiration, or even gastric perforation. Persuading a small child to drink charcoal can be difficult. More palatable preparations, with a black straw and opaque containers may help. Ultimately nasogastric administration may be necessary. Aspiration of charcoal is potentially fatal. It is essential that the patient's airway is secure before administration and that the child is observed afterwards.

CATHARTICS

Cathartics, for example sorbitol and magnesium sulphate, are given to purge the gut by drawing in fluid and reducing transit time. They are effective as single doses, given in combination with charcoal. The fluid shift can cause electrolyte imbalances and haemodynamic instability in small children. Repeat doses should be avoided in favour of whole bowel irrigation.

WHOLE BOWEL IRRIGATION (WBI)

Repeated doses of balanced electrolyte or polyethylene glycol (PEG) solutions produce a prolonged purging effect without the fluid shifts associated with cathartics. WBI is especially useful for; the removal of substances not adsorbed by charcoal, slow-release preparations and for large lumps of drugs such as packets or bezoars. Continue WBI until the rectal effluent is clear or watery-black from charcoal. Charcoal is often given with WBI although the PEG somewhat reduces its efficacy. The initial charcoal dose should be given before the PEG solution and repeat doses may be required.

MONITOR

All patients must be closely observed until they are no longer at risk from the poisoning episode. This must include repeated assessment of the ABCD. Additional monitoring, PICU admission and investigations will depend upon the type of poisoning.

NOTES ON SPECIFIC AGENTS

ACE inhibitors

- Hypotension is the major complication and may last for days.
- Haemodialysis is required for severe cases.

BACKGROUND

Even when ingestion of relatively large doses occurs, serious complications are rare in children. Hypotension is the major complication and long-acting preparations may necessitate treatment for days. Other complications include gastrointestinal disturbance, impaired consciousness, bronchospasm, hyperkalaemia and renal impairment.

MANAGEMENT

ABC. Gastric lavage is followed by activated charcoal for patients presenting early after ingestion of large quantities. Hypotension should be treated initially with intravenous fluids but inotropes and vasoconstrictors may be necessary. Naloxone may be effective and angiotensin II has also been used. Hyperkalaemia responds to insulin and dextrose but captopril, enalapril and lisinopril are all (like potassium) removed by haemodialysis, which is otherwise reserved for renal failure.

Anticoagulants (oral)

Oral anticoagulants act by interfering with the synthesis of vitamin K-dependent clotting factors. These drugs include warfarin and the 'super warfarins' (very long-acting agents used as rodenticides). Features of anticoagulant poisoning are therefore haemorrhage and bruising. Laboratory tests show a prolonged prothrombin time and treatment is with intravenous vitamin K (0.3 mg kg^{-1} to a maximum of 10 mg) and fresh frozen plasma for active bleeding.

Potentiators of warfarin include:
amiodarone, amitriptyline, anabolic steroids, aztreonam, chloral hydrate, chloramphenicol, cimetidine, ciprofloxacin, co-trimoxazole, dextrothyroxine, dipyridamole, erythromycin, fluconazole, glucagon, ketoconazole, mefenamic acid, metronidazole, miconazole, omeprazole, quinidine, salicylates, sulphonamides, tetracyclines and other broad spectrum antibiotics

Warfarin action is reduced by:
barbiturates, carbamazepine, oral contraceptives, rifampicin, vitamin K

Agents that have shown mixed effects on warfarin include phenytoin and cholestyramine.

Anticonvulsants

Many different types of drugs possess anticonvulsant activity. However they naturally display more specific patterns of toxicity.

CARBAMAZEPINE

Carbamazepine is structurally related to the tricyclics but is much less toxic. It is proconvulsant in high doses. Signs of toxicity include nausea, vomiting, drowsiness, coma, seizures, nystagmus, opthalmoplegia and dilated pupils. AV block and bradycardia can occur but serious ventricular dysrhythmias are unusual. Treatment is supportive, repeat-dose charcoal is very effective and seizures can be controlled with benzodiazepines or thiopentone. Temporary cardiac pacing may be necessary for dysrhythmias. Haemodialysis is ineffective.

PHENYTOIN

Phenytoin toxicity produces ataxia, drowsiness and coma and symptoms persist for several days. It also has negative inotropic effects and inhibits AV conduction. Supportive treatment includes repeat-dose charcoal (very effective) and lavage for large recent ingestion.

SODIUM VALPROATE

Sodium valproate toxicity produces coma, muscle spasms, hypocalcaemia and thrombocytopaenia. Liver damage and cerebral oedema may occur but are probably idiosyncratic reactions. Treatment is generally supportive, L-carnitine is probably ineffective.

Aspirin (salicylates)

- Coma or seizures are uncommon and indicate either severe toxicity or a mixed overdose.
- Urinary alkalinisation is much more important than diuresis.
- Chronic poisoning results in clinical toxicity at much lower levels than acute toxicity.

BACKGROUND

Acute aspirin poisoning is less common following the withdrawal of its routine use for children under 12 years old. However, aspirin is commonly found in the home, including non-tablet forms such as oil of wintergreen and medicinal balms for sprains and musculoskeletal injuries. These preparations may contain a high concentration of salicylate such that ingestion of only 1 to 2 teaspoons produces severe toxicity (>300 mg kg^{-1}) in small children. Doses less than 150 mg kg^{-1} are rarely toxic.

Salicylate uncouples oxidative phosphorylation and increases the metabolism of lipid, carbohydrate and amino acids. The metabolic acidosis is caused by the salicylic acid, ketones, free amino acids and lactate.

Signs of poisoning include:

- tinnitus, fever, sweating, tachycardia
- nausea and vomiting, haematemesis and dehydration
- hyperventilation because of direct brainstem stimulation
- lethargy

Non-cardiogenic pulmonary oedema may also occur. Seizures and coma are signs of severe, potentially lethal, salicylate toxicity.

The classic picture of a mixed respiratory alkalosis and metabolic acidosis is uncommon in children. They often present with a metabolic and respiratory acidosis, the latter resulting from respiratory depression caused by a reduced conscious level. Hyperglycaemia is common and may mimic diabetic ketoacidosis. Hypoglycaemia may occur in small children. Ionised hypocalcaemia is common. A multifactorial coagulopathy may be problematic. Investigations should include electrolytes, creatinine, coagulation, haemoglobin, acid–base status, salicylate level and liver function tests.

Salicylate levels (Figure 19.1):

- peak levels correlate with toxicity
- in acute overdose shows first order elimination kinetics. Late presentations may have moderate levels but severe poisoning necessitating more aggressive treatment.

Treat patients first according to their clinical status and use repeat levels as a guide to the effectiveness of treatment. Levels that rise or fail to fall, suggest the ingestion of enteric-coated salicylate or the formation of salicylate tablet bezoars. Chronic salicylate toxicity (100 mg kg^{-1} for several days) may produce severe toxicity at lower levels than those required to produce acute toxicity and paradoxically may show zero order kinetics.

MANAGEMENT

ABC. Severely poisoned children become hypovolaemic and dehydrated, and require resuscitation. Mechanical ventilation may be necessary with airway control because of the conscious level or because of non-cardiogenic pulmonary oedema.

Repeat-dose charcoal is as effective as urinary alkalinisation in reducing salicylate levels but vomiting may make it impossible to administer. Lavage or WBI should be considered for severe poisoning with enteric-coated tablets or suspected bezoar formation.

Asymptomatic children or those with levels below 400 mg L^{-1} in the first 12 hours should only require intravenous fluids and correction of electrolyte imbalances. Correct the acidosis with 1 to 2 mmol kg^{-1} of sodium bicarbonate depending on the severity. Remember that rapid correction can cause hypokalaemia, hypernatraemia and hypocalcaemia which itself may cause seizures. Aspirin is a weak acid and at low pH it is less ionised and therefore has greater tissue affinity and toxicity.

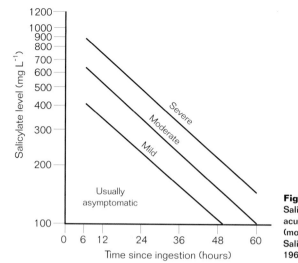

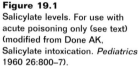

Figure 19.1
Salicylate levels. For use with acute poisoning only (see text) (modified from Done AK, Salicylate intoxication. *Pediatrics* 1960 26:800–7).

Symptomatic children with respiratory acidosis require mechanical ventilation and those with higher salicylate levels (400–700 mg L^{-1}) additionally require alkaline diuresis, which greatly enhances salicylate elimination. Alkaline diuresis can be provided by using a 5% dextrose solution, to which 40 to 80 mmol of sodium bicarbonate per 500 ml has been added, as the maintenance fluid. Titrate the bicarbonate content to maintain a urinary pH of 8 to 8.5. This fluid can also be used for replacement of any associated dehydration deficit. Forcing a diuresis with additional fluid has minimal effect on salicylate clearance and exposes the patient to the risks of fluid overload and more severe electrolyte disturbance. In addition unnecessary fluid gives a false or dilutional fall in the salicylate level. Hypokalaemia may impede urinary alkalinisation.

Severely symptomatic children or those with high levels (>700 mg L^{-1}) may require extensive resuscitation and electrolyte correction. Urinary alkalinisation should still be attempted but remember that haemodialysis (not peritoneal dialysis) rapidly removes salicylate, as well as correcting fluid and electrolyte imbalances. Indications include:

- salicylate levels above 1000 mg L^{-1} or levels which fail to fall with other therapies
- renal failure
- severe pulmonary oedema
- severe acid–base or electrolyte disturbance despite treatment
- persistent CNS signs, including coma and seizures.

Benzodiazepines

- Management of most cases is supportive.
- There is no role for flumazenil in mixed drug ingestion involving benzodiazepines.

BACKGROUND

Benzodiazepines are a common component of mixed drug overdoses in adults. Oral absorption of benzodiazepines is rapid and complete and the symptoms are primarily sedative. Many of the drugs have active metabolites which may have long half-lives (e.g. diazepam) but knowing that the metabolites to a particular agent have a short half-life does not guarantee that the symptoms of poisoning will be short lived.

MANAGEMENT

ABC. The management of benzodiazepine poisoning is supportive.

Many cases involve multiple drugs including paracetamol, tricyclics and alcohol. This must be expected, despite denials to the contrary, and treated appropriately. Under these circumstances the benzodiazepine may be suppressing seizures induced by the other drugs. It is well recognised that sudden removal of the benzodiazepine action may lead to intractable seizures and death. It is for this reason that flumazenil, a short-acting specific benzodiazepine antagonist, should not be used in benzodiazepine poisoning.

Beta-agonists

- Toxicity causes lactic acidosis and hypokalaemia.

BACKGROUND

Features of β-agonist overdose include:

- tachyarrhythmias
- severe hypokalaemia
- myocardial ischaemia and pulmonary oedema
- hyperglycaemia
- lactic acidosis
- seizures.

MANAGEMENT

- ABC
- supportive measures, lavage, charcoal
- correct hypokalaemia
- titrate a non-selective β-blocker, for example propranolol to the clinical effects; esmolol (short acting) may be preferred if there is a history of asthma
- control seizures with diazepam.

Beta-blockers

- At high doses β-blockers are relatively non-selective.
- Dangerous tachyarrhythmias can occur.

BACKGROUND

Several types are available with varying: β receptor selectivity, intrinsic sympathetic activity (ISA), membrane stabilising activity, lipid solubility, α receptor-blocking activity and duration of action. Note:

- at high doses β-blockers are relatively non-selective
- membrane-stabilising drugs may cause severe myocardial depression and arrhythmias, which are not reversed by β-agonists; sotalol has significant class III antiarrhythmic activity but may produce severe arrhythmias, including tachyarrhythmias, torsade de pointes and ventricular fibrillation

- lipid soluble drugs may cause drowsiness, coma and seizures
- drugs with high levels of ISA produce less haemodynamic disturbance and may cause hypertension
- the duration of symptoms may greatly exceed the half-life of the drug. Propranolol has a half-life of 3.9 hours, but in overdose may produce toxicity for 2 to 3 days
- the impact of toxicity may be much worse in the context of congenital heart disease
- severe toxicity is common when in combination with other drugs such as alcohol or calcium channel blockers.

The most serious of these agents is propranolol. It is non-selective, membrane stabilising and lipid soluble. Symptoms include respiratory depression, coma, seizures, bronchospasm, myocardial failure, pulmonary oedema and arrhythmias. The ECG shows QRS and QT prolongation. Hypoglycaemia and hypocalcaemia can occur.

MANAGEMENT

ABC. Patients with depressed conscious levels need airway protection. Respiratory depression requires intubation and mechanical ventilation. Bronchospasm may respond to nebulised β_2-agonists or intravenous aminophylline. Hypotensive patients require volume resuscitation and invasive monitoring. Ingestion of large quantities of β-blockers should be treated with lavage and charcoal. Atropine administered prior to lavage usefully counteracts any vagal stimulation.

Hypotension and myocardial depression are treated with sympathomimetics. Dopamine in doses up to 30 µg kg^{-1}min^{-1} may be needed. Isoprenaline and dobutamine may exacerbate hypotension. Vagolytics such as atropine (40 µg kg^{-1}) increase heart rate in about 25 per cent of cases but multiple doses run the risk of exacerbating confusion and seizures due to central anticholinergic actions. Glucagon (50–150 µg kg^{-1} followed by an infusion of 25–75 µg kg^{-1}hr^{-1}) may be effective in severe toxicity. Adverse effects include hyperglycaemia, hypokalaemia, hypercalcaemia and vomiting. To avoid potential phenol toxicity, glucagon in these doses should be made up in 5% dextrose rather than the phenol-based diluent sometimes supplied. Large doses of calcium may improve contractility, blood pressure and reduce a prolonged QRS interval. Bradycardia may respond to atropine, isoprenaline or pacing. Ventricular tachycardia may respond to potassium supplementation or magnesium. Lignocaine (lidocaine) is best avoided as it prolongs the QT interval further and increases the risk of ventricular arrhythmias. Ultimately intra-aortic balloon pump, cardiopulmonary bypass, ventricular assist device (VAD) or ECMO may be required. Without these, should cardiac arrest occur, effective CPR can be continued for several hours with ultimate complete recovery.

Calcium channel blockers

> - Common mistakes in management are inadequate gut decontamination and inadequate dosage of intravenously infused calcium.

BACKGROUND

Verapamil, diltiazem and nifedipine represent the three main groups of calcium channel blockers. Features of their toxicity include hypotension and bradycardia or asystole (most common with verapamil), hyperglycaemia and lactic acidosis. Both cardiogenic and non-cardiogenic pulmonary oedema may occur with all three groups, the latter may occur as a late phenomenon. Neurological symptoms are uncommon.

Toxicity is:

- dose related
- worse in patients with pre-existing cardiorespiratory disease
- more common with slow-release preparations after inadequate gut decontamination

- worse in the under-treated (inadequate gut decontamination, inadequate calcium infusion)
- worse with mixed ingestion (especially digoxin, β-blockers and anti-arrhythmic drugs such as flecainide).

MANAGEMENT

ABC. Vomiting is a common side effect but lavage is still required for recent ingestion of large amounts. Repeat-dose charcoal reduces the enterohepatic circulation. Slow-release preparations are better treated with WBI. Supportive treatment includes fluid resuscitation for hypotension, intravenous calcium – both bolus and infusion (large doses may be necessary), and inotropic support. Atropine is sometimes effective for bradycardia, particularly when used in combination with intravenous calcium. Glucagon may improve blood pressure and heart rate. Unresponsive bradycardia requires pacing. Cardiopulmonary bypass, ECMO and VAD are reserved for refractory hypotension or bradycardia with worsening metabolic acidosis. Otherwise in the event of cardiac arrest effective cardiopulmonary resuscitation can be continued for several hours with full recovery.

Carbon monoxide

- Normal arterial Po_2 and a normal pulse oximeter saturation reading do not exclude severe carbon monoxide poisoning therefore always give a high-flow of oxygen or a high Fio_2.

BACKGROUND

Carbon monoxide poisoning may occur in isolation (faulty gas appliances, etc.) or as part of a burn injury. Its toxicity is caused by tissue hypoxia via three mechanisms:

1 avid binding of carbon monoxide (CO) to haemoglobin (Hb), forming carboxyhaemoglobin (COHb), which reduces the haemoglobin available for oxygen carriage
2 left shift of the oxygen dissociation curve, from a P_{50} of 3.6 kPa to a P_{50} of 1.9 kPa further reducing oxygen availability to tissues
3 binding to other iron-containing proteins and enzymes, including myoglobin (producing severe muscle hypoxia) and cytochromes a and a3 (producing mitochondrial dysfunction).

The symptoms vary for acute and chronic exposure, which can lead to tolerance of higher levels of COHb. Acute symptoms include headache, dizziness, nausea, vomiting and signs such as hyperreflexia, increased muscle tone, seizures and coma. Cerebral oedema is common. Myocardial ischaemia and pulmonary oedema may occur. Muscle overactivity is associated with rhabdomyolysis.

Chronic poisoning produces 'flu-like' symptoms of malaise and headache and diagnosis requires a high level of suspicion. Blood gases reveal metabolic acidosis caused by cellular hypoxia and muscle overactivity. The Pao_2, in the absence of a smoke inhalation injury, may be normal. In addition, a pulse oximeter will show a correspondingly normal saturation. Severe carbon monoxide poisoning can be present despite a normal Pao_2 and normal saturation. Co-oximetry discriminates COHb by its absorption spectrum.

MANAGEMENT

ABC. Adequate ventilation should be assured with Fio_2 of at least 80 per cent, preferably 100 per cent. This confers a reduction in the elimination half-life of COHb of up to fourfold. Patients with impaired airway reflexes, those at risk from airway oedema or with COHb levels >20 per cent should be electively intubated and given 100% oxygen.

Muscle activity can be reduced using dantrolene 1 mg kg^{-1} (up to 10 mg kg^{-1}).

Cerebral oedema manifests with a reduced conscious level, irritability, seizures or coma and is treated with mechanical ventilation, mannitol and fluid restriction.

There are no controlled trials showing benefit from hyperbaric oxygen in carbon monoxide poisoning. However, numerous uncontrolled reports suggest benefit, particularly in the prevention of longer term sequelae. Once 100% oxygen is being administered (fourfold reduction in elimination half-life of COHb) then doubling the atmospheric pressure further reduces the elimination half-life of COHb roughly twofold. The only alternative is conservative supportive treatment and sins of omission are often more awkward for physicians than sins of commission. So indications for treatment probably include:

1 COHb level over 40 per cent when first measured
2 Pregnancy, since foetal haemoglobin binds carbon monoxide with even greater avidity than adult haemoglobin, the mother's COHb level may rapidly fall to low levels while that of the foetus may remain high
3 Coma or failure to regain full consciousness after oxygen therapy despite low COHb levels.

Corrosives

- An endoscopy must be performed if there is a clear history.
- Activated charcoal is contraindicated.

BACKGROUND

Corrosives may cause splash damage to eyes and skin. Acids produce heat on contact leading to coagulation necrosis, producing most damage to the oropharynx and stomach. The oesophagus is spared serious injury in 80 per cent of cases. Drooling of saliva, stridor and respiratory distress may develop. Evidence of perforation should be sought during clinical examination. Shock, cardiovascular collapse, pulmonary oedema, disseminated intravascular coagulation, acute renal failure, haemolysis and metabolic acidosis may all occur. Hydrofluoric acid produces severe skin necrosis and its ingestion produces hypocalcaemia because of chelation of calcium ions.

Alkali produce liquefaction necrosis on contact with the mucosa. Most of the injury is confined to the pharynx and oesophagus, less than 20 per cent of cases having significant gastric involvement. Oesophageal injury tends to be more severe than that caused by acids, with a greater chance of oesophageal perforation. Pain is not a prominent symptom even with a significant injury but drooling, vomiting and stridor can occur. Oesophageal perforation, mediastinitis and tracheal or aortic damage can occur producing severe shock and respiratory failure.

The corrosive damage caused by ingestion must be graded at endoscopy. Up to 30 per cent of children are asymptomatic despite having an injury requiring hospitalisation.

Grade 0	nil
Grade 1	mild erythema, oedema or mucosal injury only
Grade 2a	blistering with deeper tissue damage but not circumferential burns
Grade 2b	blistering but with some circumferential burns
Grade 3	transmucosal damage into peri-oesophageal tissues.

MANAGEMENT

ABC. Intubation is advisable for severe injuries or stridor and a surgical airway may be necessary. Decontaminate skin or eyes by lavage. Activated charcoal is contraindicated (it is ineffective and interferes with endoscopy). Steroids probably have no effect on oesophageal injury but may reduce the pharyngeal oedema. Antibiotics should be reserved for proven infection.

Cyanide

- The antidote is intravenous sodium nitrite (3% solution, 0.33 ml kg^{-1} up to 10 ml over 2–4 min) and sodium thiosulphate (25% solution, 1.65 ml kg^{-1} over 5 min).

BACKGROUND

Cyanide inhibits mitochondrial cytochrome oxidase, blocking oxidative phosphorylation and causing cessation of aerobic metabolism. Cyanide compounds are widely used in industry and as rodenticides, pesticides and fumigants. Cyanide is released in the combustion of polyurethane (furniture foam filling). Acetonitrile is used as nail varnish remover. Cyanide may therefore be ingested, absorbed through the skin or inhaled. Sodium nitroprusside contains 44% cyanide by weight. The risk of toxicity increases with high doses (greater than 10 μg kg^{-1} min^{-1}), prolonged infusions (several days), in the presence of renal failure or in the rare congenital absence of the enzyme rhodanase. Total doses as low as 500 μg kg^{-1} have been associated with toxicity. Toxicity may also occur after ingestion of the cyanogenic glycoside 'amygdalin' found in kernels, particularly almonds and apricots. Laetrile, sold in some health food shops contains 6% amygdalin.

Features of cyanide poisoning include:

- anxiety, palpitations, headache, weakness
- loss of consciousness, seizures
- pulmonary oedema, cardiovascular collapse, arrhythmias, hypotension
- metabolic acidosis and severe lactic acidosis
- high venous saturation and normal arterial saturation.

Cyanosis is not an initial feature as the patient is not hypoxaemic until respiratory failure ensues.

MANAGEMENT

ABC. High flow oxygen is beneficial although the mechanism is unclear. Administer sodium nitrite (3% solution, 0.33 ml kg^{-1} up to 10 ml over 2–4 min) which generates methaemoglobin, the ferric ion in it combining with hydrogen cyanide. Also give sodium thiosulphate (25% solution, 1.65 ml kg^{-1} over 5 min) which converts cyanide to thiocyanate. If after 2 hours evidence of cyanide toxicity persists, for example the patient has not regained consciousness, there is no haemodynamic improvement, lactate level and mixed venous oxygen content has not fallen, then repeat the above regime (halving the doses).

Digoxin

- Interpretation of digoxin level depends on the context of acute or chronic poisoning and whether Digibind® has been administered.
- Electrolyte abnormalities increase toxicity especially hypokalaemia.
- Digibind® is also effective for other cardiac alkaloids.

BACKGROUND

Sixty to eighty per cent of ingested digoxin is absorbed within 6 hours (up to 10 hours if a large quantity was ingested). Toxicity can result from accidental ingestion, dose changes, drug interactions or electrolyte imbalance. Potential drug interactions include erythromycin, amiodarone, quinine and diuretics. Hypokalaemia, hypomagnesaemia, hypercalcaemia and hypothyroidism all increase toxicity. Infants and young children may show serious toxicity after ingesting 0.3 mg kg^{-1}. Older children and those with pre-existing heart disease are even more sensitive.

Digoxin acts by inhibiting Na^+/K^+ ATPase, thereby increasing Ca^{2+} entry into cells. It also reduces cardiac sympathetic activity and increases parasympathetic activity by a direct vagal action. It slows AV node conduction but increases automaticity of both the atria and ventricles. Features of toxicity include:

- gastrointestinal tract – nausea, vomiting, diarrhoea
- CNS – fatigue, delirium, hallucinations, yellow vision, photophobia

- ECG – ST segment and T wave changes (inverse tick) and shortening of the QT interval
- arrhythmia – bradycardia is most common in children, with or without AV block but paroxysmal atrial tachycardia with block can still occur
- hyperkalaemia is common in acute poisoning but hypokalaemia is more common in chronic poisoning (especially with diuretics).

MANAGEMENT

ABC. Lavage is required in acute ingestion with significant toxicity and should be followed by repeated doses of activated charcoal. Correct electrolyte imbalances, including magnesium and treat arrhythmias as required. Beta-blockers may be useful for both atrial and ventricular tachycardia but since they may precipitate heart block, esmolol (short half-life) is preferred. Bradycardias respond to atropinic agents, isoprenaline and ultimately pacing. Ventricular tachycardia requires lignocaine (lidocaine), phenytoin or β-blockers. Avoid class 1a drugs (quinine, disopyramide) as these may exacerbate toxicity. Avoid DC cardioversion unless essential as there is a real risk of precipitating asystole. If DC cardioversion is necessary use the least possible energy.

In chronic intoxication, serum digoxin levels represent only 2 per cent of body stores and are 20 per cent protein bound. Management is to stop digoxin administration and treat electrolyte disturbances and arrhythmias as necessary.

Severe intoxication (acute or chronic) requires treatment with polyclonal ovine digoxin F_{ab} antibodies (Digibind®), indications for which are:

1 ingested dose over 0.3 mg kg^{-1}
2 pre-existing cardiac disease
3 a digoxin level of more than 5 ng ml^{-1} (taken at least 4 hours after ingestion) with
   - life-threatening arrhythmia
   - haemodynamic instability
   - hyperkalaemia
   - rapidly progressive toxicity.

Digibind® rapidly binds circulating digoxin (free digoxin levels drop within minutes) which is then replaced by previously tissue-bound drug. Digibind® is also effective in cases of poisoning from ingestion of other cardiac alkaloids including yew, oleander and foxglove. Total serum digoxin levels become very high after administration. F_{ab}-bound digoxin is renally excreted and haemofiltration may be required before dissociation leads to rebound toxicity.

Ecstasy (including amphetamines)

- Toxicity is usually compounded by dehydration and hyperthermia.

BACKGROUND

'Ecstasy' is a street-marketing name for 3,4 MDMA – an amphetamine derivative. Amphetamines cause suppression of appetite and confusion or euphoria, these being the usual reasons for their abuse. They also cause nausea, tachycardia, hypertension, sweating, tremor, anxiety, restlessness, mania and psychosis. Part of the action of amphetamines is via 5HT release, particularly in the hypothalamus, leading to hyperpyrexia and inappropriate ADH release. Toxicity presents in several ways:

1 hyperpyrexia and seizures, which may be confused with febrile convulsions in the relevant age group
2 hyperpyrexia and progressive multi-organ failure, including seizures, coma, acute renal and liver failure and DIC
3 coma, seizures and cerebral oedema associated with hyponatraemia
4 acute liver failure, the cause of which is unclear.

Ecstasy has mild amphetamine-like effects but its toxicity is compounded by two factors. As an illicit drug it is rarely 'pure' and it tends to be ingested to heighten pleasure at 'rave' parties to encourage relentless gymnastics and dancing in a hot environment with limited access to water. Mixed abuse with alcohol compounds dehydration. Under these circumstances life-threatening hyperpyrexia with rhabdomyolysis, convulsions, coma and DIC result.

MANAGEMENT

ABC. Rapid volume replacement may be necessary. Avoid hypotonic solutions and monitor the serum sodium, as fatal cerebral oedema from hyponatraemia is well recognised. Seizures should be rapidly controlled as they will exacerbate the hyperpyrexia and cerebral oedema. Use a benzodiazepine initially. Adequate sedation is essential to counteract the stimulant effects of the amphetamine-like drugs. Fulminant hyperpyrexia must be aggressively treated with cool intravenous fluids, exposing the patient and surface cooling. Failure to achieve rapid cooling is an indication for intubation, paralysis and ventilation (if not already done so as part of ABC), surface cooling and body cavity irrigation with cool fluids. Dantrolene 1 mg kg^{-1} (up to 10 mg kg^{-1}) is useful for control of hyperpyrexia and reduces the degree of rhabdomyolysis. The latter may precipitate acute renal failure requiring haemofiltration. Urinary alkalinisation reduces the risk of renal failure from the rhabdomyolysis. Forced acid diuresis is no longer used to increase elimination of amphetamine-like drugs. Acute liver failure is well recognised and if it occurs the patient should be referred to a PICU with a regional hepatology service.

Ethylene glycol

- Drunkenness without the smell of ethanol but with a metabolic acidosis should suggest ethylene glycol toxicity.
- 4-methylpyrazole (loading 15 mg kg^{-1} over 30 min, then 10 mg kg^{-1} 12 hourly for 4 doses then 15 mg kg^{-1} 12 hourly until ethylene glycol levels are less than 200 mg L^{-1}) has replaced ethanol in the treatment of severe poisoning.

BACKGROUND

Ethylene glycol is used as antifreeze, it is not toxic but is metabolised by alcohol dehydrogenase to the toxic metabolites glycoaldehyde, glycolate, glyoxylate and oxalate. These products cause severe lactic acidosis and a syndrome of neurotoxicity, nephrotoxicity and cardiorespiratory failure. Doses above 0.11 ml kg^{-1} produce toxicity and 1.5 ml kg^{-1} is lethal.

Three phases of toxicity are seen.

1 Apparent drunkenness without the smell of ethanol, nausea, vomiting, haematemesis, slurred speech, ataxia, seizures, cranial nerve palsies, drowsiness and coma. A worsening metabolic acidosis is usual. The oxalate chelates calcium leading to hypocalcaemia and tetany. Lumbar puncture may show a pleocytosis suggestive of meningoencephalitis. Urine microscopy will show oxalate crystalluria.

2 If the patient survives the initial phase, pulmonary oedema, cyanosis and cardiac failure develop because of direct toxicity of the metabolites and oxalate crystal deposition in the tissues.

3 Those patients who survive phase two may then develop renal failure.

A high index of suspicion is needed to diagnose ethylene glycol poisoning. Clues include apparent drunkenness with no smell of alcohol, a severe metabolic acidosis (with anion gap more than 20), lactic acidosis, an osmolar gap (the gap between measured and calculated osmolality) more than 10 mosmol kg^{-1}, ionised hypocalcaemia and oxalate crystalluria.

MANAGEMENT

ABC. Blood levels can be measured but assays may not be easily available. Treatment is guided by clinical signs and biochemical markers. Supportive measures include cardiorespiratory support, correction of acidosis with sodium bicarbonate, correction of hypocalcaemia and renal support. Ethylene glycol is not adsorbed by charcoal and lavage is ineffective. Ethanol and 4-methylpyrazole are inhibitors of the metabolism of ethylene glycol, and they preferentially bind to alcohol dehydrogenase. This prolongs the half-life of ethylene glycol (from 3 hours to 17 hours in the case of ethanol), allowing renal (or dialysis) removal. Indications for such treatment include:

- clear history (give the treatment immediately)
- severe acidosis or other symptoms irrespective of ethylene glycol level
- peak serum level over 20 mg dL^{-1}.

The dose of ethanol is 700 mg kg^{-1} (about 2 ml kg^{-1} of a standard 40% spirit) orally or intravenously followed by infusion, or repeat oral doses of 125 mg kg^{-1}hr^{-1}. Regular ethanol levels must be maintained between 100 and 150 mg dL^{-1}. Treatment continues until ethylene glycol levels are undetectable. This dose of ethanol produces inebriation with its attendant risks of impaired airway reflexes, aspiration and hypoglycaemia. Thiamine and pyridoxine should be given as co-factors. The preferred option is 4-methylpyrazole because it causes less central nervous system depression but, like many agents, it has not been specifically tested in children.

Early haemofiltration may be safer than trying to achieve a high urine output which risks fluid overload and pulmonary oedema. Indications include:

- acute renal failure or marked oxaluria
- persistent metabolic acidosis despite administration of bicarbonate
- severe electrolyte imbalances
- blood ethylene glycol levels over 50 mg dL^{-1}.

If it is used in conjunction with ethanol then ethanol must also be added to the replacement fluid.

Iron

- A low serum iron level taken more than 6 hours after ingestion does not exclude significant poisoning.

BACKGROUND

The toxicity of iron is directly related to the dose of elemental iron ingested, this varies between preparations, ferrous gluconate 12%, ferrous sulphate 20%, ferrous fumarate 33%. A dose of elemental iron of less than 20 mg kg^{-1} is unlikely to produce toxicity, 20 to 60 mg kg^{-1} (mild), over 60 mg kg^{-1} (moderate to severe) and over 200 mg kg^{-1} (lethal).

Symptoms develop within hours of ingestion. Vomiting, diarrhoea, gastrointestinal bleeding, shock, encephalopathy, seizures, fever and leucocytosis may be followed by a transient recovery phase, but further gastrointestinal symptoms of shock, acidosis, coma, multi-organ failure (and death) ensue. Survivors often develop gastric and intestinal strictures.

The presence of symptoms implies significant ingestion and a plain abdominal X-ray may reveal radio-opaque tablets. The serum iron level peaks 2 to 6 hours after ingestion and rapidly falls after 6 hours. Thus a high early level can predict toxicity but the negative predictive power of a low level is poor, particularly if the history of the time of ingestion is uncertain.

MANAGEMENT

ABC. Lavage should be performed for a large ingestion, with airway protection if there is any possibility of encephalopathy. Emesis should be avoided for the same reasons.

Charcoal does not adsorb iron but is indicated for possible multiple drug ingestion. Both whole bowel irrigation and endoscopic tablet removal should be considered if a large number of iron tablets are seen on X-ray. Desferrioxamine (15 mg kg⁻¹hr⁻¹ to a maximum of 8 g per 24 hr) should be considered for:

- ingestions of more than 100 mg kg⁻¹
- severe gastroenteritis
- serum iron over 500 µg dL⁻¹ at any time
- serum iron 300–500 µg dL⁻¹ at 4 to 6 hours
- symptoms of hyperglycaemia, acidosis or encephalopathy.

Desferrioxamine will turn the urine orange/red by the production of ferrioxamine. Treatment should be continued for 12 to 24 hours after the urine colour returns to normal.

Lead

- If there is a clear history of severe poisoning start intravenous chelation therapy without waiting for results of lead levels.
- Encephalopathy may be associated with raised intracranial pressure.

BACKGROUND

Sources include paintwork, piping, lead shot, pottery glazing, surma (eye makeup) and car fumes. Chronic low level lead poisoning is associated with intellectual impairment. As levels rise, pica, anorexia, vomiting and constipation occur. Severe acute lead poisoning leads to encephalopathy (drowsiness, convulsions, coma and death). Rapid treatment is essential to stand any chance of avoiding long-term sequelae such as developmental delay epilepsy, blindness and hemiparesis. Major symptoms are unlikely with blood lead levels below 1.2 µmol L⁻¹ (25 µg dL⁻¹), although levels as low as 0.5 µmol L⁻¹ (10 µg dL⁻¹) may produce some long-term intellectual impairment. Chronic poisoning produces hypochromic anaemia with basophilic stippling and increased long-bone density with transverse bands at bone ends.

MANAGEMENT

ABC. Control seizures. Raised intracranial pressure is possible so careful fluid and electrolyte management are required. Chelation therapy is relatively safe and should not be delayed for the results of lead levels if there is a strong suspicion of severe acute lead poisoning. Mild poisoning is treated with oral D-penicillamine.

Indications for intravenous therapy (calcium edetate disodium 40 mg kg⁻¹ intravenously over 1 hr every 12 hr for 5 days) include:

- lead levels above 2.7 µmol L⁻¹ (55 µg/dL)
- lead levels between 1.2 and 2.7 µmol L⁻¹ (25–55 µg dL⁻¹) and high levels of urinary lead, >9.7 µmol L⁻¹ (200 µg dL⁻¹), in the 8 hours after first dose of intravenous therapy
- severe symptoms in the absence of lead levels.

If the patient is encephalopathic, dimercaprol is added as a deep intramuscular injection.

Methanol

- Ethanol therapy is reserved for early presentations.
- Early haemodialysis or filtration for patients with papilloedema.

BACKGROUND

Methanol is used in household products such as windscreen wash and antifreeze. The formation of formaldehyde and formic acid make it highly toxic (just 5 ml of pure methanol may be lethal to a small child). Methylated spirits contains 5% methanol and 95% ethanol; its ingestion does not result in methanol poisoning but will produce toxicity because of its ethanol content. After poisoning the patient is initially inebriated, and has breath smelling of alcohol. Irritability, nausea, vomiting, CNS depression, fixed dilated pupils, photophobia, papilloedema, convulsions, coma and respiratory failure follow. Permanent blindness is common. A Parkinson's disease-like syndrome is occasionally seen after apparent recovery. A severe metabolic acidosis, caused by lactic and formic acid accumulation, a raised anion gap and raised osmolar gap are suggestive of ingestion of either ethylene glycol or methanol.

MANAGEMENT

ABC. Lavage and charcoal are ineffective. Supportive treatment includes correction of acidosis (very large quantities of sodium bicarbonate may be needed) together with ethanol for early presentations. After 4 hours the toxic metabolites have already formed and ethanol may worsen the acidosis. Folinic acid (10–15 mg m^{-2} dose every 6 hours) may reduce the risk of blindness. Early haemodialysis or haemofiltration should be considered for:

- ingestion of large quantities of methanol in the absence of a level
- severe acidosis
- severe hypernatraemia (secondary to large amounts of bicarbonate)
- methanol level >50 mg dL^{-1}
- neurological or visual symptoms or papilloedema.

Mushrooms

- There is a danger of fulminant hepatorenal failure.
- Symptoms that start more than 6 hours after ingestion suggest potentially fatal ingestion.

BACKGROUND

The most common mushroom accidentally ingested is *Amanita phalloides* (95% of cases). This mushroom contains RNA polymerase inhibitors (amatotoxins) which induce fulminant hepatorenal failure. However, recreational drug-abusing teenagers ingest a diversity of species in search of hallucinogenic effects. Poisoning can generally be classified by the time taken from ingestion to the onset of symptoms and early symptoms may be severe but the truly ominous ones in terms of mortality risk are those that start late.

Early symptoms (within 2 hours) indicate toxicity (usually self-limiting) in one of three patterns

1. muscarinic – vomiting, diarrhoea, abdominal cramps, miosis, bradycardia
2. CNS – ataxia, muscle cramps, hallucinations, mydriasis, photophobia
3. direct gastrointestinal – cramps, diarrhoea, vomiting.

Late symptoms (starting more than 6 hours after ingestion) usually mean ingestion of potentially fatal mushrooms. Initial abdominal pain, muscle cramps, nausea and vomiting, with severe watery or bloody diarrhoea give way to hepatorenal failure along with fever, convulsions, hypoglycaemia, encephalopathy, coma and death.

Investigations should include serial measurements of urea and creatinine, liver function tests (ALT, AST and GGT) and coagulation profile.

MANAGEMENT

ABC. For all cases of mushroom ingestion the initial management is the same:

- reduce absorption (charcoal, lavage)
- identify the mushroom if possible
- correct fluid and electrolyte disturbances
- observe.

For potentially fatal poisonings:

- give supportive treatment
- correct hypoglycaemia
- control seizures
- discuss with a poisons advice unit.

Cases of hepatorenal failure should be referred to a unit with a paediatric hepatology service that includes a liver transplant programme.

Neuroleptics

- Neuroleptic malignant syndrome is rare.
- Multiple drug interactions are possible.

BACKGROUND

This class of drug includes the phenothiazines, butyrophenones and thioxanthines. Their most significant therapeutic effect is to block central dopamine receptors. Features of toxicity include drowsiness, coma, seizures, hypotension, extrapyramidal signs including tremor, oculogyric crisis and abnormal temperature control. Cardiac arrhythmias are unusual but AV conduction abnormalities, QT prolongation and ventricular tachycardia may be seen, particularly with haloperidol. Toxicity persisting for more than 2 weeks can produce cholestatic jaundice and longer term toxicity can produce corneal opacities. Neuroleptics have anticholinergic side effects, potentiate the sedative effects of other drugs and compound the hypotensive effects of other drugs.

Neuroleptic malignant syndrome is an idiosyncratic reaction occurring up to 7 days after starting a new neuroleptic. It consists of hyperthermia, altered consciousness, muscular rigidity and autonomic dysfunction.

MANAGEMENT

ABC. Management is generally supportive. Lavage after recent large ingestion and use activated charcoal. Control seizures with benzodiazepines, phenytoin or thiopentone. Hypotension responds to intravenous fluids, vasoconstrictors and inotropes. Correct electrolyte imbalances and acidosis. The first choice antiarrhythmic is lignocaine (lidocaine). Temporary pacing may be necessary for AV block. The treatment of an oculgyric crisis is benztropine 0.02 mg kg^{-1} or procyclidine 0.1 mg kg^{-1} intravenously or intramuscularly.

Treatment of the neuroleptic malignant syndrome involves stopping the neuroleptic, cooling (which may require elective paralysis and ventilation) and dantrolene. Rhabdomyolysis may necessitate urine alkalinisation, fluid resuscitation and haemofiltration or dialysis.

Opioids

- Gastric lavage may be useful up to 10 hours after ingestion.
- The effects of naloxone are shorter than those of the opioid.
- Combined tablets containing opioids have more toxic effects than might be expected from their individual ingredients.

BACKGROUND

Opioids produce a characteristic syndrome of depressed consciousness, coma, respiratory depression and pinpoint pupils. Other signs include hypotension, cardiac failure, cardiac arrhythmias, non-cardiogenic pulmonary oedema, seizures, renal failure and rhabdomyolysis. Opioids are common drugs of abuse, being injected, smoked or ingested and hence overdose is common in drug-abusing age groups. Medical staff must take precautions when dealing with intravenous drug abusers who may be HIV positive or carrying hepatitis B and C.

MANAGEMENT

ABC. Use gastric lavage for enteral ingestion. Because of the effects of opioids on gastrointestinal motility, tablets may be recovered several hours after ingestion. Repeated doses of activated charcoal should follow lavage if bowel sounds are present.

Naloxone (0.1 mg kg^{-1} up to maximum of 2 mg) is a competitive antagonist and will usually produce marked, rapid improvement in conscious level and respiration. Partial effects should prompt repeat doses. Failure to fully arouse a patient after administration of naloxone suggests a mixed overdose, an overdose of a partial opioid agonist/antagonist (pentazocine, buprenorphine, etc.) or hypoxic brain damage. Naloxone lasts 30 to 60 minutes and repeat doses, or an infusion (10–20 μg kg^{-1}hr^{-1}) will be required. Patients must be closely monitored for signs of resedation or signs of acute withdrawal such as seizures and arrhythmias.

Diphenoxylate combined with atropine (Lomotil®) is used as an antidiarrhoeal medication. The lethal dose for children can be as little as one tablet. Diphenoxylate produces biphasic respiratory depression which may last up to 30 hours. Therefore, all children should be admitted to hospital and closely observed if ingestion is suspected. The combination of atropine produces a syndrome of respiratory depression, excitation or depressed consciousness, dry skin, urinary retention, fever, tachycardia and flushing. Miosis rather than mydriasis, occurs. Gastric lavage may recover tablets up to 10 hours after ingestion. Naloxone may be useful.

Dextropropoxyphene and paracetamol (co-proxamol) is often readily available. The potential for paracetamol poisoning and opioid toxicity combine with acute cardiac failure, lethal arrhythmias and seizures, probably because of a toxic metabolite. Naloxone does not reverse these latter effects.

Organophosphates/carbamates

- Symptoms of poisoning depend on the portal of entry.
- Atropine and pralidoxime are the principal therapies.

BACKGROUND

These substances may be ingested, inhaled or absorbed through the skin. They are found in the home as treatments for skin infestations or as pesticides. Transcutaneous absorption is well recognised from treated carpets or contaminated linens. Organophosphate (OP) compounds produce longer lasting effects than carbamates, because of slower hydrolysis and a tendency to form irreversible OP-cholinesterase bonds (ageing) that permanently inactivate the enzyme. Being lipid soluble, they penetrate the blood–brain barrier. Carbamates produce less severe and more short-lived effects than organophosphates because of the reversible inactivation of cholinesterases. Effects are caused by central and peripheral overactivity of cholinergic (nicotinic and muscarinic) transmission. The commonest findings are miosis, excessive salivation, nausea and vomiting, muscle weakness, fasciculations, tachycardia, hypertension, hyporeflexia, lethargy, respiratory distress and respiratory failure. Seizures occur in over 20 per cent of cases. Aspiration pneumonitis is not uncommon because of either reduced airway reflexes or the aspiration of the petroleum distillate used to carry the organophosphate or carbamate.

The initial symptoms are often peripheral muscarinic and related to the portal of entry. Ingestion is associated with vomiting, nausea, diarrhoea and abdominal cramps. Inhalation of the substance produces coughing, wheezing, salivation, lacrimation, respiratory distress, a tight chest and pulmonary oedema. Nicotinic signs include muscle fasciculation followed by paralysis, double vision and respiratory failure. Central muscarinic signs include tachycardia, anxiety, restlessness, convulsions and coma.

MANAGEMENT

ABC. Intubation and assisted ventilation is frequently necessary. Control seizures with diazepam or barbiturates. Atropine is the mainstay of organophosphate or carabamide poisoning, 0.02 mg kg⁻¹ repeated every 10 to 20 minutes until secretions stop or signs of atropine toxicity develop (dry mouth, vasodilatation and tachycardia). Most children need less than five doses but occasionally children need up to 50 doses over a 24-hour period. Tachycardia is a common feature of organophosphate or carbamate poisoning in children. If the diagnosis is likely and the child has a tachycardia before atropine is administered, atropine will *slow* the tachycardia via a central antimuscarinic action.

Pralidoxime (25 mg kg⁻¹ over 30 min followed by 10–20 mg kg⁻¹hr⁻¹ guided by control of symptoms for at least 18 hr) inhibits the binding of the organophosphate and displaces it, provided it has not aged (ageing is the irreversible inhibition of cholinesterase activity). Whilst atropine improves muscarinic function, pralidoxime restores nicotinic function improving muscle weakness and respiratory function. Pralidoxime is not necessary in carbamate poisoning as hydrolysis occurs spontaneously.

Paracetamol

> • Acidosis, hypoglycaemia, coagulopathy and oliguria are ominous signs of fulminant hepatorenal failure.
> • Late presentations must all be treated with N-acetylcysteine.

BACKGROUND

Paracetamol poisoning is common in teenagers but is uncommon in small children, because of the relatively large amount required for toxicity. Liver metabolism of the drug produces a toxic intermediary that depletes glutathione and then accumulates causing hepatic necrosis. The livers of young children have a greater sulphonation ability (less reliant on glutathione) but hepatic toxicity is still dose related. The toxic dose in children is 140 mg kg⁻¹ although toxicity can follow sustained dosage of 100 mg kg⁻¹day⁻¹ over several days. Toxicity is increased in the presence of:

• liver enzyme induction (chronic alcohol use, phenytoin, phenobarbital, etc.)
• malnutrition, including anorexia and HIV disease.

Patients in these categories are *high risk* and treatment thresholds are therefore lower (see Figure 19.2).

Initial nausea and anorexia are not universal but may last for up to 6 hours. Symptoms may abate for up to 48 hours. Hepatic dysfunction then follows with nausea, vomiting and lethargy, or fulminant hepatorenal failure and death. If the patient survives then recovery takes several weeks.

MANAGEMENT

ABC. Laboratory investigations should include an assessment of acid–base status, prothrombin time (a true liver *function* test) and blood sugar. Urea, electrolytes, creatinine and liver enzymes are also useful. Paracetamol levels should be taken as indicated below.

N-acetylcysteine (NAC) is the mainstay of treatment. Despite warnings about the risk of anaphylactic reactions, hypokalaemia is a more common side effect. The standard regime:

• 150 mg kg⁻¹ in 5% dextrose over 15 min, followed by
• 50 mg kg⁻¹ in 5% dextrose over 4 h, followed by
• 100 mg kg⁻¹ in 5% dextrose over 16 h.

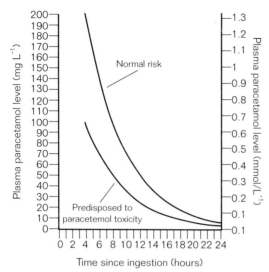

Figure 19.2
Paracetamol levels. The two curved lines have been drawn to be used as thresholds for intervention. The lower threshold is for patients with existing hepatic risk factors.

For presentation within 8 hours of ingestion:
- prevent further absorption by giving activated charcoal. Lavage is unnecessary
- check paracetamol level
- start standard NAC regime if indicated by levels or there is a delay in obtaining results
- stop NAC regime if paracetamol levels are below appropriate treatment line. If levels are high (Figure 19.2) check bloods and continue NAC regime
- otherwise check bloods (including a repeat paracetamol level) on completion.

If the patient is then asymptomatic and the investigations are normal then no further treatment is required. If they remain symptomatic or investigations are abnormal then continue NAC at 6 mg kg⁻¹ hr⁻¹ and contact a regional PICU with a paediatric hepatology service.

For presentation 8 to 15 hours after ingestion:
- check paracetamol level and bloods
- start a standard NAC regime immediately before paracetamol level results
- if level is below the treatment line and the patient is asymptomatic with normal laboratory results then stop NAC. If the level is above treatment line continue NAC regime
- after completing NAC regime, recheck bloods. If the results are abnormal or the patient is symptomatic, continue NAC at 6 mg kg⁻¹ hr⁻¹ and contact a regional PICU with a paediatric hepatology service.

For presentation more than 15 hours following ingestion or if the time since ingestion is not known:
- start standard NAC regime immediately
- check bloods before and after NAC regime, if either are abnormal or the patient is symptomatic then contact a regional PICU with a paediatric hepatology service and continue NAC at 6 mg kg⁻¹ hr⁻¹ at the end of the regime
- repeat laboratory investigations at least 12 hourly.

Regional PICUs with a paediatric hepatology service are likely to want to accept/transfer patients with:

- prothrombin time in seconds greater than number of hours following ingestion (e.g. a PT of 36 seconds, 30 hours after ingestion)
- prothrombin time greater than 50 seconds at any stage

- acidosis
- rising creatinine or oliguria
- encephalopathy.

Both oral methionine (36 mg kg^{-1} 4 hourly for 4 doses) and NAC are effective in preventing toxicity in early poisoning. Their actions are not fully understood but they include the regeneration of glutathione. NAC has also been shown to modify the course of severe paracetamol poisoning, including fulminant hepatic failure, even when given more then 24 hours after ingestion. Oral methionine should be avoided in favour of NAC in:

- severe poisoning
- late presentations (>10 hours after ingestion)
- patients with vomiting (common)
- patients with possible delayed gastric emptying (such as multiple drug ingestion)
- patients receiving activated charcoal.

Paraquat

- Blood levels fall quickly and may be low after ingestion of a lethal dose.
- Pulmonary fibrosis is universally fatal.

BACKGROUND

Most deaths from paraquat poisoning occur with the concentrated solutions (Gramoxone®), usually taken by deliberate ingestion, but transcutaneous absorption does occur. Many household weedkillers contain a less concentrated form of paraquat (e.g. Weedol®) and poisoning with these less concentrated products is much less common but it can occur in children. Ingestion of large quantities causes death within hours because of myocardial depression and pulmonary oedema. Smaller quantities produce nausea, vomiting and diarrhoea. Severe painful ulceration of the oropharynx and oesophagus develop over days with dysphagia, dyspnoea and cough. Acute renal failure is common. Evolving breathlessness over days to weeks indicates the development of progressive, universally fatal pulmonary fibrosis.

MANAGEMENT

ABC. Include skin decontamination and repeated doses of activated charcoal (which has superseded Fuller's earth) for ingestion. Paraquat is rapidly cleared from the blood so late presentations may have low levels despite a potentially lethal dose. A high initial level is almost universally fatal but some success has been achieved in these cases using decontamination, charcoal haemoperfusion, cyclophosphamide and high-dose steroids. The decision for aggressive further treatment should be made in conjunction with a poisons unit. Once pulmonary fibrosis ensues, sympathetic terminal care may be more appropriate than further aggressive therapy.

Petroleum distillates

- There is a high risk of aspiration leading to lipoid pneumonia.
- Do not lavage routinely and never without airway protection.

BACKGROUND

Injury is caused through aspiration leading to lipoid pneumonia. Following ingestion the risk of aspiration is high because these substances:

- depress the conscious level and may rarely cause seizures (CNS toxicity may occur with doses above 1 ml kg^{-1})
- have a low viscosity and surface tension.

MANAGEMENT

ABC. Protect the airway if the conscious level is depressed. Do not lavage unless there has been a recent ingestion of a large amount of the substance or there is evidence of CNS toxicity. If lavage is considered it must be preceded by intubation using an endotracheal tube without a leak. Charcoal is ineffective. Steroids are ineffective.

Quinine

- Prevention of absorption using repeat-dose charcoal is highly effective.

BACKGROUND

Quinine is an antimalarial drug. Both quinine and its optical isomer, quinidine, have sodium channel blocking, α-blocking and anticholinergic properties. Quinine is rapidly and completely absorbed from the gastro-intestinal tract and has a large volume of distribution. It increases refractory periods of muscle and reduces excitability of the motor end-plate. The elimination half-life ranges from 7 to 12 hours. 95 per cent is hepatic metabolised and 5 per cent is excreted unchanged in the urine. Quinine increases digoxin levels, enhances warfarin and potentiates neuromuscular blockade. Toxicity ('cinchonism') causes myocardial depression, conduction defects (prolonged PR and QT intervals), broad complex tachycardia, electro-mechanical dissociation, visual field defects, fixed dilated pupils, blindness (usually temporary), tinnitus, deafness, abdominal pain, vomiting, headache, sweating and hypotension. Atypical reactions include hypersensitivity, bone marrow suppression and haemolysis.

MANAGEMENT

ABC. Gastric lavage and repeated doses of activated charcoal both reduce absorption and increase plasma elimination. Hypotension requires fluid resuscitation and inotropes, with or without glucagon. Common arrhythmias may respond to correction of electrolyte abnormalities. Hypokalaemia indicates severe poisoning but hyperkalaemia will increase toxicity. Phenytoin and lignocaine (lidocaine) may also prove useful but bradyarrhythmias may require pacing. Since myocardial depression and toxicity are reversible, prolonged CPR and extracorporeal cardiac support are reasonable approaches to life-threatening hypotension, arrhythmia or asystole. Acid diuresis is no longer used. Bilateral stellate ganglion blocks for eye toxicity are ineffective and should not be attempted.

Other antimalarials and dapsone

BACKGROUND

Many antimalarials are oxidising agents and hence cause methaemoglobinaemia which manifests as profound cyanosis despite normal or elevated PaO_2 (if FiO_2 is increased). The pulse oximeter tends to read around 85 per cent irrespective of the PaO_2 or the degree of cyanosis. A co-oximeter gives correct oxyhaemoglobin and methaemoglobin readings. Other features of poisoning include nausea, vomiting, visual disturbances (chloroquine), and ventricular arrhythmias (halofantrine).

MANAGEMENT

ABC. Give activated charcoal with or without lavage. Methaemoglobinaemia of >30 per cent requires methylene blue, 1 to 2 mg kg^{-1} intravenously over 5 min, but severe cases (e.g. with metabolic acidosis) will require exchange transfusion.

Solvent abuse

BACKGROUND

Freely available household products such as aerosol propellants, glue, nail polish remover, hair spray, gasoline and typewriter correction fluid, contain agents with toxic effects that are open to abuse. The chemical agents include aliphatic hydrocarbons, alkyl halides, alkyl nitrites, aromatic hydrocarbons, ethers, esters and ketones. These agents are extensively lipid soluble, have a high volume of distribution and slow clearance. Seventy per cent of deaths from solvent abuse occur in the 14 to 16 year age group. When abused the solvents are inhaled directly or from soaked cloth or plastic bags to rapidly achieve a state of disorientation, part of which is due to hypoxia. Impairment however lasts up to an hour, is associated with anaesthesia to injuries and can induce persistent psychosis.

Sudden death is usually caused by cardiac arrhythmia or hypoxia but acute effects can include carbon monoxide poisoning, hepatorenal failure and methaemoglobinemia. Myopathy, rhabdomyolysis, metabolic acidosis and electrolyte disturbance also occur. The diagnosis may be implied by mucosal, pulmonary and skin irritation which follow acute exposure.

MANAGEMENT

ABC. Protect the airway if the conscious level is depressed. Charcoal is ineffective. Lipoid pneumonia, seizures and arrhythmias are treated on their merits but the latter two can recur at any time until clearance is complete. High lipid solubility however makes clearance very slow and not amenable to dialysis or charcoal perfusion.

Theophylline

> • Failure of levels to fall rapidly implies a slow-release preparation or bezoar formation, necessitating whole bowel irrigation and repeat-dose or continuous activated charcoal.

BACKGROUND

Many theophylline preparations are slow release with the risk of prolonged and continuing toxicity. Acute poisoning occurs at levels above 80 μg ml^{-1}. It is characterised by nausea, vomiting, haematemesis, tachycardia, hypotension, dysrhythmias and seizures. Metabolic derangement is common, including lactic acidosis, hyperglycaemia, hypokalaemia and hypophosphataemia. Chronic poisoning often results from drug-dose errors, drug interactions or reduced hepatic clearance. It is more common in younger children and the metabolic derangement is less severe. Seizures tend to occur at lower levels than with acute poisoning (40 μg ml^{-1}). The symptoms of theophylline poisoning vary between acute and chronic poisoning and infants are at greater risk than older children.

Theophylline levels correlate well with toxicity in acute poisoning (>80 μg ml^{-1}) and less well in chronic poisoning, but seizures may be seen with levels of 40 μg ml^{-1}. Levels will initially rise after ingestion but should then fall. If they do not fall or continue to rise then ingestion of slow-release tablets or formation of a bezoar should be suspected.

MANAGEMENT

ABC. Gastric lavage should be considered for recent ingestion of a large quantity of tablets and WBI for slow-release tablets or bezoar formation. Activated charcoal is very effective and repeated doses or a continuous nasogastric infusion (0.25 – 0.5 g kg^{-1}hr^{-1}) should be given. The H$_2$ antagonist ranitidine (NOT cimetidine), may improve the tolerance to charcoal. Ondansetron may be effective for problematic vomiting but phenothiazine antiemetics should be avoided as they further lower the seizure threshold.

Haemodialysis, plasmafiltration and plasmapheresis, and charcoal haemoperfusion are all effective at removing theophylline. Exchange transfusion is an alternative in neonates. Indications include:

• recurrent seizures
• refractory hypotension, ventricular dysrhythmias
• severe metabolic derangement, worsening metabolic acidosis

- levels >100 µg ml⁻¹ in acute poisoning, less if there is intractable vomiting
- levels >60 µg ml⁻¹ in chronic poisoning (>6 months old)
- levels of 30 to 40 µg ml⁻¹ in acute or chronic poisoning (less than 6 months old)
- early symptoms/signs suggesting the prospect of major toxicity, particularly for those children with pre-existing liver or cardiac disease.

NB Repeat-dose activated charcoal should be commenced while haemodialysis is being organised.

Phenytoin is often ineffective and may even worsen seizures, which should be treated with diazepam and phenobarbital. Intractable seizures require intubation, ventilation and thiopental infusion. Arrhythmias should only be treated if they cause haemodynamic instability and the first step in their treatment is to treat electrolyte and acid–base imbalances. Supraventricular tachycardia may respond to β-blockers, which usually increase blood pressure but occasionally produce severe hypotension. Adenosine might be useful but is unproven in this context. Ventricular arrhythmias may respond to lignocaine (lidocaine) or β-blockers. Otherwise hypotension is commonly caused by excessive vasodilatation and may respond to volume and noradrenaline (norepinephrine) by infusion.

BETA-BLOCKERS

N.B. Where theophylline was being used for reversible airways disease, β-blockers should be either avoided or used with great care and in the smallest possible dose necessary to achieve the desired clinical effect. Propanolol (0.02 mg kg⁻¹ repeated as necessary up to a total dose of 0.1 mg kg⁻¹), is the drug of choice for supraventricular and ventricular arrhythmias. It also improves blood pressure by inhibiting the theophylline-induced hypotension. In addition, it reduces the metabolic effects of theophylline. Esmolol may be safer in patients with reversible airways disease but will have little effect on the metabolic derangement. Esmolol is very short acting; give 500 µg kg⁻¹, over 1 min followed by an infusion of 50 µg kg⁻¹min⁻¹. As theophylline levels fall the infusion rate should be reduced.

Tricyclic antidepressants

- Tricyclic overdose is suggested by the combination of Coma, Convulsions and Cardiac signs.
- Alkalinisation should be used in all cases.

BACKGROUND

The toxic dose is 10 to 20 mg kg⁻¹, which for a small child may be as little as 1 to 2 tablets. Central effects cause coma which may ensue rapidly. Anticholinergic effects include tachycardia, mydriasis, urinary retention, dry mucous membranes and increased gut transit time. Sodium channel blockade and blockage of neurotransmitter uptake cause seizures. Membrane stabilisation may also cause prolongation of the PR, QRS and QTc intervals of the ECG. Heart block, sinus tachycardia, ventricular ectopics, idioventricular rhythm, ventricular tachycardia, torsade de pointes, fibrillation, electromechanical dissociation and asystole may all result. Hypotension from myocardial dysfunction is aggravated by α-blockade and noradrenaline (norepinephrine) depletion. Patients demonstrating coma, seizures or prolongation of the QRS interval >100 milliseconds are at risk of the more life-threatening complications.

MANAGEMENT

ABC. Hypoventilation, reduced airway reflexes or haemodynamic instability are indications for intubation and mechanical ventilation. Mild hyperventilation to a $PaCO_2$ of 4 kPa will help alkalinisation (see below). Extreme hyperventilation should be avoided as it will depress cardiac output further.

Reduce absorption using repeated doses of activated charcoal. The tendency to increased transit time may make gastric lavage effective for up to 10 hours post-ingestion but since lavage could push the stomach contents into the duodenum (increasing drug absorption) it must be followed by more charcoal and cathartics.

Alkalinisation encourages ionisation of the drug, reducing lipid solubility and tissue affinity and thereby reduces toxicity, particularly the more life-threatening cardiac effects. All patients who have ingested a potentially toxic dose should receive 1 mmol kg^{-1} of sodium bicarbonate, by intravenous infusion over 1 hour. Symptomatic patients require more aggressive alkalinisation to maintain a plasma pH of 7.45 to 7.55.

Convulsions must be treated to avoid hypoxia, hypercarbia and acidosis. Control is usually easy with intravenous diazepam. Intubation and mechanical ventilation may be necessary for airway protection and treatment of associated cerebral oedema. Phenytoin should be reserved for intractable seizures or seizures in combination with ventricular arrhythmias.

Many of the cardiac arrhythmias are relatively benign requiring attention to electrolyte disturbances (including potassium, calcium and magnesium), alkalinisation and observation. Anti-arrhythmics are reserved for intractable, life-threatening arrhythmias when simple measures have failed. Lignocaine (lidocaine) and phenytoin (Class 1b drugs) are the safest but are negative inotropes and may worsen the myocardial depression. Class 1a, 1c, 2, 3 and 4 drugs are contraindicated, as they will either worsen the arrhythmia or are potent myocardial depressants. Physostigmine at this stage may cause seizures. Torsade de pointes may respond to slow magnesium infusion. Other manifestations of myocardial depression may include electromechanical dissociation.

Hypotension that is unresponsive to volume should be treated with noradrenaline (norepinephrine) and if recalcitrant may respond to glucagon (1 mg kg^{-1} bolus and a further 1 mg kg^{-1} over 6 hr). In the event of cardiac arrest, cardiopulmonary resuscitation can be continued for several hours if necessary, with a full recovery. Intractable life-threatening arrhythmias, severe myocardial depression and uncontrollable acidosis are sound indications for ECMO.

During recovery a period of acute confusion, lasting up to 48 hours, is not uncommon. Benzodiazepines may be useful rarely supplemented by physostigmine (if seizures and dysrrhythmias are over).

20 Issues Surrounding Death on the PICU

- **Withdrawal of intensive care**
- **Brain stem death (organ donation)**
- **Dying without a diagnosis**

WITHDRAWAL OF INTENSIVE CARE

PIC beds are a limited resource and have to be used to their maximum benefit. It is not part of the intensive care unit's role to delay an inevitable death. However it is very much part of the medical and nursing role to care for the dying and the bereaved. In paediatric intensive care, issues relating to childhood mortality cannot be avoided. A typical unit with a thousand admissions a year and a crude mortality rate of 7 per cent will see 70 deaths a year which is about six a month, or more than one a week.

Common scenarios

It is inevitable that on occasion patients reach the intensive care unit during resuscitation or treatment that ultimately proves to have been unsuccessful. Additionally many children at the point of death from incurable disease abruptly encounter medical and nursing staff who have never met them or their families before. These introductions occur in what appears to be a medical emergency. Even in these enlightened times, few of the families or children have been adequately prepared in advance for the encounter. It is rarely possible or appropriate for new medical or nursing acquaintances to make decisions about withholding escalation of care when the child is dying and the issues have not been discussed in advance. Thus these patients can be admitted to the PICU through what may later appear to have been inappropriate resuscitation. PICU patients may also deteriorate during their stay, or they may encounter complications that drastically alter the prospects for intact survival. Such circumstances demand re-evaluation of further management. It is the duty of the paediatric intensivist to question the merits of further intensive care and address the issues surrounding its potential withdrawal.

When to withdraw intensive care

The consensus within the medical profession over when to withdraw medical care is not complete but it does cross national boundaries. A useful framework for considering when to withdraw attempts at curative medical treatment was provided by the Royal College of Paediatrics and Child Health in the UK in 1997. The college recognised five situations where such action might be considered.

1　The **brain dead** child.
2　The **permanent vegetative state** (permanent was defined as 12 months following traumatic brain injury and 6 months following PVS from other causes). .
3　The **no chance** situation where the child has such severe disease that life-sustaining treatment delays death without significant alleviation of suffering.
4　The **no purpose** situation where, although survival may be possible with treatment, the degree of physical or mental impairment will be so great that it is unreasonable to expect the child to bear it. The child in this situation will never be able to take part in decisions regarding treatment or its withdrawal.
5　The **unbearable** situation where the child and family feel that in the face of progressive and irreversible disease further treatment is more than can be borne.

Counselling – who needs it?

The first effort in such situations is always to counsel the child where appropriate, as well as the parents, carers and family of the child. This process takes time, empathy and effort. However the potentially and imminently bereaved in these situations are not just the immediate family. The intensivist will frequently have to address the feelings of other health professionals involved in the case. The professional detachment of physicians and nurses is rarely complete and during the stress of an intensive care admission, self-cognisance and objectivity may quite naturally be impaired. Some staff may have difficulty reconciling the reality of the situation with their own spiritual or religious beliefs. For others the recognition of the impending death of a patient may represent an intolerable testament to their own (or medicine's) limitations or fallibility. All these individuals may have to progress through the numbness, denial and anger of a grief reaction before accepting that intensive care must logically be withdrawn.

Whose decision?

Under circumstances such as these, the patient is the prime consideration and one frequently has to advocate on their behalf without claiming sole rights to the moral high ground. However, the needs of the family are equally important and it is wholly appropriate, indeed essential, to incorporate them in fundamental management decisions. Nevertheless it is advisable to be clear from the outset that the family are not individually or solely responsible for the decision. Rather that it is a medical decision or at least one made on the basis of medical advice. In this format the decision can be easier for the family to live with subsequently. Often parents or guardians do not resist the withdrawal of intensive care. Some vigorously attempt to curb what they see as the distasteful resuscitative efforts of medical and nursing staff and occasionally they are more rational than the physicians. Other families, for religious, empathic or even selfish reasons, want therapy to persist until their own definition of death supervenes and they are unable to countenance moderation on any front under any circumstances.

From the two paragraphs above it is clear that the counselling process can develop in a variety of ways. Without the consensus of all involved, progress can be very slow and it is abhorrent to impose one's own personal morality on these situations to the exclusion of others. Nevertheless when facing intensive care in the context of brain death, persistent vegetative state or a no chance, no purpose or unbearable situation, appropriate withdrawal is not a democratic or corporate decision process so much as a collective moral, ethical and humanitarian responsibility.

There is a clear procedural (but not moral, ethical or humanitarian) distinction between decisions involving an inevitable mortality and those involving discussions about the potential quality of future life (or lack of it). In the case of the latter there is enormous variation among individuals in terms of what degree of compromised outcome is considered tolerable.

Even when dealing with the recognition of inevitable mortality, it may take the individuals involved different lengths of time to reach the same conclusions. The decision should not be rushed even though the commonest scenario is for the intensivist to reach this conclusion first. If the assessment is correct then death may supervene during the decision-making process. Ultimately if health care professionals are at loggerheads with a family then there is recourse to the legal system, but the need to go to such lengths is excessively rare.

Medical futility: what treatments are withdrawn?

There is no moral, ethical, professional or legal responsibility to pursue futile medical treatment. In this regard all aspects of intensive care are 'medical treatments' including the administration of oxygen, mechanical ventilation, inotrope administration, artificial feeding, etc. and as such should not be pursued if futile. The concept of 'futility' in medical treatment has both medico-legal and philosophical ramifications but a practical definition is required for intensive care. In this regard Schneiderman *et al.*(*Annals of Internal Medicine* 1990: 949–54) provide a pragmatic approach that the reader may find useful. Schneiderman's submission was that when physicians conclude (either through personal experiences, experience shared with colleagues or consideration of published empirical data) that in the last 100 cases a medical treatment has been useless (i.e. has not altered the outcome), they should regard that treatment as futile. Such judgements were to be made on the basis of benefits (defined as impacts on the patient as a whole) and not effects (defined as influences on parts of the body or physiology). Of course mortality prediction models, which are tools of intensive care audit, have *no* conceivable application in these decisions.

The procedure for withdrawal of care from patients receiving a classic public perception of intensive care (i.e. mechanical ventilation) should involve sufficient analgesia and sedation while other drugs, for example inotropes, are discontinued. The ventilator should be switched off and the patient extubated. Compromises in terms of not withdrawing some of these futile therapies while withdrawing others are, in general terms, anathema since the obligation is to avoid prolonging suffering. However, the withdrawal of intensive care is not the withdrawal of all medical or nursing care, and some of the patients due these considerations will not be receiving the 'classic public perception of intensive care' alluded to above. Palliative treatments are not futile and are not judged by the same outcomes. It is wholly appropriate, indeed obligatory, to continue palliative aspects of medical support during the withdrawal of intensive care. The ethos of palliative care is not a complete paradigm shift from the care that preceded it. It should be instituted prior to the withdrawal of intensive care and it demands a similar level of commitment and attention to detail.

The imminently bereaved family and friends may have strong opinions about certain aspects of palliative therapy that the intensivist may not have anticipated and it is always wise to ask if there are any specific requests. The emphasis is to satisfy physical needs for symptom relief and pain control, along with emotional, social and spiritual needs. Many families appreciate a religious ceremony or blessing on the PICU around this time and they should be offered one even if they have not professed their religious faith up to that point. If the required duration of palliative care is expected to be prolonged then discharge from the PICU to a lower dependency area of the hospital or to a more homely environment may be preferable, with agreement that the patient is not to be readmitted to the PICU in the event of deterioration.

Who withdraws care?

The paediatric intensivist needs both an empathic and a pragmatic approach to these situations. Intensive care staff see more childhood deaths than most paediatric practitioners and are in a position to assure attention to 'quality of death' issues which may not occur to people who experience the situation less often. It is therefore wholly appropriate that these tasks fall to the intensivist.

BRAIN STEM DEATH (ORGAN DONATION)

A question that is often asked is whether one should wait until a diagnosis of brain stem death can be made in order to withdraw intensive care. The answer is no. A diagnosis of brain stem death is a fundamental prerequisite for organ donation but it is not an essential criterion for intensive care withdrawal. Brain stem death is an unusual mode of death in paediatrics and the definitions involved are rarely applied to neonates who are less suitable for organ donation than older children anyway. Because of the implications of organ donation, brain death is covered by regulations that vary between countries.

It is recommended that the diagnosis of brain death is made by two independent consultants testing alone or together on two separate occasions. The diagnosis should not usually be considered until at least 6 hours after the onset of coma or, if cardiac arrest was the cause of the coma, until 24 hours after the circulation has been restored. Both consultants must be satisfied that potentially reversible causes for the patient's condition have been adequately excluded. These include depressant drugs, neuromuscular blocking agents, hypothermia and metabolic or endocrine disturbances. The clinical tests for brain stem death are:

- pupils should not react to light
- corneal reflex should be absent
- there should be no eye movement on caloric testing
- there should be no motor responses in the cranial nerve distribution in response to stimulation of face, limbs or trunk, therefore there should be no conjugate eye movements in response to head turning (oculomotor reflex should be absent, i.e. doll's eye sign present)
- there should be no gag reflex
- there should be no cough reflex
- there should be no respiratory movements seen during apnoea testing.

The test for apnoea should be long enough for the $PaCO_2$ to rise to 6.7 kPa or above. This usually will require pre-oxygenation or apnoeic oxygenation using continual low flow oxygen via a catheter inserted into the trachea. For patients with compensated respiratory acidosis, or in whom hypoxic respiratory drive is suspected, the clinicians need to satisfy themselves that a sufficient respiratory stimulus has been provided.

Many patients will have been receiving barbiturate therapy prior to suspicion of brain stem death. After withdrawal, drug levels must be allowed to fall below a threshold before brain stem death tests can proceed. The level of this threshold has not been defined by consensus, but thiopentone levels of less than 40 mg L^{-1} are unlikely to adequately explain apparent brain stem death.

In some protocols (e.g. in the USA) brain stem death tests are routinely supplemented with a requirement to demonstrate that the EEG, or serial EEGs, is/are isoelectric. However an isoelectric EEG is not inevitably the result of brain death. Hypothermia and drugs can produce a reversible flat EEG and mains and other electrical interference can frustrate attempts to make the recording anyway. Attempts to document severely reduced or absent cerebral blood flow are similarly unhelpful in making the diagnosis of brain death.

Maintenance of the organ donor

Cardiovascular deterioration in brain dead patients can generally be averted pending organ harvest with attention to intravascular volume, appropriate catecholamine therapy and treatment of diabetes insipidus.

DYING WITHOUT A DIAGNOSIS

If a child dies without a diagnosis, then there are statutory obligations with regard to the reporting and further investigation of the case. A post mortem on medical grounds could provide an answer and in the UK will form an essential part of the coroner's enquiries into the case. Referral to the coroner is also mandatory:

- if there is any suspicion that violence, neglect or injury contributed to the death
- if death occurs within 24 hours of hospital admission
- if there has been recent surgery.

In the latter two scenarios if an adequate explanation can be offered the coroner may decline to hold an inquest.

It is also important to consider whether there is any possibility that a genetic cause was involved since this makes further counselling of the parents essential. Chromosomal analysis is unlikely to be successful on all but the freshest post mortem blood samples and karyotype should be sought antemortem where indicated. Furthermore if there is any possibility of an inborn error of metabolism, then attempts should be made to pursue the diagnosis. A standard protocol should be arranged in collaboration with the local laboratory to obtain blood and urine, and skin, liver and muscle biopsies soon after death. Samples for electron microscopy need to be frozen in liquid nitrogen and those for histology placed in formalin.

Index

Note: Page references in italics refer to Figures; those in bold refer to Tables

efficiency 32–3, 40
efficiency index 40
elastance 143
electrolytes 88–92, 129
electromechanical dissociation 16
elemental diets 107
emesis, induced 298
emphysema, pulmonary interstitial 76
encephalopathy 131, 261
   hepatic 255–8, 255
   hypoxic ischaemic 76
   post-asphyxial 76
endocardial fibroelastosis 195
endocarditis 261
endothelium derived relaxation factor 271
endotoxin 262, 274
endotracheal tube 64, 66–7, 66
energy expenditure on activity (AEE) 100
energy requirements 102, 102
enoximone 185
enteral drug administration 115–16, 115
enteral feeding 106–9
enteritis, radiation-induced 107
eosinophils 262
ephedrine 185
epiglottitis 162
epsilon aminocaproic acid (EACA) 203
Equity of intensive care 33, 34
erythromycin 120, 252
esmolol 209, 320
ethylene glycol 309–10
etomidate 58
evoked potentials 229
exotoxins 274
exponential functions 291–3, 292
extracorporeal membrane oxygenation
   (ECMO) 187–8
   in ARDS 164
   in near-drowning 21–2
   neonatal 32, 80–1
   protocol 158–60
extrahepatic bilary atresia 74

failure to thrive 194–5
falciparum malaria 261
Fallot's tetralogy 173, 191, 209–10, 209
Fanconi's syndrome 130
fat
   parenteral 110
   requirements 103–4
fatty acids, essential 104
feeds/feeding
   baby, choosing between 108
   enteral 106–9
   parenteral 109–11
   thermic effect of (TEF) 100
fentanyl 55, 63–4, 68
fever, treatment of 261
fibrinogen deficiency 247
Fick equation 172, 271
Fick principle 140, 289

Fick's law of diffusion 272
flail chest 19
flecainide 179, 305
Flora's Z statistic 37
flow 284–8
   laminar 284–6
   measurement of 288–9
   mixed 286
   turbulent 286
fluconazole 252
Fontan 216–17, 216
foreign body 22
   in airway 162
   cardiac arrest and 10
   in oropharynx 11
   tracheitis 162
fosphenytoin 232
fraction of inspired oxygen (FiO2) 27
free radicals 274
free water clearance (CH20) 239
fresh frozen plasma (FFP) 94–5
Friedreich's ataxia 195
fructose intolerance 130
frusemide 231
fulminant hepatic failure 254–5
functional residual capacity (FRC) 138
futility 324–5
fuzzy logic 2

galactosaemia 130, 131
gas flows
   continuous 288
   intermittent 288
gas volumes 288
gastric lavage 298
gastro-intestinal haemorrhage 252–3
gastro-oesophageal reflex 252
Gay-Lussac law 27
gelatins 97
Gibbs Donnan effect 271
Glasgow Coma Scale (GCS) 13, 14, 233,
   233–4
Glenn procedure 213, 217
glomerular filtration rate (GFR) 85, 237,
   240–1, 241
glucagon 185
glucocorticoids 253
glucose
   in inborn errors of metabolism 130
   parenteral 109–10
glucose-6–phosphate dehydrogenase
   deficiency 131, 250
glutaric acidemia type ii 129
glyceryl trinitrate 186
glycosaminoglycans 271
Guillain–Barrè syndrome 237, 247, 288

haematoma
   intracranial 222
   subdural 19
haemochromatosis, neonatal 131